WOUND CARE CERTIFICATION
STUDY GUIDE

SECOND EDITION

WOUND CARE CERTIFICATION STUDY GUIDE

SECOND EDITION

EDITOR:

Jayesh B. Shah, MD

CO-EDITORS:

Paul J. Sheffield, PhD & Caroline E. Fife, MD

IN PARTNERSHIP WITH

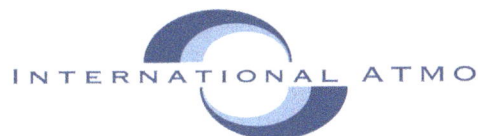

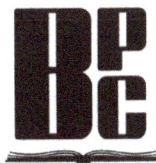

INTERNATIONAL ATMO

BEST PUBLISHING COMPANY

First edition 2011
Second edition 2016

International Standard Book Number: 978-1-930536-83-8

Library of Congress catalog card number: 2010917802

Best Publishing Company
631 US Highway 1, Suite 307
North Palm Beach, FL 33408

Printed in the United States

TABLE OF CONTENTS

FOREWORD

Certification in wound care is a formal recognition of a master level of knowledge in the field. It is a way to increase one's professional image and give both patients and colleagues the confidence that the clinician managing the patient's wound is truly qualified. This book is a study guide that reviews the basic principles that candidates must understand to obtain wound care certification. Dr. Jayesh B. Shah has organized each chapter to focus on key information that the various wound care certifying agencies consider important in their examinations.

The contributing authors were chosen because they are wound care experts, certified in wound care, and/or instructors of key elements in wound management. Dr. Shah approached me and my company, International ATMO, Inc., to augment our wound care course by creating a review course for physicians and nurses who planned to take a wound care certification examination. Dr. Shah assembled the faculty, and with the contributions of wound care consultants Dr. Diane Krasner and Deborah Sheffield, we created our first offering of the Review Course for Wound Care Certification in 2008. Dr. Shah and I co-directed the course many times, and numerous physician and nurse attendees subsequently obtained their wound care certifications.

In 2009, Dr. Shah perceived the need for this wound care certification review as a study guide to help candidates prepare for various wound specialty certification examinations. In 2011, the first edition of the *Wound Care Certification Study Guide* was published by Best Publishing Company in partnership with International ATMO, Inc. This second edition is presented in a format that makes it easy for candidates to review the topics and identify areas of strength and areas that need further study. The information is organized by key points to review. The reader will find more details and additional study questions in the second edition of *Wound Care Practice* (Best Publishing Company, 2007).

Paul J. Sheffield, PhD
Co-Editor
May 15, 2015

PREFACE

The statistics on the growing number of non-healing wounds is alarming. It is encouraging to see emerging wound care specialists—physicians, podiatrists, nurses, physical therapists, enterostomal therapists, occupational therapists, and many others who have chosen wound care as their full time profession. The evidence-based treatments and technologies in the field of wound care today guide healthcare professionals with the management of challenging wounds. While such awareness exists, a thorough knowledge of wound care basics to identify the multiple factors contributing to a wound is crucial.

I am delighted to put the second edition of the *Wound Care Certification Study Guide* forward and hope it will prove to be a valuable tool in the preparation of any certification exams related to wound care. With the curriculums of the wound care certifying associations in mind, this book is designed to provide a quick, concise review from an exam-oriented perspective.

The chapters are in an outline format to allow for the quick review of topics. From my more than 15 years of clinical experience in wound care, I have designed the wound assessment pathways in Chapter 32 to assist with the treatment of patients with wounds. New to this edition is an introductory chapter on hyperbaric oxygen therapy. The original chapters have been updated with the latest information, and hundreds of new images and sample questions have been added to make this book a comprehensive resource for any clinician preparing for wound care examinations.

The reader is encouraged to have an in-depth understanding of wound care by reviewing the second edition of *Wound Care Practice* by Drs. Sheffield and Fife before proceeding with this review.

Jayesh B. Shah, MD
Editor

CONTRIBUTOR LIST

Gregory Anstead, MD, PhD
Director, Immunosuppression and Infectious Diseases Clinics
South Texas Veterans Health Care System
Professor, Department of Medicine Division of Infectious
Diseases University of Texas Health Science Center
San Antonio, Texas

Jesse Cantu, RN, BSN, CWS, FAACWS
Wound Care Consultant
San Antonio, Texas

Elias R. Cheleuitte, DPM, FACFAS
Podiatric Surgeon, affiliation to Baptist Health System
San Antonio, Texas

Caroline E. Fife, MD, CWSP, FAAFP, FUHM
Medical Director, CHI St. Luke's Wound Clinic
The Woodlands, Texas
Professor of Geriatrics, Baylor College of Medicine
Houston, Texas
Chief Medical Officer, Intellicure, Inc.
The Woodlands, Texas

Jane Fore, MD, FAPWCA, FACCWS
Internal Medicine, Wound Healing and Hyperbaric Medicine
Tri-State Wound Healing and Hyperbaric Center
Clarkston, Washington

Frederick Gale, MD, FACS
Surgical Director, Inpatient Skin Management and Risk
Reduction Team
Tufts Medical Center, Boston, Massachusetts
Wound Specialist, The Center for Vascular, Wound Healing, and
Hyperbaric Medicine
Tufts Medical Center, Boston, Massachusetts

Rose L. Hamm, PT, DPT, CWS, FACCWS
Assistant Professor of Clinical Physical Therapy, Division of
Biokinesiology and Physical Therapy
Ostrow School of Dentistry, University of Southern California
Keck Hospital of USC, Los Angeles, California

Ellen Heiderich, RN,CWS, CHT
Clinic Manager, Peterson Wound Healing Center
Kerrville, Texas

Javier La Fontaine, DPM, MS
Associate Professor, Department of Plastic Surgery
UT Southwestern Medical Center
Dallas, Texas

Kathren McCarty DPM, MS, FACFAS
Podiatrist, Private practice
San Antonio, Texas

Yvette Ponce-Hall, CHT
Safety Director, Northeast Baptist Wound Healing Center
San Antonio, Texas

E. Patricia Rios, RN, MSN, CHRN-C
Program Director, Northeast Baptist Wound Healing Center
San Antonio, Texas

Dianne Rudolph, RN, GNP-BC, DNP, CWOCN
Nurse Practitioner, South Texas Veterans Health Care
Administration, Kerrville, Texas
Adjunct Faculty, School of Nursing, University of Texas Health
Science Center, San Antonio, Texas
Adjunct Faculty, School of Nursing, University of Texas Health
Science Center, Houston, Texas

Jayesh B. Shah, MD, CWSP, FAPWCA, FACCWS
Adjunct Assistant Professor
Department of Family & Community Medicine
University of Texas Health Science Center at San Antonio
San Antonio, Texas
President, South Texas Wound Associates, PA
Medical Director, Wound Healing Center
Northeast Baptist Hospital
Co-Medical Director, Wound Healing Center
Mission Trail Baptist Hospital
San Antonio, Texas

Neha J. Shah, MPT, CLT
Staff Lymphedema Therapist
Health Link, North Central Baptist Hospital
San Antonio, Texas
Office Manager
South Texas Wound Associates, PA
San Antonio, Texas

Prachi J. Shah
Freshman, University of Texas at San Antonio
Research Assistant, South Texas Wound Associates, PA
San Antonio, Texas

Paul J. Sheffield, PhD, CAsP, CHT, FASMA, FUHM
President, International ATMO, Inc.
San Antonio, Texas

Rasa Silenas, MD
Physician, South Texas Wound Associates
Northeast Baptist Hospital
San Antonio, Texas

Richard Simman, MD, FACS, FACCWS
Professor Department of Pharmacology and Toxicology,
Division of Plastic and Reconstructive Surgery
Wright State University Boonshoft School of Medicine
Dayton, Ohio

Rajendra Singh, MD
Assistant Professor and Director, Immunodermatology
Departments of Dermatology and Pathology
Icahn School of Medicine at Mount Sinai
Mount Sinai, New York

DEDICATION

To my loving and supportive wife, Neha, for her understanding and patience with my hectic schedule.

To my two beautiful children, Prachi and Aj, for giving me the space to write and edit this book, and for giving me the emotional support to persevere through a challenging year.

To my mother, Jaivanti, for keeping me spiritually uplifted.

To my late father, Bipinchandra, for inspiring me to be a physician: his spirit is with me every day.

To my wonderful team of wound care staff and colleagues at Northeast Baptist Wound Healing Center and Mission Trail Baptist Wound Healing Center in San Antonio, for helping me care for patients with non-healing wounds.

And finally, to my patients and their caregivers, for their trust in me.

Jayesh B. Shah, MD
Editor

THE "WHAT" AND "HOW" OF CERTIFICATION EXAMS

1

Jayesh B. Shah, MD, CWSP, FAPWCA, FACCWS
Caroline E. Fife, MD, CWSP, FAAFP, FUHM
Paul Sheffield, PhD, CAsP, CHT, FASMA, FUHMP

INTRODUCTION

This study guide has been developed to encourage participants to obtain recognized credentials in wound care, which should subsequently result in improved medical practice, competence, and patient outcomes. This chapter is designed to help you determine which certification exam best fits your situation and provides ten "pearls" to help pass the certification exam.

I. Wound care certification (certificate of added qualification)

A. Physicians should be aware that neither the American Board of Medical Specialties (ABMS) nor its osteopathic counterpart, the Bureau of Osteopathic Specialists (BOS), recognizes wound care as a specialty or subspecialty; thus, none of the certification options can be considered an actual board certification. Wound care certification is perhaps better described as a certificate of added qualification. Certification identifies a standard of knowledge essential for developing a comprehensive wound management background; advances cooperation and resource exchange among the various disciplines and organizations involved in treatment of patients with chronic wounds; encourages continued professional growth and development of individuals and the field of wound management; and establishes a code of ethics, responsibility, and high professional standards by all certified individuals.

B. The wound care certification testing agencies and their corresponding certifications listed in this chapter reflect a compilation of information about the exams available to the authors at the time of this writing. It is highly recommend that all prospective applicants do their own research at the individual certification exam websites, which are provided in the following table. In addition to the degree/ license requirement, there is an application fee for each of the exams. Some exams require annual maintenance fees and/or have practice requirements. Prospective candidates are advised to contact the individual organizations for further details.

C. Table 1.1 summarizes the credentials in wound care that are currently available.

II. Hyperbaric medicine certification (board certification and certificate of added qualification, or CAQ)

A. Increasing numbers of wound care practices are adding hyperbaric oxygen therapy as a treatment option for difficult wounds. A list of accepted indications for hyperbaric oxygen is available on the Undersea and Hyperbaric Medical Society (UHMS) website at www.uhms.org.

B. Wound care specialists are often asked to supervise HBOT treatments. Many Medicare Administrative Carriers (MACs) and private payers have begun to specify the physician training required for reimbursement of physician-supervised HBOT. Physicians are encouraged to read their Local Carrier Determinations (LCDs) as requirements vary, though most require ACLS certification and at least a recognized 40-hour introductory course. Some payers require that a minimum number of treatments or hours of HBOT be precepted by a credentialed physician and/or that the physician obtains a CAQ in hyperbaric medicine to be reimbursed for the supervision of HBOT.

C. The American Board of Medical Specialties (ABMS) recognizes subspecialty board certification in undersea and hyperbaric medicine (UHM) that is offered by both the American Board of Preventive Medicine (ABPM) and the American Board of Emergency Medicine (ABEM). UHM subspecialty board certification is now only possible for physicians who complete a one-year Accreditation Council for Graduate Medical Education (ACGME) approved fellowship in UHM and thus is unlikely to be an option for most physicians.

D. Physician CAQs in hyperbaric medicine are available from the UHMS, the American Osteopathic Board of Preventive Medicine (AOBPM), and the American Board of Wound Healing (ABWH).

E. Hyperbaric nurse and hyperbaric technologist certification is available from the National Board of Diving and Hyperbaric Technology (NBDHMT). The American Board of Wound Healing (ABWH) offers a certified hyperbaric and wound specialist certificate.

F. Table 1.2 summarizes the credentials in hyperbaric medicine that are currently available.

Table 1.1: Wound care credentials.

CERTIFYING BODY	CERTIFICATIONS AVAILABLE	DEGREE/LICENSE REQUIRED
ABWM– American Board of Wound Management	**CWCA**– Certified Wound Care Associate	LVN/LPN, RN, PT, certified HCA, administrators, dietitians, sales and marketing professionals, researchers
	CWS– Certified Wound Specialist	Bachelor's, master's, doctoral degree
	CWSP– Certified Wound Specialist Physician	MD, DO, DPM
More information can be found at: http://www.abwmcertified.org/ American Board of Wound Management, 1155 15th Street NW, Suite 500, Washington, DC 20005 Phone: (202) 457-8408; Fax: (202) 530-0659		
ABWMS– American Board of Wound Medicine and Surgery	**Diplomate**	MD, DO
More information can be found at: http://www.abwms.org/ American Board of Wound Medicine and Surgery, PO Box 133, Aspers, PA 17304 Phone: (717) 677-0165; Fax: (717) 398-0396		
ABWH– American Board of Wound Healing	**PCWC**– Physician Certification in Wound Care	MD, DO, DPM
	CHWS– Certified Hyperbaric and Wound Specialist	Hyperbaric technician, diver medical technician, medical assistant, respiratory therapist, certified nurse aide, EMT/paramedic, life support technician, physician assistant, registered nurse or LPN, nurse practitioner, physician, veterinarian, podiatrist
More information can be found at: https://abwh.net/home American Board of Wound Healing, 9875 South Franklin Drive, Suite 300, Franklin, WI 53132 Phone: (414) 269-5464; Fax: (414) 269-5464		
CMET– Council for Medical Education and Testing	**CMET**—Physician Certified in Wound Healing	MD, DO, DPM
More information can be found at: http://www.councilmet.org/ Council for Medical Education and Testing, 3524 Yadkinville Road, Suite 235, Winston-Salem, NC 27106 Phone: (336) 923-5065		
WOCNCB– Wound, Ostomy, and Continence Nursing Certification Board	**CWOCN**–Certified Wound Ostomy Continence Nurse **CWON**– Certified Wound Ostomy Nurse **CWCN**– Certified Wound Care Nurse **COCN**– Certified Ostomy Care Nurse **CCCN**– Certified Continence Care Nurse **CFCN**– Certified Foot Care Nurse	Bachelor's-prepared RN
	CWOCN-AP–Certified Wound Ostomy Continence Nurse-Advanced Practice **CWON-AP**– Certified Wound Ostomy Nurse-Advanced Practice **CWCN-AP**– Certified Wound Care Nurse-Advanced Practice **COCN-AP**– Certified Ostomy Care Nurse-Advanced Practice **CCCN-AP**– Certified Continence Care Nurse-Advanced Practice	Master's-prepared APRN
More information can be found at: https://www.wocncb.org/ WOCNCB Office, 555 East Wells Street, Suite 1100, Milwaukee, WI 53202-3823 Phone: (888) 496-2622; Fax: (414) 276-2146		

Table 1.1: Wound care credentials, continued.

CERTIFYING BODY	CERTIFICATIONS AVAILABLE	DEGREE/LICENSE REQUIRED
NAWCO– National Alliance of Wound Care and Ostomy	**WCC**– Wound Care Certified	RN
	DWC– Diabetic Wound Certified	LPN/LVN, RN, NP, PT, PTA, OT, MD, DPM, DO, PA
	LLE– Lymphedema Lower Extremity Certified	RN, LPN/LVN, NP, PT, PTA, OT, MD, DO, PA
	OMS– Ostomy Management Specialist	LPN/LVN, RN, NP, PT, PTA, OT, MD, DPM, DO, PA
More information can be found at: http://www.nawccb.org National Alliance of Wound Care and Ostomy, 717 St. Joseph Drive, Suite 297, St. Joseph, MI 49085 Phone (888) 929-4575 or (877) 922-6292; Fax: (800) 352-8339		

Table 1.2: Hyperbaric credentials.

PHYSICIAN BOARD CERTIFICATION IN UNDERSEA & HYPERBARIC MEDICINE		
CERTIFYING BODY	CERTIFICATIONS AVAILABLE	DEGREE/LICENSE REQUIRED
ABPM– American Board of Preventive Medicine	**Subspecialty Certification in UHM** Recognized by American Board of Medical Specialties (ABMS)	MD
		Must have completed a one-year ACGME-approved fellowship in Undersea and Hyperbaric Medicine
More information can be found at: https://www.theabpm.org/uhm.cfm American Board of Preventive Medicine, 111 West Jackson Blvd, Suite 1110, Chicago, IL 60604 Phone: (312) 939-2276; Fax: (312) 939-2218 E-mail: abpm@theabpm.org		
ABEM– American Board of Emergency Medicine	**Subspecialty Certification in UHM** Recognized by American Board of Medical Specialties (ABMS)	MD (Diplomates of the ABEM)
		Must have completed a one-year ACGME-approved fellowship in Undersea and Hyperbaric Medicine
More information can be found at: https://www.abem.org/public/home American Board of Emergency Medicine, 3000 Coolidge Road, East Lansing, MI 48823-6319 Phone: (517) 332-4800; Fax: (517) 332-2234 Email: abem@abem.org		
PHYSICIAN CERTIFICATE OF ADDED QUALIFICATION IN HYPERBARIC MEDICINE		
AOBPM– American Osteopathic Board of Preventive Medicine	**Certificate of Added Qualification in UHM**	DO (Diplomates of the AOA or COA)
		Must have completed a one-year AOA or ACGME-approved fellowship in Undersea and Hyperbaric Medicine
More information can be found at: http://www.aobpm.org American Osteopathic Board of Preventive Medicine, 142 East Ontario Street, Floor 4, Chicago, IL 66011 Phone: (800) 621-1773 ext. 8229; Fax: (312) 202-8495		
UHMS– Undersea & Hyperbaric Medical Society	**Certificate of Added Qualification in UHM**	MD, DO, or equivalent
More information can be found at: https://www.uhms.org Undersea and Hyperbaric Medical Society, 631 US Highway 1, Suite 307, North Palm Beach, FL 33408 Phone: (919) 490-5140; Fax: (919) 490-5149 Email: uhms@uhms.org		
ABWH– American Board of Wound Healing	**Certificate of Added Qualification in HM**	MD, DO (Members of ACHM)
More information can be found at: https://abwh.net/home American Board of Wound Healing, 9875 South Franklin Drive, Suite 300, Franklin, WI 53132 Phone: (414) 269-5464; Fax: (414) 269-5464		

Table 1.2: Hyperbaric credentials, continued.

NURSE & TECHNOLOGIST CERTIFICATION IN HYPERBARIC MEDICINE		
CERTIFYING BODY	**CERTIFICATIONS AVAILABLE**	**DEGREE/LICENSE REQUIRED**
NBDHMT– National Board of Diving and Hyperbaric Technology	**CHRN** (Certified Hyperbaric Registered Nurse) **ACHRN** (Advanced Certified Hyperbaric Registered Nurse) **CHRNC** (Certified Hyperbaric Registered Nurse Clinician)	RN
	CHT (Certified Hyperbaric Technologist) **CHT-ADMIN** (CHT with management or administrative duties)	RT, PA, EMT/paramedic, RN, LPN, NP, MD, DO, active duty military corpsman
More information can be found at: http://www.nbdhmt.org or https://www.uhms.org/education/credentialing/certification-cht-chrn-dmt.html Address: NBDHMT, 9 Medical Park, Suite 330, Columbia, SC 29203 Phone: (803) 434-7802; Fax: (866) 451-7231 Email: nbdhmt@aol.com		
ABWH– American Board of Wound Healing	**CHWS**– Certified Hyperbaric and Wound Specialist	RN, LPN, NP, PA, MD, DO, DPM, DMT, RT, CNA, EMT/ paramedic, medical assistant, hyperbaric technician, life support technician, veterinarian
More information can be found at: https://abwh.net/home American Board of Wound Healing, 9875 South Franklin Drive, Suite 300, Franklin, WI 53132 Phone: (414) 269-5464; Fax: (414) 269-5464		

III. Test-taking strategies

Test pass rates vary, but about 15-20% of applicants fail their certification exam. There are three important factors that affect one's test performance: studying the right material, managing stress/test anxiety, and practical experience. Studying the reference materials on which the exam is based is the most important factor. The certification agencies want to know you understand the "textbook answer" to their questions. Managing test anxiety is the second most important factor. Even the most intelligent and studious individuals may do poorly on exams if they are overwhelmed by test anxiety. The best way to overcome test anxiety is to practice taking tests. Practice exams, like the one found in Chapter 33, are your best weapon against test anxiety. Practical experience, while a prerequisite to some wound care certifications, may actually impair test performance. It may be counterintuitive to think your experience can harm you, but it is important to recognize that the exam is not based on the wound care knowledge that has proven successful for you, unless that knowledge also happens to be the textbook answer to the question at hand. It is imperative you know the textbook answers, not the common practice in your facility.

The following is a list of suggestions for proper study techniques and general preparation considerations.
A. At least two months before the exam:
1. Carefully follow all the test registration procedures.
2. Know the test instructions, duration, topics, question types, and number of questions.
3. Familiarize yourself with the testing facility protocol. Do they allow any personal effects, e.g., phones, calculators, ear plugs into the testing environment? If not, will they provide you with a location to store these items? What happens if you have to go to the bathroom in the middle of the test?
4. Set up a flexible study schedule and stick to it.
5. Study during the time of day you are most alert, relaxed, and stress free. Most test applicants work, so no more than one or two hours a day should be set aside for studying.
6. Focus on your weakest knowledge base. Do not study the material you are familiar with; study the topics you don't know or don't frequently use.
7. Find a study partner for reviewing and clarifying questions.
8. Practice, practice, practice.
B. The day before the exam:
1. Get a good night's sleep. Do not try to cram the night before the test.
2. Know the exact physical location of the testing site. Drive the route to the site prior to the test day.
3. Keep your cool—play with your kids or go out for an evening walk.
4. Select and set aside what you need to take to the testing center.
C. The day of the exam:
1. Consider taking ear plugs; the testing center could be noisy.
2. Eat a well-balanced meal, but don't overeat.
3. Wear comfortable, loose-fitting, layered clothing; the examination room may be cold or hot.
4. Take along the required documents to the testing center. This may include forms of identification or a document showing your reservation.
5. Arrive early, be prepared to wait, and be patient.
6. Stay positive.

D. Ten "pearls" to ace the test:
1. Read the entire question carefully. Scan all the answers, and read the question again. Make sure that you did not misread the question.
2. Once you have selected your answer, always go back and check it against the question. Make sure your choice answers the question—all answers may be correct statements, but the correct choice is the one that directly answers the question.
3. Do not disregard any information in the question. Information in the question is there for a reason; it is not there to throw you off.
4. If you only know the answer to part of the question, the best action is to eliminate the choices you know to be incorrect and make a best educated guess from the remaining answers.
5. If you've read the question and don't know the answer, skip over the question and return to it later, if you have that option. Reading the remainder of the test may jog your memory or allow the answer to pop into your head when you aren't stressing over it. If skipping the question is not an option, as with some electronic tests, don't waste time on it. Pick an answer and move on to the next question.
6. Don't read too much into the question. Test writers are not writing questions to throw you off. Be practical and understand that the question is there to test a specific objective. Try to imagine what the test writer had in mind and was actually trying to ask. Don't overcomplicate the problem by creating theoretical relationships or explanations that will warp time or space. These are normal problems rooted in reality. The applicable relationship or explanation may not be readily apparent, and you may have to figure it out. Use common sense to interpret anything that isn't clear.
7. Avoid answer choices that have definitive words like "exactly," "always," and "never." These extreme statements do not leave room for exception. In medicine, almost everything has an exception. Avoid any answer choices with slang.
8. Time management is crucial: don't spend too much time on any one question. Pace yourself and check the clock every 30 minutes to make sure that you are on target with your time.
9. Don't panic: if you don't know the answer to a question, it is not the end of the world. You do not have to know all the answers to pass the test.
10. Finally:
    a) Prepare early—do not procrastinate!
    b) Study multiple books.
    c) Find a good source of practice tests and try to simulate the exam three weeks before the test.
    d) Concentrate on your weakest areas.
    e) About 80-85% of the test-takers pass their exam. You are more likely to pass than to fail.

IV. Wound care resources

1. Krasner DL, Rodeheaver GT, Sibbald RG. *Chronic Wound Care: A Clinical Sourcebook for Healthcare Professionals*. 4th ed. Wayne: HMP Communications; 2007.
2. Armstrong D, Lavery L, editors. *Clinical Care of the Diabetic Foot*. Alexandria: American Diabetes Association; 2005.
3. Hess C. *Clinical Guide: Skin and Wound Care*. 5th ed. Philadelphia: Lippincott Williams & Wilkins; 2004.
4. Veves A, Giurini JM, LoGerfo FW, editors. *The Diabetic Foot*. 2nd ed. Totowa: Humana Press; 2006.
5. Joseph WS. *Handbook of Lower Extremity Infections*. 2nd ed. New York: Churchill Livingstone; 2002.
6. Campbell DR, Kozak GP, Frykberg RG. *Management of Diabetic Foot Problems*. 2nd ed. Philadelphia: W.B. Saunders Company; 1995.
7. Baranoski S, Ayello E. *Wound Care Essentials: Practice Principles*. Philadelphia: Lippincott Williams & Wilkins; 2003.
8. Baranoski S, Ayello E. *Wound Care Essentials: Practice Principles*. 2nd ed. Philadelphia: Lippincott Williams & Wilkins; 2008.
9. Falabella A, Kirsner R, editors. *Wound Healing*. New York: Informa Healthcare; 2005.
10. Sheffield PJ, Fife CE, Smith APS, editors. *Wound Care Practice*. North Palm Beach: Best Publishing Company; 2004.
11. Sheffield PJ, Fife CE, editors. *Wound Care Practice*. 2nd ed. North Palm Beach: Best Publishing Company; 2007.
12. Masturzo A, Beltz WR, Cook R, et al. Wound care certification: the grin without a cat. Wound Healing Society Education Committee Chair Commentary. *Wound Rep Reg*. 2013; 21:494-7.
13. American Board of Wound Management (CWS) Exam. http://www.abwmcertified.org/abwm-certified/cws/cws-how-to-prepare.
14. American Board of Wound Management (CWCA) Exam. http://www.abwmcertified.org/abwm-certified/cwca/cwca-how-to-prepare.
15. American Board of Wound Management (CWSP) Exam. http://www.abwmcertified.org/abwm-certified/cwsp/cwsp-how-to-prepare.
16. American Board of Wound Management Foundation CWCA, CWS, CWSP practice exams (registration fee is required): http://www.abwmfoundation.org/practice-exams/.
17. Certified Wound and Ostomy Care Nurse (CWOCN) Exam. https://www.wocncb.org/certification/wound-ostomy-continence/eligibility. http://www.wocncb.org/certification/foot-care-certification/eligibility. https://www.wocncb.org/certification/advance-practice-certification/eligibility.
18. WOCNCB Examination Handbook. http://www.wocncb.org/pdf/WOCNCB_handbook.pdf.

19. Council for Medical Education & Testing (CMET) Physicians Wound Care Certification Exam: https://www. councilmet.org/index.php/exam-overview.html.

20. National Alliance of Wound Care and Ostomy (NAW-CO) Wound Care Certified (WCC) Exam: http://www. nawccb.org/wound-care-certification.

V. Hyperbaric resources

21. Kindwall EP, Whelan HT. *Hyperbaric Medicine Practice.* 3rd ed. North Palm Beach: Best Publishing Company; 2008.

22. Kindwall EP, Niezgoda JA. *Hyperbaric Medicine Procedure: The Kindwall HBO Handbook.* 9th ed. Aurora Health Care; 2006. American College of Hyperbaric Medicine (www. ACHM.org).

23. Larson-Lohr V, Norvell H, Josefsen L, Wilcox J, editors. *Hyperbaric Nursing and Wound Care.* North Palm Beach: Best Publishing Company; 2011.

24. Neuman TS, Thom SR. *Physiology and Medicine of Hyperbaric Oxygen Therapy.* Philadelphia: Saunders Elsevier; 2008.

25. Sheffield DA, Sheffield RB. *CHT and CHRN Certification Exam Review Course.* 2nd ed. San Antonio: International ATMO; 2013.

26. Workman WT, editor. *Hyperbaric Facility Safety: A Practical Guide.* North Palm Beach: Best Publishing Company; 2000.

CELL STRUCTURE AND FUNCTION 2

Jayesh B. Shah, MD, CWSP, FAPWCA, FACCWS
Prachi J. Shah

INTRODUCTION

This chapter describes the basic cellular components and their functions. The discussion includes steps in preparing slides and methods of examination.

OBJECTIVES

Participants should be able to describe three major types of cell functions, list the components of cytoplasm, list the components of the cell membrane, and contrast mitosis with meiosis.

I. Cells

A. Cells are the building blocks of all plants and animals.
B. Cells are produced by the division of preexisting cells.
C. Cells are the smallest units that perform all vital physiological functions.
D. Each cell maintains homeostasis at the cellular level, tissue level, organ, organ system, and organization levels, which reflects the combined and coordinated actions of many cells.
E. Cytology
   1. The study of structure and functions of cells.
F. Interstitial fluid
   1. Extracellular fluid that surrounds the cell in a tissue.
G. Cell membrane
   1. The cell's outer boundary is the cell membrane or plasma membrane.
   2. The membrane functions include physical isolation, regulation of exchange with the environment, sensitivity, and structural support.
   3. The cell membrane is a phospholipid bilayer and contains lipids, proteins, and carbohydrates.
   4. Membrane proteins can act as anchors, identifiers, enzymes, receptors, or channels.
H. Membrane permeability
   1. Permeability is the ease with which substances can cross the cell membrane.

2. Diffusion is the net movement of material from an area where its concentration is relatively high to an area where its concentration is lower.
3. Osmosis is the diffusion of water across a membrane in response to differences in solute concentration.
4. Osmotic pressure is the pressure that must be applied to a solution to prevent inward flow of water across a semipermeable membrane.
5. Hydrostatic pressure is the bulk flow of water molecules across a membrane. It can oppose osmotic pressure.
6. Tonicity is the effect of osmotic solutions on living cells.
7. Isotonic solutions do not cause an osmotic flow.
8. Hypotonic solutions cause water to flow into a cell to make it swell and can lead to hemolysis.
9. Hypertonic solutions cause water to flow out of a cell to make it shrink and can lead to crenation.
10. Filtration is water that is forced across a membrane because of hydrostatic pressure and can lead to crenation.
11. Facilitated diffusion is a carrier-mediated transport. Compounds are transported across a membrane after binding to a receptor site of a carrier protein.
12. Active transport mechanisms consume ATP but are independent of concentration gradients.
13. Vesicular transport involves material movement into or out of a cell in vesicles.
14. Endocytosis is an active process that helps movement of material into the cell.
    a) Receptor-mediated endocytosis by means of coated vesicles
    b) Pinocytosis—cellular drinking
    c) Phagocytosis using pseudopodia
15. Exocytosis is the ejection of materials from the cytoplasm.
16. Transmembrane potential is the potential difference between the two sides of a cell membrane.
17. Resting potential is the transmembrane potential in an undisturbed cell.

II. Cytoplasm

A. Definition

1. Cytoplasm is a general term for material located inside the cell membrane and outside the membrane surrounding the nucleus. It contains cytosol (intracellular fluid) and organelles.

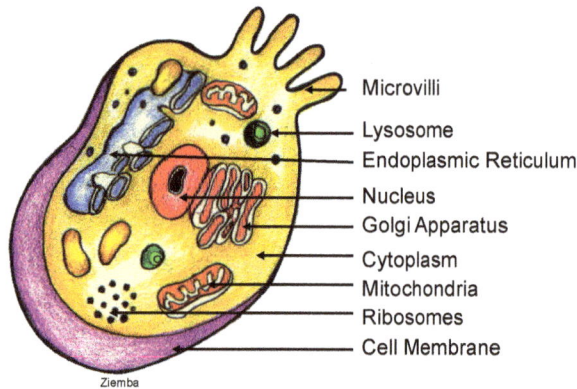

Figure 2.1: Cell structure. Courtesy of Tina Ziemba.

B. Components (Figure 2.1)

1. Nonmembranous organelles are always in contact with the cytosol. They include the cytoskeleton, microvilli, centrioles, cilia, flagella, and ribosomes.
2. The cytoskeleton gives the cytoplasm strength and flexibility. It has the following components:
   a) Microfilaments—actin
   b) Intermediate filaments (thick)—myosin
   c) Microtubules—tubulin
3. Microvilli are small projections of the cell membrane that increase the surface area exposed to the extracellular environment.
4. The centrioles direct the movement of chromosomes during cell division and organize the cytoskeleton.
5. The centrosome is the cytoplasm surrounding the centrioles.
6. The cilia is anchored by a basal body and beats rhythmically to move fluids or secretions across the cell surface.
7. The flagella moves a cell through surrounding fluid rather than moving fluid past a stationary cell.
8. Ribosomes are composed of light and heavy ribosomal subunits that contain ribosomal RNA (rRNA).
9. Ribosomal RNA (rRNA) is an intracellular factory that manufactures proteins.
10. Mitochondria are responsible for 95% of ATP production in a cell.
11. Endoplasmic reticulum is a network of intracellular membranes that function in synthesis, storage, transport, and detoxification.
12. The Golgi Apparatus moves material via transfer vesicles, forms secretory vesicles and new membrane components, and packages lysosomes.
13. Lysosomes are vesicles filled with digestive enzymes.
14. Perioxomes carry enzymes that absorb and neutralize toxins.
15. The nucleus is the control center of cellular operations.
16. Chromosomes consist of DNA bound to histones.
17. Chromatin is a tangle of filaments formed by chromosomes.
18. Cell division is the reproduction of cells.
19. Apoptosis is the genetically controlled death of cells.
20. Mitosis refers to the nuclear division of somatic cells.
21. Mitosis proceeds in four stages: prophase, metaphase, anaphase, and telophase.
22. Meiosis refers to nuclear division of sex cells.
23. Interphase—most somatic cells spend the majority of their time in this phase, which includes DNA replication. A variety of growth factors can stimulate cell division and growth.
24. Four types of cell junctions:
    a) Tight junction—there is partial fusion of the lipid portions of the two cell membranes.
    b) Desmosomes—cell adhesion molecules and proteoglycans linking the opposing cell membranes.
    c) Hemidesmosomes—cell adhesion molecules and proteoglycans link cells to the basement membrane.
    d) Gap junctions—two cells held together by an interlocking of membrane proteins.

C. Methods of examining slides

1. Light microscopy: a light microscope can magnify cellular structures about 1,000 times and can show details as fine as 0.25 micrometer.
   a) Steps for preparing slides
      i) Embed the tissue sample.
      ii) Section the block with a machine called a microtome.
      iii) If embedded in wax, you can remove the wax with solvent.
      iv) Add special dyes to stain your slides.
      v) Put a cover slip on your slide and look through the microscope.
2. Electron microscopy: an electron microscope can magnify structures up to approximately 500,000 times.

RESOURCES

1. Martini FH. *Fundamentals of Anatomy and Physiology.* 4th ed. Englewood Cliffs: Prentice-Hall; 1998.

2. Martini FH. *Fundamentals of Anatomy and Physiology: Applications Manual.* 4th ed. Englewood Cliffs: Prentice-Hall; 1998.

3. Moore KL, Dalley AF. *Clinically Oriented Anatomy.* 4th ed. Philadelphia: Lippincott Williams & Wilkins; 1999.

SAMPLE QUESTIONS

1. Diffusion of water across a membrane in response to differences in solute concentration is the process of:
    a) Osmosis
    b) Diffusion
    c) Permeability
    d) Facilitated diffusion

2. Cell adhesion molecules and proteoglycans, which link cells to basement membranes, are called:
    a) Desmosomes
    b) Hemidesmosomes
    c) Tight junction
    d) Microvilli

3. Crenation happens when a cell is in:
    a) A hypotonic solution that causes water to flow into the cell
    b) An isotonic solution that does not cause any osmotic flow
    c) A hypertonic solution that causes water to flow out of the cell
    d) A hypertonic solution that causes water to flow into the cell

4. The genetically controlled death of cells is called:
    a) Mitosis
    b) Meiosis
    c) Apoptosis
    d) Interphase

5. Cell membranes contain:
    a) Lipids
    b) Carbohydrates
    c) Protein
    d) All of the above

6. An active process that helps the movement of material into cells is called:
    a) Mitosis
    b) Apoptosis
    c) Facilitated diffusion
    d) Endocytosis

7. Light microscopy can magnify cellular structure up to:
    a) 10 times
    b) 100 times
    c) 1,000 times
    d) 10,000 times

8. Electron microscopy can magnify cellular structure up to:
    a) 100,000 times
    b) 200,000 times
    c) 250,000 times
    d) 500,000 times

9. Which of the following statements about meiosis is accurate?
    a) It refers to the nuclear division of sex cells.
    b) It refers to the nuclear division of somatic cells.
    c.) It proceeds in four stages: prophase, metaphase, anaphase, and telophase.
    d.) It refers to the genetically controlled death of cells.

10. Lysosomes are:
    a) Vesicles filled with digestive enzymes
    b) Vesicles filled with protelytic enzymes
    c) Vesicles filled with proteases
    d) Vesicles filled with matrix metalloproteases

See answers on page 11.

NOTES

ANSWER KEY

1. a) Osmosis is the diffusion of water across a membrane in response to differences in solute concentration. Diffusion is the net movement of material from an area where its concentration is relatively high to an area where its concentration is lower. Permeability is the ease with which a substance can cross the cell membrane, and facilitated diffusion is a carrier-mediated transport.

2. b) Cell adhesion molecules and proteoglycans, which link cells to basement membranes, are called hemidesmosomes.

3. c) Crenation happens when a hypertonic solution causes water to flow out of the cell.

4. c) The genetically controlled death of cells is called apoptosis.

5. d) The cell membrane contains lipids, carbohydrates, and proteins.

6. d) Endocytosis is an active process that helps the movement of material into cells.

7. c) Light microscopy can magnify cellular structure by 1,000 times.

8. d) Electron microscopy can magnify cellular structure by 500,000 times.

9. a) Meiosis refers to the nuclear division of sex cells.

10. a) Lysosomes are vesicles filled with digestive enzymes.

ANATOMY OF SKIN 3

Jayesh B. Shah, MD, CWSP, FAPWCA, FACCWS
Prachi J. Shah

INTRODUCTION

This chapter describes the functions of the skin, layers of the skin (epidermis, dermis, and hypodermis), the function of dermal cells (mast cells, neutrophils, macrophages, and lymphocytes), and skin changes in the elderly.

OBJECTIVES

Participants should be able to discuss the primary functions of the skin, list the layers of the skin, discuss the function of dermal cells, and describe the changes in aging skin.

I. Anatomy of skin
A. Healthy skin is tough, pliable, elastic, slightly moist, and well-hydrated.
B. Skin is the largest organ of the body.
1. Approximately 18 square feet in area (1.7 square meters)
2. Weight is approximately 12 pounds (5.5 kilograms)
C. Skin is naturally populated with microorganisms, including *Staphylococcus aureus*, *Staphylococcus epidermis*, and some forms of *Streptococcus*.
D. Substances in sweat and sebum and the acidic pH (4.5–5.5) of the skin help prevent these organisms from becoming pathogenic.

II. Functions of skin
A. Protection
B. Sensing the environment
C. Water retention
D. Thermoregulation
E. Synthesis of vitamin D
F. Expression of emotion

III. Layers of skin (Figure 3.1)
A. Epidermis
1. Outermost layer
2. Varies in thickness
3. No blood supply of its own
4. Minor injuries affect this layer (abrasion or sunburns)

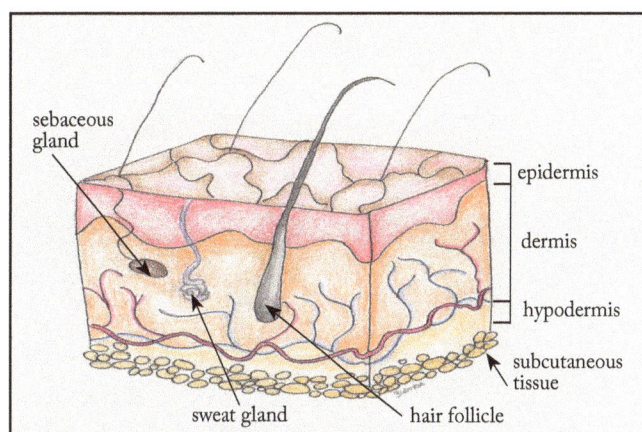

Figure 3.1: Layers of the skin. Courtesy of Tina Ziemba.

5. Composed of several layers of cells—90% are keratinocytes (synthesize keratin)
   a) Keratins
      i) Insoluble fibrous proteins
      ii) Extremely resistant to changes in pH, temperature, and enzymatic digestion
      iii) Two broad categories
         (1) Hard (hair, nails)
         (2) Soft (found in cells of the stratum corneum)
B. Dermis
C. Hypodermis

IV. Layers of epidermis (Figure 3.2)
A. Stratum corneum
1. The outermost layer is thick with rows of dead cells.
2. These cells contain soft keratin, which keeps the skin elastic and protects underlying cells from drying out.
3. Movement from the basal layer to the stratum corneum takes about two to three weeks.
4. Complete epidermal renewal can occur between 45–75 days.
B. Stratum granulosum
1. The thin middle layer initiates keratinization (production of keratin), a process that starts the death of

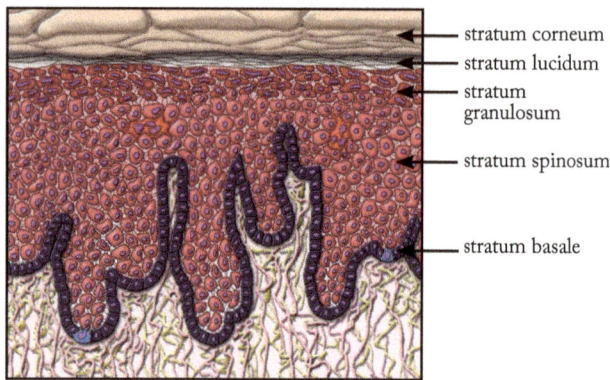

Figure 3.2: Layers of the epidermis.
Courtesy of Dr. Rajinder Singh.

epithelial cells (the cell type that makes up skin).
C. Stratum lucidum
   1. Protects against sun ultraviolet-ray damage. A thick layer appears only in frequently used areas such as the palms of the hands and soles of the feet.
   2. Thick skin epidermis has all five strata.
   3. Thin skin, which covers thinner epidermal areas such as eyelids, has three or four of the five strata; it never has stratum lucidum.
   4. Replaces shed stratum corneum.
D. Stratum spinosum
   1. Spiny prickle cells (multisided cells) that interlock to support the skin.
   2. Langerhans cells—on infected skin, local Langerhans cells will take up and process microbial antigens to become fully functional antigen-presenting cells.
   3. Contain desmosomes (contact areas) between cells.
E. Stratum basale/stratum germinativum
   1. Rests on a basement membrane attached by hemidesmosomes (the layer between the dermis and epidermis).
   2. Receives blood supply and nourishment from dermis.
   3. Outer layer cells die and desquamate.
   4. Melanocytes (can regenerate).

V. Key cells in the epidermis
A. Keratinocytes: 90% of cells in the epidermis
B. Corneocytes: differentiated keratinocytes surrounded by cornified envelope
C. Melanocytes: produce melanin; variation in skin color is related to the amount and distribution of melanin synthesized and stored in keratinocytes
D. Merkel cells: found in basal layer
   1. Attached to keratinocytes by desmosomes.
   2. Thought to function as touch receptors.
E. Langerhans cells: bone marrow derived
   1. Important in immune function of skin.
   2. Recognize foreign invaders.
   3. Implicated in skin graft rejection.

VI. Basement membrane zone (BMZ)
A. Dermal-epidermal junction
B. Contains fibronectin, type IV collagen, heparin sulfate, proteoglycan, and glycosaminoglycan
C. Has rete ridges
D. Anchors epidermis to dermis

VII. Layers of skin: dermis (Figure 3.1)
A. Made up of collagen and elastin fibers
B. Provides strength, bulk support, and elasticity
C. Rich in nerve and blood supply
D. Contains appendages
E. Collagen forms up to 30% of the volume or 70% of the dry weight
   1. A family of proteins (19 types known)
      a) Type I—tendons, ligament, bones, skin (90%)
      b) Type II—major component of cartilage
      c) Type III—found in arteries, intestine, uterus
      d) Type IV—found in basement membrane of epidermis
      e) Other 15 types are much lower in quantity
F. Dermal layers
   1. Papillary layer
      a) Lies immediately below the basement membrane
      b) Has loose connective tissue composed of collagen and reticular fibers
      c) Contains pain touch receptors
   2. Reticular layer
      a) Has dense connective tissue
      b) Contains a complex of cutaneous blood vessels

VIII. Dermal cells
A. Mast cells: primarily distributed in the papillary dermis
   1. Often seen near blood vessels and nerves
   2. Also found in subcutaneous fat and connective tissue
   3. Involved in the presence of subacute and chronic inflammatory disease
   4. Part of the skin immune system
B. Neutrophils
   1. First inflammatory cells to respond to the soluble mediators released by platelets and the coagulation cascade
   2. Phagocytosis
   3. Recruit and activate fibroblasts and epithelial cells
   4. Persistent presence of bacteria in a wound may contribute to chronicity through the continued recruitment of neutrophils and their release of proteases, cytokines, and reactive oxygen species
   5. Usually neutrophils are depleted in the wound after two to three days by the process of apoptosis and are replaced by tissue monocytes
C. Macrophages
   1. Circulating monocytes
   2. Seen at wound site 24 hours after injury

3. Activated in response to chemokines, cytokines, growth factors, and soluble fragments of extracellular matrix components
4. Functions of macrophages:
   a) Phagocytosis
   b) Regulate proteolytic destruction of wound tissue by secreting inhibitors for the proteases
   c) Release a wide variety of growth factors and cytokines
   d) Recruit and activate fibroblasts
   e) Promote angiogenesis

D. Lymphocytes
   1. Part of immune system with three major cell types: T cells, B cells, and natural killer (NK) cells.
   2. T cells produce cytokines that direct the immune response and produce toxic granules that kill pathogen-infected cells.
   3. B cells produce antibodies that neutralize foreign objects like bacteria and viruses.
   4. NK cells defend the host from both tumors and virally infected cells.

IX. Layers of skin: hypodermis or subcutaneous tissue (Figure 3.1)

A. Below the dermis
B. A receptacle for the storage and formation of fat
C. Insulates, supports, and cushions other tissues
D. Nutritional storage depot

X. Skin changes in the elderly

A. Decreased
   1. Dermal thickness
   2. Fatty layers
   3. Collagen and elastin fibers
   4. Size (depth) of rete ridges
   5. Sensation and metabolism
   6. Sweat glands
   7. Subcutaneous tissue
   8. Circulation
B. Increased
   1. Time for epidermal regeneration
   2. Damage to skin from the sun

RESOURCES

1. Martini FH. *Fundamentals of Anatomy and Physiology.* 4th ed. Englewood Cliffs: Prentice-Hall; 1998.
2. Martini FH. *Fundamentals of Anatomy and Physiology: Applications Manual.* 4th ed. Englewood Cliffs: Prentice-Hall; 1998.
3. Moore KL, Dalley AF. *Clinically Oriented Anatomy.* 4th ed. Philadelphia: Lippincott William & Wilkins; 1999.
4. McCulloch JM, Kloth LC, Feeder JA, editors. *Wound Healing: Alternatives in Management.* Philadelphia: FA Davis Company; 1995.
5. Baronoski S, Ayello EA. *Wound Care Essentials: Practice Principles.* 2nd ed. Philadelphia: Lippincott William & Wilkins; 2008.
6. Sheffield PJ, Fife CE, editors. *Wound Care Practice.* 2nd ed. North Palm Beach: Best Publishing Company; 2007.

SAMPLE QUESTIONS

1. The first cells to reach the site of wound injury are:
   a) Platelets
   b) Neutrophils
   c) Macrophages
   d) Lymphocytes

2. All of the following are part of the skin immune system except:
   a) Lymphocytes
   b) Langerhans cells
   c) Mast cells
   d) Merkel cells

3. Which is the most common type of collagen found in skin?
   a) Type I collagen
   b) Type II collagen
   c) Type III collagen
   d) Type IV collagen

4. All of the following cells are found in the epidermis except:
   a) Melanocytes
   b) Merkel cells
   c) Langerhans cells
   d) Mast cells

5. All the following skin changes occur in an elderly patient except:
   a) Increase in size of rete ridges
   b) Decrease in sweat glands
   c) Decrease in circulation
   d) Increase in time of epidermal regeneration

6. Which of the following layers of epidermis is not always present in skin?
   a) Stratum corneum
   b) Stratum granulosum
   c.) Stratum lucidum
   d) Stratum basale

7. Melanocytes are present in which layer of epidermis?
   a) Stratum basale
   b) Stratum spinosum
   c) Stratum lucidum
   d) Stratum granulosum
   e) Stratum corneum

8. All of the following are functions of macrophages except:
   a) Phagocytosis
   b) Secretion of MMPs
   c) Secretion of growth factors
   d) Secretion of lactic acid
   e) Formation of provisional matrix

9. The basement membrane zone contains all of the following except:
   a) Glycosaminoglycan
   b) Proteoglycan
   c) Heparin sulphate
   d) Fibronectin
   e) Type I collagen

10. Neutrophils are depleted in the wound within:
    a) 24 hours
    b) 2 to 3 days
    c) 4 to 5 days
    d) 6 to 14 days

See answers on page 18.

NOTES

ANSWER KEY

1. a) The first cells to reach the wound site are platelets.

2. d) Lymphocytes, Langerhans cells, and mast cells are part of the skin immune system. Merkel cells are touch receptors, not part of the immune system.

3. a) Type I collagen is the most common collagen found in the skin.

4. d) Key cells found in the epidermis are keratinocytes, corneocytes, melanocytes, Merkel cells, and Langerhans cells. Mast cells are found in the dermis, not in the epidermis.

5. a) In elderly patients, skin experiences a decrease in the size of rete ridges, in sweat glands, and in circulation. Elderly skin also requires increased time for epidermal regeneration.

6. c) Thin skin, which covers thinner epidermal areas such as eyelids, does not have stratum lucidum.

7. a) Melanocytes are present in the stratum basale layer of the epidermis.

8. e) Macrophages secrete MMPs, growth factors, and lactic acid, but they do not help in the formation of provisional matrix. Platelets are the cells that help in the formation of provisional matrix.

9. e) The basement membrane zone contains fibronectin, type IV collagen, heparin sulfate, proteoglycan, and glycosaminoglycan. It does not contain type I collagen.

10. b) Neutrophils are depleted in wounds within 2 to 3 days.

CELLULAR COMPONENTS IN WOUND HEALING

4

Jayesh B. Shah, MD, CWSP, FAPWCA, FACCWS

INTRODUCTION

This chapter describes the cellular components involved in wound healing, including chemokines, cytokines, growth factors, integrins, matrix metalloproteases (MMPs), and tissue inhibitors of MMPs, as well as the cellular components of extracellular matrix (collagen, glycosaminoglycans, proteoglycans, and fibrin). Nitric oxide is described as the key mediator of cutaneous physiology and regulator of wound healing.

OBJECTIVES

Participants should be able to list the five cellular components involved in wound healing, discuss the roles of the six growth factors relevant to wound healing, and state the function of matrix metalloproteases (MMPs) in wound healing.

I. Review of cellular components of wound healing

A. Chemokines
   1. Chemokines are named from a contraction of chemoattractive cytokines.
   2. Regulate the trafficking of leukocyte populations during normal health and development.
   3. Direct recruitment and activation of neutrophils, lymphocytes, macrophages, eosinophils, and basophils during inflammation.
B. Cytokines (Table 4.1)
   1. Small polypeptides.
   2. Have powerful action on chemotaxis, proliferation, and differentiation of inflammatory and noninflammatory cells.
   3. Cytokines are major signaling molecules in the immune system.
C. Growth factors (GFs)
   1. Growth factors are complex proteins released by cells that stimulate:
      a) Chemotaxis
      b) Mitosis
      c) Angiogenesis
      d) Apoptosis

Table 4.1: Cytokines involved in wound healing.

CYTOKINE	CELL SOURCE	BIOLOGICAL ACTIVITY
Pro-inflammatory cytokines		
TNF-α	Macrophages	PMN margination and cytotoxicity, ± collagen synthesis; provides metabolic substrate
IL-1	Macrophages Keratinocytes	Fibroblast and keratinocyte chemotaxis, collagen synthesis
IL-2	T lymphocytes	Increases fibroblast infiltration and metabolism
IL-6	Macrophages PMNs Fibroblasts	Fibroblast proliferation, hepatic acute-phase protein synthesis
IL-8	Macrophages Fibroblasts	Macrophage and PMN chemotaxis, keratinocyte maturation
IFN-γ	T lymphocytes Macrophages	Macrophage and PMN activation; retards collagen synthesis and cross-linking; stimulates collagenase activity
Anti-inflammatory cytokines		
IL-4	T lymphocytes Basophils Mast cells	Inhibition of TNF, IL-1, IL-6 production; fibroblast proliferation, collagen synthesis
IL-10	T lymphocytes Macrophages Keratinocytes	Inhibition of TNF, IL-1, IL-6 production; inhibits macrophage and PMN activation

      e) Growth factor production by other cells
      f) Production and degradation of extracellular matrix
   2. Role of growth factors in healing
      a) Mediates all cellular functions
      b) Mechanism is usually local
      c) Bind to cell receptors
   3. Growth factors most involved in wound healing (Table 4.2)
      a) PDGF (platelet-derived growth factor)
         i) Found in the platelets but also macrophages, fibroblasts, and other cell types

Table 4.2: Major growth factor families.

GROWTH FACTOR FAMILY	CELL SOURCE	ACTIONS
Transforming growth factor β TGF-β1, TGF-β2, TGF-β3	Platelets Fibroblasts Macrophages	Fibroblast chemotaxis and activation ECM deposition • Collagen synthesis • TIMP synthesis • MMP synthesis Reduces scarring • Collagen • Fibronectin
Platelet-derived growth factor PDGF-AA, PDGF-BB, VEGF	Platelets Macrophages Keratinocytes Fibroblasts	Activation of immune cells and fibroblasts ECM deposition • Collagen synthesis • TIMP synthesis • MMP synthesis Angiogenesis
Fibroblast growth factor Acidic FGF, Basic FGF, KGF	Macrophages Endothelial cells Fibroblasts	Angiogenesis Endothelial cell activation Keratinocyte proliferation and migration ECM deposition
Insulin-like growth factor IGF-I, IGF-II, Insulin	Liver Skeletal muscle Fibroblasts Macrophages Neutrophils	Keratinocyte proliferation Fibroblast proliferation Endothelial cell activation Angiogenesis • Collagen synthesis ECM deposition Cell metabolism
Epidermal growth factor EGF, HB-EGF, TGF-α Amphiregulin, Betacellulin	Keratinocytes Macrophages	Keratinocyte proliferation and migration ECM deposition
Connective tissue growth factor CTGF	Fibroblasts Endothelial cells Epithelial cells	Mediates action of TGF-βs on collagen synthesis

ii) Chemotactic for fibroblasts, smooth muscle cells, monocytes, and neutrophils

iii) Has profound effects on extracellular matrix

b) Vascular endothelial growth factors (VEGF) modulate blood vessel formation.

c) Fibroblast growth factors (FGF) help with collagen synthesis and ECM deposition.

d) Transforming growth factor beta (TGF–β) is a potent stimulant for collagen deposition.

e) EGF (epidermal growth factor)

 i) Stimulates cell growth, proliferation, and differentiation by binding to its receptor EGFR

f) IGF (insulin-like growth factor)

 i) Proteins with high sequence similarity to insulin

 ii) Part of a complex system that cells use to communicate with their physiologic environment

D. GF receptors

1. Initiate effect by binding to and activating specific, high affinity receptor-proteins located on the target cell's surface.

2. Activation of receptors stimulate cellular processes.

3. Different cells secrete different GFs and can express several different receptors.

E. Functions of integrins (family of cell surface receptors)

1. Enable cells to detect and interact with components of the extracellular matrix.

2. Platelet interactions with collagen during hemostasis.

3. Leukocyte extravasation during early inflammation.

4. Endothelial cell budding and ingrowth during angiogenesis.

5. Epithelial cell migration.

6. Fibroblast movement through granulation tissue.

F. Matrix metalloproteases (MMPs)

1. MMPs are a family of protein degrading enzymes.

2. Synthesized and secreted by multiple cell types (neutrophils, macrophages, fibroblasts, endothelial cells, and epithelial cells).

3. Secreted in response to biochemical signals (TNF, IL-1, IL-6).

4. Play an important role in wound healing.

5. Besides wounds, MMPs are increased and are pathogenic in diseases such as:

 a) Cystic fibrosis

 b) Rheumatoid arthritis

 c) Osteoarthritis

 d) Atherosclerosis

 e) Aneurysms

 f) Tumor growth

 g) Periodontal disease

G. Tissue inhibitors of MMPs (TIMPs)

1. Reversibly bind MMPs in 1:1 ratio to inactivate MMPs.

2. Secreted locally by cells.

3. Four TIMPs known.

4. Each TIMP can bind more than one type of MMP.

H. Extracellular matrix (ECM)

1. Matrix components:

 a) Collagen (refer to Chapter 3, page 14)

 b) Glycosaminoglycans (GAGs)

  i) Provide bulk and maintain hydration in ECM.

 c) Proteoglycans (GAG + 1 or more proteins)

  i) Provide protein anchoring and regulate collagen fibril formation.

 d) Fibrin/fibronectin/vitronectin

  i) Helps create scaffolding during hemostasis.

  ii) Sometimes called a provisional matrix.

  iii) Binds and stores growth factors.

  iv) Fibronectin coats the fibrin network and plays a role in cellular attachment.

  v) Fibronectin facilitates movement of cells into the wound site.

I.   Role of nitric oxide (NO)
1.   Key mediator of cutaneous physiology and regulator of wound healing.
2.   NO is formed from L-arginine by three isoforms of nitric oxide synthase (NOS).
3.   Oxygen and L-arginine are combined by NOS to form NO and citrulline.
4.   Inducible isoform (iNOS) is synthesized early in the inflammatory phase of wound healing primarily by macrophages.
5.   NO synthesis occurs for 10-14 days after wounding and gradually decreases.
6.   Multiple cells participate in NO synthesis, including fibroblasts.
7.   NO crosses cell membranes without mediation of channels or receptors enhancing its ability to act as a cellular signal for wound healing.
8.   Arginine and NO administration improves healing.

RESOURCES

1.   McCulloch JM, Kloth LC, Feeder JA, editors. *Wound Healing: Alternatives in Management*. Philadelphia: FA Davis Company; 1995.
2.   Sheffield PJ, Fife CE, Smith APS, editors. *Wound Care Practice*. North Palm Beach: Best Publishing Company; 2004.
3.   Sheffield PJ, Fife CE, editors. *Wound Care Practice*. 2nd ed. North Palm Beach: Best Publishing Company; 2007.
4.   Krasner DL, Rodeheaver GT, Sibbold RG. *Chronic Wound Care: A Clinical Sourcebook for Healthcare Professionals*. 3rd ed. Wayne: HMP Communications; 2001.
5.   Bowker JH, Pfeifer MA, editors. *Levin and O'Neal's The Diabetic Foot*. 7th ed. Philadelphia: Mosby/Elsevier Health Sciences; 2008.
6.   Baronoski S, Ayello EA. *Wound Care Essentials: Practice Principles*. 2nd ed. Philadelphia: Lippincott William & Wilkins; 2008.

SAMPLE QUESTIONS

1. Platelet-derived growth factors are derived from:
   a) Platelets
   b) Macrophages
   c) Fibroblasts
   d) All of the above

2. Growth factors stimulate:
   a) Chemotaxis
   b) Meiosis
   c) Angiogenesis
   d) Apoptosis
   e) a, c, d
   f) a, b, c

3. MMPs are secreted by all of the following cells except:
   a) Neutrophils
   b) Macrophages
   c) Fibroblasts
   d) Endothelial cells
   e) Platelets

4. Nitrous oxide synthesis increases after wounding for:
   a) 10-14 days
   b) 14-28 days
   c) 2-3 months
   d) 6 months

5. Arginine and nitric oxide administration improves healing.
   a) True
   b) False

6. All of the following statements about fibronectin are true except:
   a) Fibronectin helps to form a provisional matrix.
   b) Fibronectin helps create scaffolding during hemostasis.
   c) Fibronectin binds and stores growth factors.
   d) Fibronectin provides protein anchoring and regulates collagen fibril formation.

7. All of the following statements regarding MMPs are true except:
   a) MMPs are a family of protein degrading enzymes.
   b) MMPs and growth factors both help with tissue deposition.
   c) MMPs are secreted in response to biochemical signals.
   d) Gelatinase and collagenases are examples of MMPs.

8. MMPs are increased in:
   a) Chronic wounds
   b) Rheumatoid arthritis
   c) Osteoarthritis
   d) Tumor growth
   e) All of the above

9. Vascular endothelial growth factor is a potent stimulant of collagen deposition.
   a) True
   b) False

10. Which of the following statements about fibroblast growth factors is true?
    a) FGFs are secreted by macrophages, endothelial cells, and fibroblasts.
    b) FGFs help in angiogenesis.
    c) FGFs help in endothelial cell activation.
    d) FGFs help in extracellular matrix deposition.
    e) All of the above are true.

See answers on page 24.

NOTES

ANSWER KEY

1. d) Platelet-derived growth factors are derived from platelets, macrophages, and fibroblasts.

2. e) Growth factors stimulate chemotaxis, angiogenesis, mitosis, and apoptosis. They do not stimulate meiosis.

3. e) MMPs are secreted by multiple cells, including neutrophils, macrophages, fibroblasts, and endothelial cells, but not by platelets.

4. a) Nitrous oxide synthesis increases during wounding for 10-14 days.

5. a) Arginine and nitric oxide administration improves wound healing.

6. d) Fibronectin helps form provisional matrix, creates scaffolding during hemostasis, and binds and stores growth factors.

7. b) MMPs are a family of protein-degrading enzymes. Growth factors help with tissue deposition while MMPs cause tissue destruction. MMPs are secreted in response to biochemical signals. Gelatinase and collagenases are both examples of MMPs.

8. e) MMPs are increased in chronic wounds, rheumatoid arthritis, osteoarthritis, tumor growth, and many other conditions.

9. b) Transforming growth factor beta is a potent stimulant for collagen deposition, not vascular endothelial growth factor.

10. e) FGFs are secreted by macrophages, endothelial cells, and fibroblasts. FGFs help in angiogenesis, endothelial cell activation, and extracellular matrix deposition.

PHYSIOLOGY OF WOUND HEALING 5

Jayesh B. Shah, MD, CWSP, FAPWCA, FACCWS

INTRODUCTION

This chapter describes the five phases of wound healing (vascular phase, inflammatory phase, migratory phase, proliferative phase, and maturation phase). The major cellular players in each phase are identified as well as their roles in healing.

OBJECTIVES

Participants should be able to list the five phases of wound healing, discuss the key cellular components in each phase of wound healing, and describe wound remodeling and maturation.

I. Series of events in normal and chronic wound healing

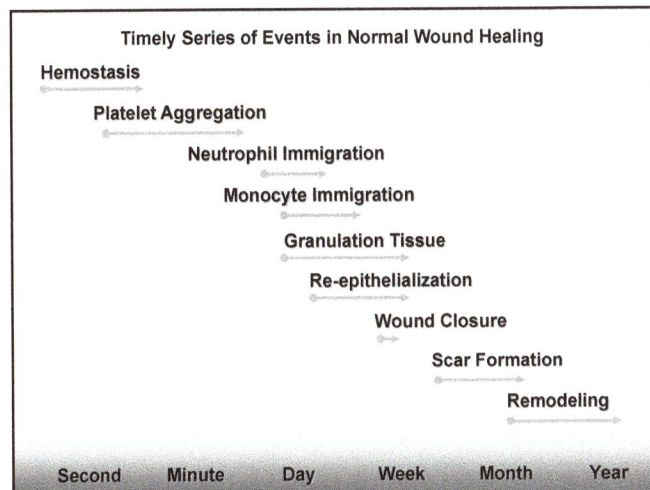

Figure 5.1a: Timely series of events in normal wound healing. Courtesy of Dr. Caroline Fife.

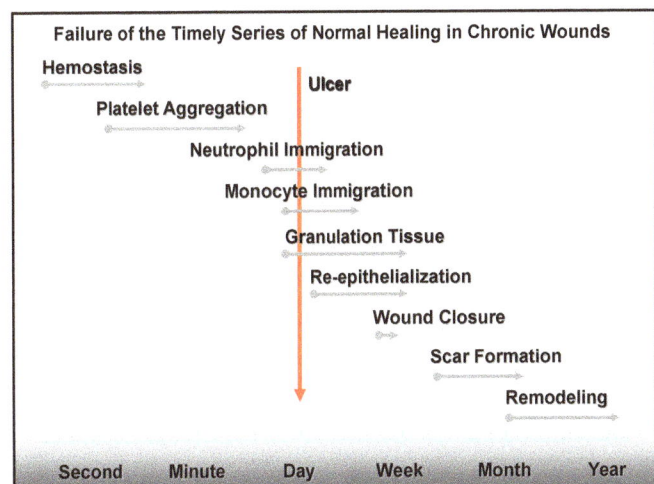

Figure 5.1b: Failure of the timely series of normal healing in chronic wounds. Courtesy of Dr. Caroline Fife.

II. Phases of wound healing

A. Vascular (hemostasis) phase (immediate response—first 24 hours) (Figure 5.2)
   1. Bleeding→vasoconstriction and retraction of damaged end vessels→formation of platelet plug→histamine mediated vasodilation→increased capillary permeability (transudative fluid), rounding of endothelial cells→periwound edema
   2. Major players during vascular phase
      a) Platelets
         i) Promote hemostasis
         ii) Initiate wound healing cascade
         iii) Form provisional matrix
      b) Coagulation
         i) Vessel rupture: platelet aggregation, coagulation (Figure 5.3a)
         ii) Platelets degranulate, release cytokines and growth factors
         iii) Fibrin clot forms (Figure 5.3b)
B. Inflammatory phase (1–3 days) (Figure 5.4)
   1. Inflammation: attraction/activation of infiltrating cells

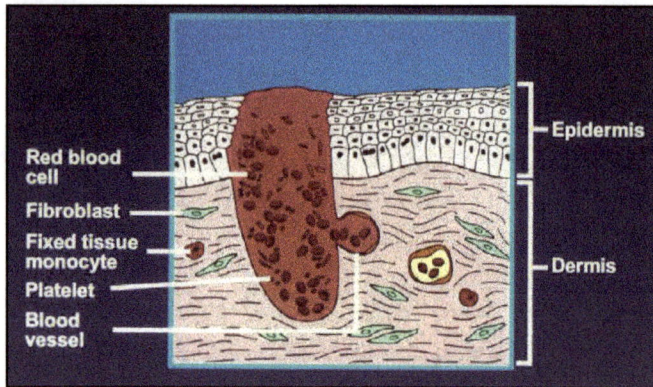

Figure 5.2: Vascular (homeostasis) phase. Courtesy of Chin et al., *Wound Care Practice*. 2007.

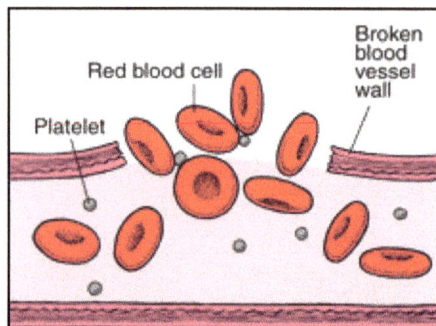

Figure 5.3a: Vessel rupture. Courtesy of Kerstein MD. *Adv Wound Care*. 1997/Martin P. *Science*. 1997.

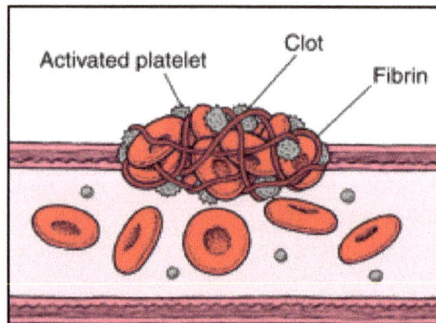

Figure 5.3b: Fibrin clot formation. Courtesy of Kerstein MD. *Adv Wound Care*. 1997/Martin P. *Science*. 1997.

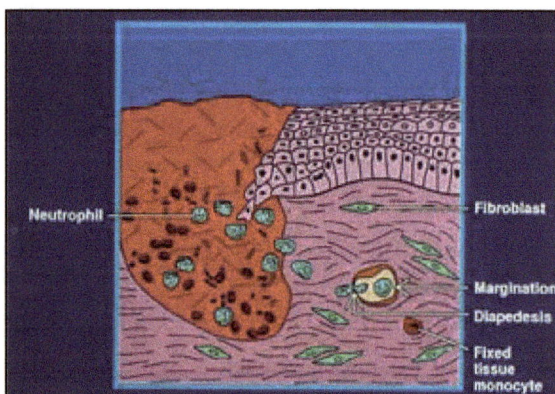

Figure 5.4: Inflammation phase. Courtesy of Chin et al., *Wound Care Practice*. 2007.

a) Extends from injury to ~ 3-4 days
b) Platelets adhere, vital release of GFs
c) PMNs combat bacteria; complement activated
d) Monocytes attracted, become macrophages
   i) Debridement/matrix turnover
   ii) Major source of GFs
e) The clean-up crew
   i) When monocytes leave the blood stream and move to an area of injury (chemotaxis), they become tissue macrophages.
   ii) These phagocytes ingest and destroy invading bacteria, foreign particles, and cellular debris (phagocytosis).
   iii) These are the clean-up crew for injured tissue.
f) Macrophages also secrete growth factors that attract and activate more cells involved in tissue repair.
g) Mast cells control vasodilation of blood vessels, which also increases permeability (this causes the redness, pain, and warmth).
h) This inflammatory response continues until all foreign material is gone and the wound is repaired.
i) Proteases are part of normal healing.
   i) Proteases are matrix metalloproteases (MMPs)
     (1) Collagenases—MMP-1
     (2) Gelatinases—MMP-2
     (3) Stromelysins—MMP-3
   ii) Assist leukocyte diapedesis and transmigration
   iii) Kept in balance by inhibitors
2. Key player in inflammatory phase: leukocytes
a) Leucocytes are the first inflammatory cells to reach the site of injury.
b) Leucocytes depend on oxygen for effective phagocytosis.
   i) There are two mechanisms of phagocytosis
     (1) Oxygen independent mechanisms (slow)
       Indirect effect because of:
       (a) Changes vacuole pH
       (b) Hydrolytic enzymes
       (c) Cationic proteins
       (d) Lactoferrin binding proteins
     (2) Oxygen dependent mechanism (fast)
       Direct effect because of:
       (a) Increased oxygen tension
       (b) Oxygen free radical formation
       (c) Free radical release
       (d) Free radical bind with bacterial cell walls
       (e) Oxidative killing mechanism
         ((1)) Respiratory burst

((2)) Free radical burst
((3)) Degranulation
((4)) Margination
(f) The killing capacity of leukocytes is reduced by 50% when oxygen tensions are below 30 mmHg in wounded tissues. A 30 mmHg oxygen tissue tension is needed for human tissue function (40 mmHg if measured transcutaneously).
((1)) Physiologically significant for human tissue function
((2)) Required for generating ATP for cell replication
((3)) Required for collagen synthesis(hydroxylation)

C. Migratory phase (day 4–5)
1. Key events
   a) Ongoing phagocytosis.
   b) Fibroblasts form from perivascular mesenchymal cells.
   c) Fibroblasts migrate into the wound area along fibrin strands of the wound clot.
   d) Macrophages signal for angiogenesis via angiogenesis factor.
2. Key player during migration phase: macrophages
   a) Most versatile player
   b) Arise from fixed tissue monocytes as well as from circulating monocyte precursors
   c) Functions of macrophages (refer to Chapter 3, pages 14-15)
      i) Release a variety of growth factors
      ii) Induce fibroblast proliferation
      iii) Chemotaxis
      iv) Collagen deposition
      v) Secrete collagenase
      vi) Release large amounts of lactate–angiogenic factors
      vii) Phagocytosis

D. Proliferative phase (6–14 days) (Figure 5.5)
1. Key events
   a) Fibroblasts synthesize ground substance and collagen.
   b) Appreciable amount of collagen is present by day 7.
   c) Capillaries invade the wound, bringing nutrients to metabolically active fibroblast.
   d) During this stage fibrin, debris, and leukocytes are nearly absent.
   e) Granulation tissue is formed.
   f) Angiogenesis
   g) Epithelialization
2. Key player: fibroblasts
   a) Derived from undifferentiated mesenchymal cells or existing fibroblasts.

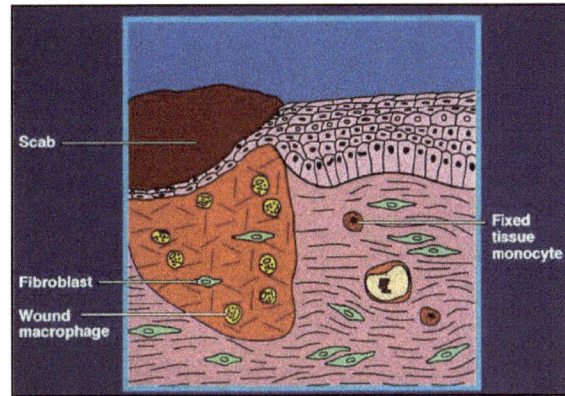

Figure 5.5: Proliferative phase. Courtesy of Chin et al., *Wound Care Practice.* 2007.

   b) Differentiation stimulated by the mitogenic factor from the macrophage; fibroblasts move into the wound along pre-existing fibrin strands.
   c) Integrin expression vital to migration of fibroblasts.
   d) Migration of fibroblasts stimulated by a variety of cytokines (PDGF and TGF-β).
   e) Migration can be impeded by residual debris in/on the wound.
   f) TGF-β stimulates fibroblasts to secrete MMPs to facilitate migration.
   g) Function dependent on adequate oxygen.
   h) Tissue oxygen tension of 30 mmHg is required (40 mmHg if measured transcutaneously).
      i) Generate ATP for cell replication
      ii) Collagen synthesis (hydroxylation)
   i) Without molecular oxygen, the amino acids (proline and lysine) can not be hydroxylated.
   j) Without hydroxylation, the fibroblasts cannot form precollagen strands.
3. Wound healing neovascularization (angiogenesis)
   a) Process
   New vessels originate from vessels at wound margin stimulated by:
      i) Macrophage angiogenesis factor
         (1) Relative hypoxia
         (2) Lactic acid
      ii) The developing collagen matrix and the wound clot provide the scaffolding and support for new capillary growth.
      iii) The relatively hypoxic wound center and lactic acid stimulate macrophage angiogenesis factor release.
      iv) The normoxic periphery provides the oxygen substrate for effective collagen synthesis.
   b) Key player: endothelial cells
      i) Migrate into new tissue to form capillary structures.
      ii) Endothelial cells also secrete growth factors.

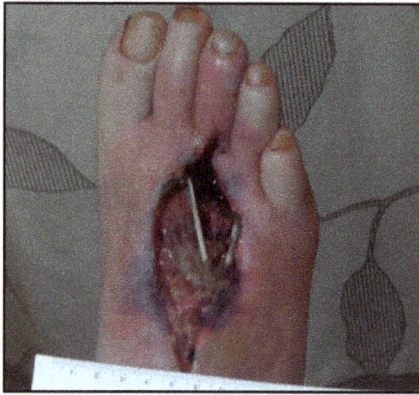

Figure 5.6a: Infected and ischemic diabetic wound.

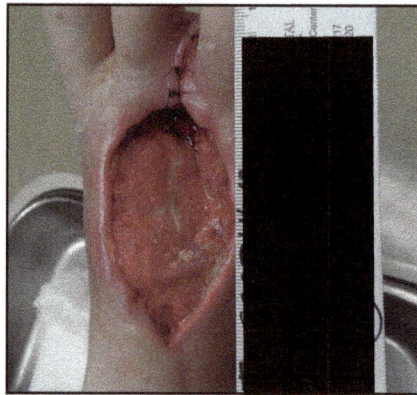

Figure 5.6b: Wound after third toe amputation and debridement.

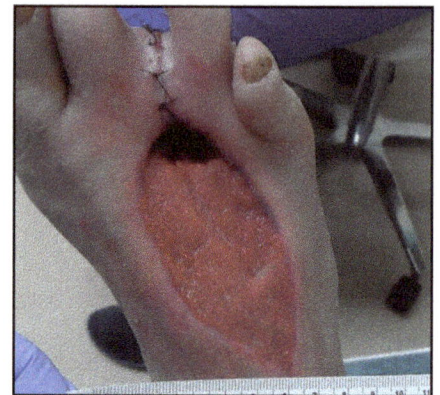

Figure 5.6c: Wound after negative pressure wound therapy.

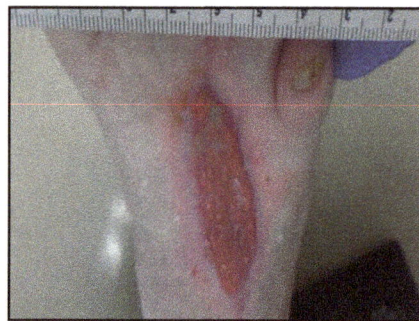

Figure 5.6d: Wound epithelializing from edges subsequent to epidermal bubble harvest skin application.

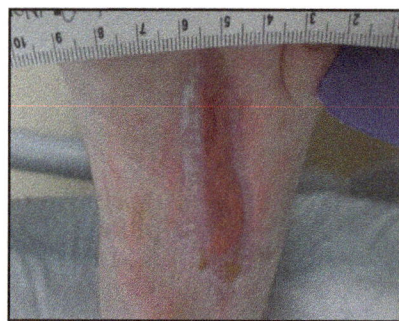

Figure 5.6e: Epithelialization in the wound.

      iii) Stimulate production of fibronectin and collagen.

      iv) Produce enzymes that degrade tissue protein, which helps with cell migration.

4. Wound healing process (Figures 5.6a–5.6e)

  a) Wound contraction

    i) Force comes from myofibroblasts located in centrally granulating mass, which is responsible for wound contraction.

    ii) Contraction may account for 50-70% of wound closure.

    iii) Rate of contraction varies between anatomic locations, averaging 0.6 to 0.7 mm per day.

    iv) Epithelialization and contraction often proceed simultaneously and independently.

  b) Key player: myofibroblast

    i) Fibroblast-to-myofibroblast differentiation represents a key event during wound healing and tissue repair.

    ii) The high contractile force generated by myofibroblasts is beneficial for physiological tissue remodeling but detrimental for tissue function when it becomes excessive, such as in hypertrophic scars.

    iii) Myofibroblast differentiation is a complex process regulated by at least a cytokine (TGF-β1), an extracellular matrix component (the ED-A splice variant of cellular fibronectin), as well as the presence of mechanical tension.

    iv) The myofibroblast is a key cell for connective tissue remodeling that takes place during wound healing and fibrosis development.

5. Wound healing epithelialization

  a) Process

    i) Epidermal covering (keratinocytes) reconstituted from wound margin and hair follicle remnants

    ii) Keratinocytes migrate across the wound.

    iii) During and after migration, differentiation and stratification of the neodermis occurs.

    iv) Epithelialization is aided by a moist environment and inhibited by scab.

    v) Epithelial cells are held in check by chalone inhibition factor.

    vi) Epithelial cells only migrate over granular tissue.

    vii) Eschar impedes epithelialization.

    viii) Epithelial cells enzymatically lyse eschar.

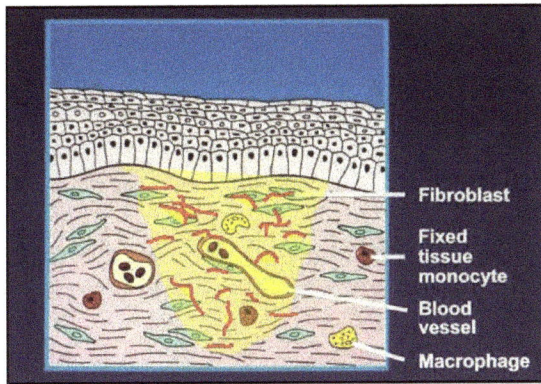

Figure 5.7: Maturation (remodeling) phase. Courtesy of Chin et al., *Wound Care Practice*. 2007.

    b) Key players: keratinocytes
        i) Keratinocytes detach from their site of origin, migrate over the wound site, reattach, differentiate, and finally proliferate.
        ii) Keratinocytes secrete MMPs and other collagenases, which act to degrade tissue proteins, allowing them to migrate.
        iii) Keratinocytes secrete growth factors.

E. Maturation phase (weeks—months—years) (Figure 5.7)
1. Immature collagen remodels into mature collagen.
2. Collagen matures along lines of stress.
3. Normal circulation is reestablished.
4. Any remaining eschar sloughs off.
5. Collagen will continue to remodel for up to two years.
6. Over time collagen cross-linking occurs.
7. Immature type III collagen is replaced by stronger type I dermal collagen.
8. Collagen fibers orient along lines of tension.
9. A wound scar is never as strong as undamaged skin (85%).
10. Wound maturation may continue for two years.

RESOURCES

1. McCulloch JM, Kloth LC, Feeder JA, editors. *Wound Healing: Alternatives in Management*. Philadelphia: FA Davis Company; 1995.
2. Chin GA, et al. Biochemistry of wound healing in wound care practice. In: Sheffield PJ, Fife CE, editors. *Wound Care Practice*. 2nd ed. North Palm Beach: Best Publishing Company; 2007.
3. Chaurasia BD. *Handbook of General Anatomy*. Delhi: CBS Publishers & Distributors; 1985.
4. Moore KL, Dalley AF. *Clinically Oriented Anatomy*. 4th ed. Philadelphia: Lippincott William & Wilkins; 1999.
5. Krasner DL, Rodeheaver GT, Sibbald GR. *Chronic Wound Care: A Clinical Source Book for Healthcare Professionals*. 3rd ed. Wayne: HMP Communications; 2001.
6. Bowker JH, Pfeifer MA, editors. *Levin and O'Neal's The Diabetic Foot*. 7th ed. Philadelphia: Mosby/Elsevier Health Sciences; 2008.
7. Hunt TK, Zabel DD. Critical care of wounds and wounded patients. In: Ayres SM, Grenvik A, Holbrook PR, et al., editors. *Textbook of Critical Care*. 3rd ed. Philadelphia: WB Saunders Co; 1995: 1475-86.
8. Witte MB, Barbul A. General principles of wound healing. *Surg Clin North Am*. 1997 Jun;77(3):509-28.
9. Martin P, Hopkinson-Woolley J, McCluskey J. Growth factors and cutaneous wound repair. *Prog Growth Factor Res*. 1992; 4:25-44.
10. Martin P. Wound healing: aiming for perfect skin regeneration. *Science*. 1997; 276:75-81.
11. Kerstein MD. The scientific basis of healing. *Adv Wound Care*. 1997; 10(3):30-6.

SAMPLE QUESTIONS

1. All of the following are the functions of macrophages except:
   a) Phagocytosis
   b) Cell recruitment and activation
   c) Angiogenesis
   d) Promotion of hemostasis

2. The killing capacity of leukocytes is reduced by _____ if tissue oxygen tension is less than 30 mmHg.
   a) 100%
   b) 75%
   c) 50%
   d) 25%

3. The cells responsible for wound contraction are:
   a) Fibroblasts
   b) Myofibroblasts
   c) Endothelial cells
   d) Keratinocytes

4. After a wound is completely healed, skin regains strength to_____% by the process of remodeling and maturation.
   a) 100
   b) 85
   c) 75
   d) 50

5. Angiogenesis is stimulated by:
   a) Relative hypoxia
   b) Hyperoxia
   c) Lactic acid
   d) Both a and c
   e) Both b and c

6. Hypertrophic scars can happen because of:
   a) Excessive MMPs
   b) Excessive growth factors
   c) Excessive myofibroblasts
   d) All of the above

7. A tissue oxygen tension of 30 mmHg (40 mmHg if measured transcutaneously) is:
   a) Physiologically significant for human tissue function
   b) Required for generating ATP for cell replication
   c) Required for collagen synthesis
   d) All of the above

8. All of the following statements about phagocytosis are true except:
   a) The oxygen independent mechanism of phagocytosis is a slow pathway.
   b) The oxygen independent mechanism of phagocytosis is a fast pathway.
   c) Oxygen free radicals are released during oxygen dependent mechanisms and bind to bacterial cell walls.
   d) All of the above are true statements.

9. The first inflammatory cells to reach a site of injury are:
   a) Platelets
   b) Leucocytes
   c) Macrophages
   d) Fibroblasts

10. Epithelial cells only migrate over good granulation tissue.
   a) True
   b) False

See answers on page 32.

NOTES

ANSWER KEY

1. d) Functions of macrophages include phagocytosis, cell recruitment and activation, and angiogenesis. Platelets help with hemostasis.

2. c) The killing capacity of leukocytes is reduced by 50% in tissue if the oxygen tension is less than 30 mmHg.

3. b) The cells responsible for wound contraction are myofibroblasts.

4. b) After the wound is completely healed, skin regains strength to 85% by the process of remodeling and maturation.

5. d) Angiogenesis is stimulated by relative hypoxia and lactic acid.

6. c) Hypertrophic scars can happen because of excessive myofibroblasts and a decrease in MMPs.

7. d) A tissue oxygen tension of 30 mmHg (40 mmHg if measured transcutaneously) is required for physiologically significant human tissue function, generating ATP for cell replication, and collagen synthesis.

8. b) The oxygen independent mechanism of phagocytosis is a slow pathway.

9. b) The first inflammatory cells to reach a site of injury are leucocytes.

10. a) Epithelial cells only migrate over good granulation tissue.

PATHOPHYSIOLOGY OF WOUND HEALING 6

Caroline E. Fife, MD, CWSP, FAAFP, FUHM

INTRODUCTION

This chapter addresses causes of non-healing. The discussion includes pathophysiology of venous stasis ulcers, arterial insufficiency ulcers, diabetic foot ulcers, and pressure ulcers. Also discussed is the pathophysiology of wounds caused by radiation injury, electrical injury, chemical burns, mechanical injury, ischemia/reperfusion injury, foreign bodies, thermal injury, and compromised skin grafts and flaps.

OBJECTIVES

Participants should be able to explain the causes of non-healing, discuss the pathophysiology of ulcers, and discuss the pathophysiology of selected injuries.

I. Introduction

A. Wound pH
   1. The pH is a measure of the acidity or alkalinity of an aqueous solution (on a scale of 0-14).
   2. The skin surface has an acidic pH of around 4.5-5.5.
      a) The body's internal environment maintains a near-neutral pH of 7.
   3. Open wounds tend to have a neutral or alkaline pH, predominantly in the range of 6.5-8.5.
      a) Since chronic wounds can be described as having permanently elevated protease levels, resulting in a prolonged inflammatory state, one strategy to promote healing may be to decrease the proteolytic activity to the normal levels observed in acute wounds (post-48 hours) by use of a pH modulator.
   4. A weakly acidic environment may promote healing in open wounds by inhibiting the action of proteases.
B. Acute wounds
   1. Cells are viable and able to respond to growth stimuli.
   2. Sufficient growth factors are released in the wound environment.
   3. Cells proliferate and can migrate and synthesize components of new tissue.

C. Chronic versus acute wounds
   1. Normal acute wounds are caused by surgery or trauma and usually heal and close rapidly.
   2. A chronic non-healing wound has been defined as a wound that fails to proceed through the orderly and timely series of events required to produce a durable, structural, functional, and cosmetically acceptable closure.

II. Causes of non-healing

A. Chronic wounds
   1. Growth factors may be deficient.
   2. Increased bacteria.
   3. Decreased oxygen.
   4. Cells are senescent, unable to respond to growth factors.
   5. Cells may be slow to proliferate and migrate (<0.5 mm/week wound closure rate).
B. Inflammation
   1. Inflammation is necessary to initiate healing.
   2. Chronic, non-progressive inflammation is inhibitory to healing.
      a) The cytokine environment of chronic wounds is more pro-inflammatory than in acute wounds.
      b) The ratio of cytokines TNF alpha and IL-1b to their inhibitors is increased.
C. Proteases
   1. Proteases are significantly elevated in chronic wound fluid.
      a) Normally tightly controlled in early healing.
      b) Matrix metalloproteases (MMPs) elevated up to 116-fold.
      c) Decrease when wounds start to heal.
D. Abnormal matrix
   1. Keratinocytes inhibited
      a) Abnormal collagen, fibronectin, glycosaminoglycans (GAGs).
      b) Fibronectin inhibits attachment, migration, and proliferation.
      c) Keratinocytes accumulate at the wound edge.

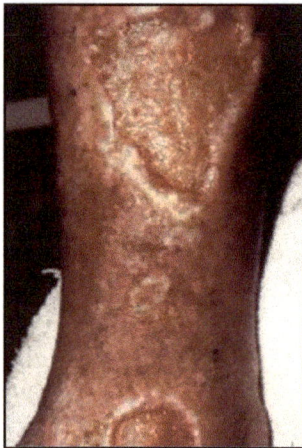

Figure 6.1: Venous stasis ulcer.

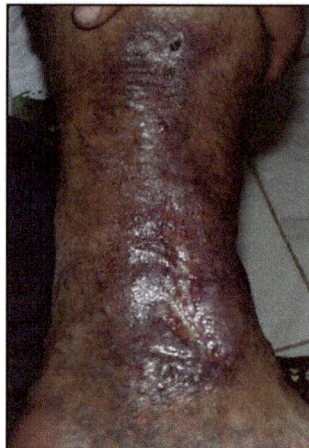

Figure 6.2: An example of phlebolymphedema.

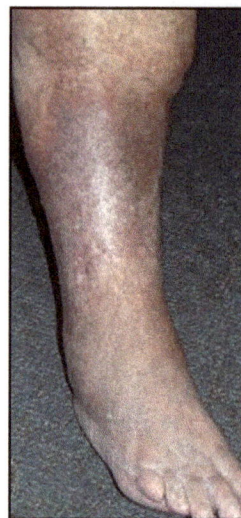

Figure 6.3a: Increased pigmentation.

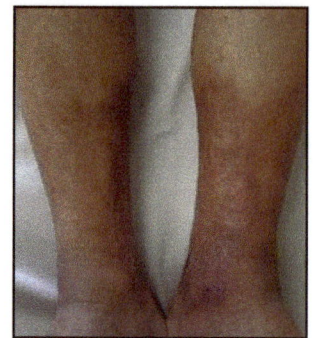

Figure 6.3b: Thickening and hardening of the skin.

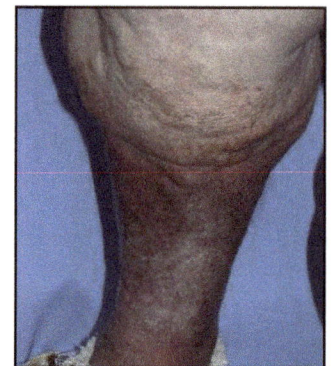

Figure 6.3c: Small white scarred areas (atrophie blanche). Also note "inverted champagne bottle" leg deformity.

III. Ulcers by etiology

A. Venous stasis ulcer characteristics (Figure 6.1)
   1. Venous stasis is almost always associated with:
     a) Edema
     b) Hemosiderin deposits
     c) Stasis dermatitis
     d) Lipodermatosclerosis (late)
   2. Venous stasis ulcers, in appearance, are:
     a) Irregular in shape, but have well-defined borders
     b) Contrary to textbooks, may be painful
     c) Never occur on the plantar feet
     d) Almost never have an eschar
     e) Never involve deep structures of the leg
     f) Almost never cause osteomyelitis
   3. Leukocyte trapping
     a) Valvular incompetence causes venous reflux.
     b) Leukocytes accumulate and become activated.
     c) Activated white cells release oxygen radicals, collagenases, and elastases, which injure surrounding tissue.
   4. Terms
     a) Phlebolymphedema is used to describe the edema caused by chronic venous insufficiency or varices, varicose phlebitis, and complications involving venous pressure flow rates (Figure 6.2).
     b) Lipodermatosclerosis (Figures 6.3a–6.3c)
       i) Lipodermatosclerosis literally means "scarring of fat and skin," and a typical description is the "inverted champagne bottle" leg. It is a type of panniculitis (inflammation of subcutaneous fat).
       ii) Lipodermatosclerosis findings:
         (1) Pain
         (2) Hardening of the skin
         (3) Localized thickening
         (4) Moderate redness
         (5) Increased pigmentation
         (6) Small white scarred areas (atrophie blanche)
         (7) Increased edema in the leg
         (8) Varicose veins
         (9) Leg ulcers

B. Arterial ulcer characteristics (Figure 6.4)
   1. Location: distal, bony prominences
   2. Size: small, "punched out," partial to full thickness
   3. Wound bed: dry, pale pink, gray-yellow to black, may be necrotic (gangrenous tissue)
   4. Drainage: usually minimal, unless infected
   5. Painful
   6. Gangrenous tissue

C. Diabetic foot ulcers (Figure 6.5)
   General considerations (14, 15)
   1. Diabetic foot ulcers are most commonly seen on weight-bearing surfaces.
   2. Foot deformities common in patients with diabetes can accentuate bony prominences and predispose the patient to pressure and the development of ulcers.
   3. Common locations of diabetic foot ulcers include the plantar surface at the hallux, first metatarsal joint, heel, nail fold, nail bed, and on the bottoms, tips, or between toes.
   4. Ulcers may be small at the surface but have large subcutaneous abscesses.
   5. Always probe a diabetic foot ulcer with a sterile swab/probe to determine the depth of wound and the possibility of bone involvement.

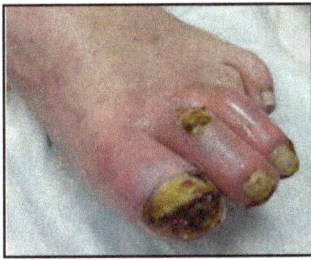

Figure 6.4: Arterial ulcer (note gangrenous changes of great toe).

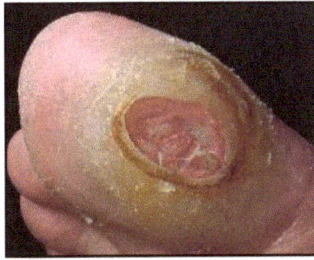

Figure 6.5: Diabetic foot ulcer.

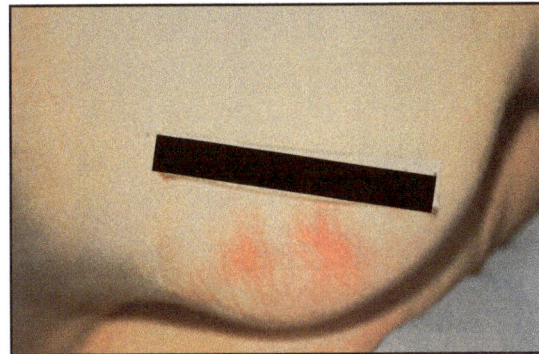

Figure 6.7a: NPUAP: Stage I pressure ulcer (left buttock); intact skin with non-blanchable redness on buttock.

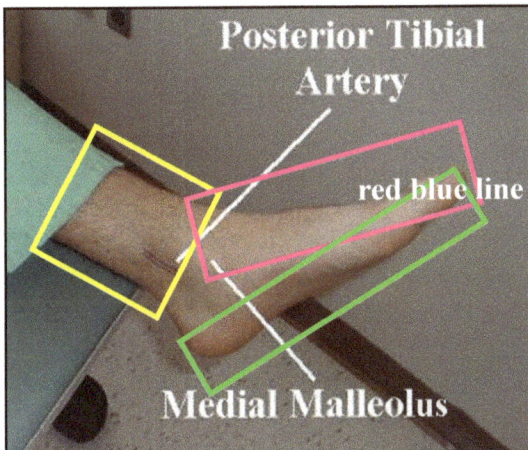

Figure 6.6: Usual location of leg ulcer types. Yellow: venous ulcers; proximal to the malleolus. Pink: arterial ulcers; distal to the malleolus. Green: diabetic neuropathic ulcers; inferior to the red blue line.

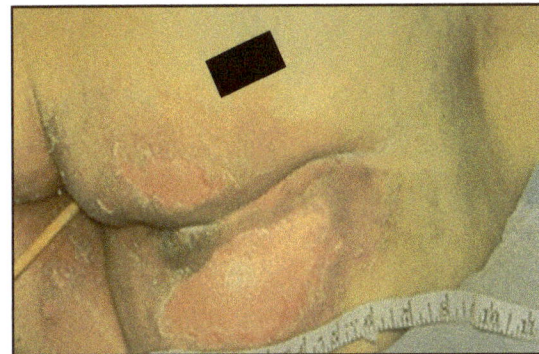

Figure 6.7b: NPUAP: Stage II pressure ulcer (both buttocks); partial thickness loss of dermis presenting as a shallow open ulcer.

6. Usual location of leg ulcer types (Figure 6.6)
   a) Venous ulcers: proximal to the malleolus (yellow box)
   b) Arterial ulcers: distal to the malleolus (pink box)
   c) Diabetic neuropathic ulcers: inferior to the "red blue" line (green box)
D. Pressure ulcers (Figures 6.7a–6.7d)
E. Radiation wounds
   1. Radiation leads to:
      a) Hypoxic—hypovascular—hypocellular matrix (fibroblast and endothelial damage due to radio-therapy [XRT]), which leads to:
      b) Tissue breakdown—lysis exceeds synthesis (in-ability to regenerate vascular bed with hypoxia, PO_2 <20–30% of non-radiated tissue), which leads to:
      c) Non-healing (demand exceeds supply)
   2. Spectrum of late effects of radiation (Figures 6.8a–6.8c)
F. Electrical injury
   1. The three major mechanisms of electricity-induced injury are:
      a) Electrical energy causing direct tissue damage, altering cell membrane resting potential, and eliciting muscle tetany

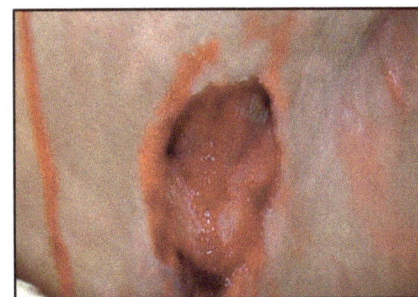

Figure 6.7c: NPUAP: Stage III pressure ulcer (sacrum). Full thickness tissue loss, subcutaneous fat may be visible but bone, tendon, or muscle is not exposed.

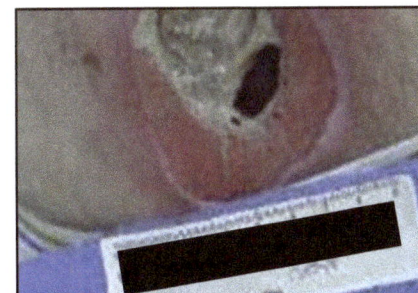

Figure 6.7d: NPUAP: Stage IV pressure ulcer (left buttock). Full thickness tissue loss with exposed bone, tendon, or muscle.

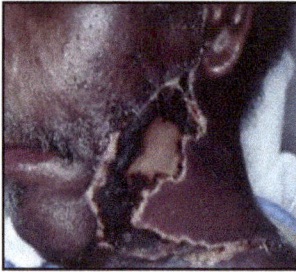

Figure 6.8a: Facial reconstruction of cancer-related deformities in irradiated tissues.

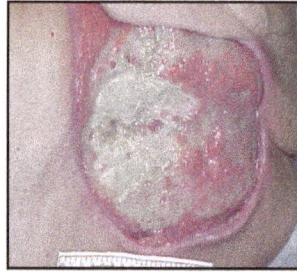

Figure 6.8b: Radiation wound on sacrum started after radiation therapy for uterine cancer.

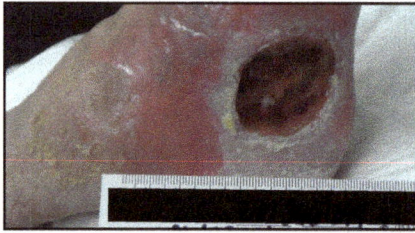

Figure 6.9a: Chemical burn secondary to dopamine extravasation.

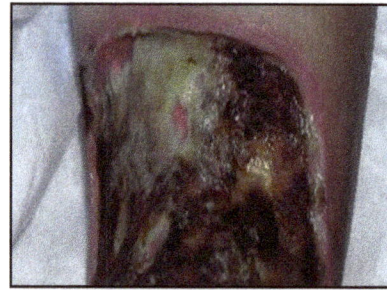

Figure 6.8c: Leg wounds s/q radiation for squamous cell cancer.

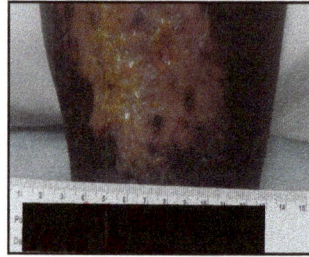

Figure 6.9b: Chemical burns secondary to paint.

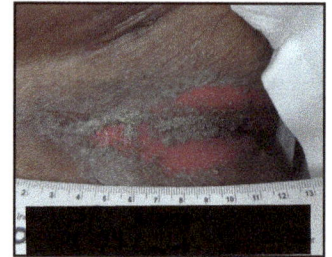

Figure 6.9c: Chemical burns secondary to applying medication for skin tag.

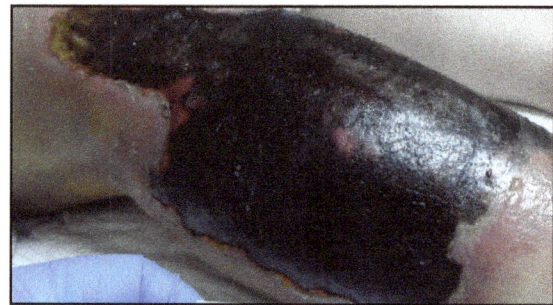

Figure 6.10: Mechanical (crush) injury; here the right leg was crushed under a car during a motor vehicle accident.

b) Conversion of electrical energy into thermal energy, causing coagulative necrosis
c) Mechanical injury from falls or violent muscle contraction

2. Factors that determine the degree of injury include:
   a) Magnitude of energy delivered
   b) Resistance encountered
   c) Type of current and current pathway
   d) Duration of contact

3. Tissue damage is directly proportional to the magnitude of current delivered.

4. Current flow (amperage) is directly related to voltage and inversely related to resistance.

5. Electrical shock is classified as high voltage (>1,000 volts) or low voltage (<1,000 volts).
   a) As a general rule, high voltage is associated with greater morbidity and mortality.

G. Chemical burns (Figures 6.9a–6.9c)
1. Five categories of corrosive and irritant products: acids, bases, oxidizers, reducing agents, and solvents.
2. Aggressiveness of a chemical agent is proportional to its concentration; the more concentrated it is, the more aggressive it is.
3. The factors which determine the severity of burn are:
   a) Type of chemical
   b) Chemical temperature
   c) Chemical concentration

H. Mechanical (crush) injury (Figure 6.10)
1. A crush injury occurs when a body part is subjected to a high degree of force or pressure, usually after being squeezed between two heavy objects.

2. Manifestations are caused by the destruction of muscle tissue and the influx of myoglobin, potassium, and phosphorus into the circulation.
3. Can cause compartment syndrome.

I. Ischemia/reperfusion injury
1. After ischemia, PMNs adhere to the venous endothelial lining.
2. Activation produces oxygen free radicals using the oxygen delivered when perfusion is restored.
3. Vasoactive substances cause constriction of adjacent arterioles resulting in a secondary reduction in blood flow.

J. Foreign bodies
1. Certain non-visible foreign bodies may be managed expectantly. Small foreign bodies of relatively nonreactive materials, such as metals, may be left in place and simply followed.
2. Pain, functional impairment, or infection from foreign bodies would warrant their removal.
3. Metal and glass >2 mm are usually seen on plain x-rays; wood is seldom seen well on x-rays.

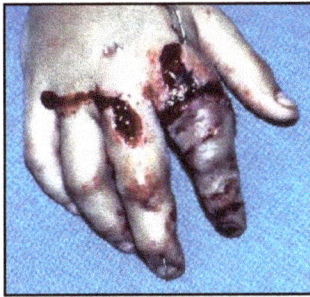

Figure 6.11a: Reimplanted finger with distal ischemia.

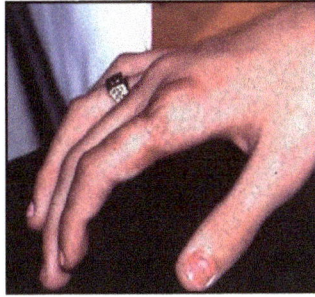

Figure 6.11b: Reimplanted finger after HBOT.

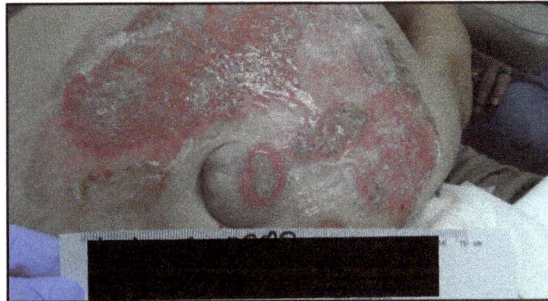

Figure 6.12: Thermal injury caused by hot water.

4. Use of antibiotics should be based on the degree of bacterial contamination, the presence of infection-potentiating factors (such as soil), the mechanism of injury, and the presence or absence of host predisposition to infection.

5. In general, decontamination is far more important than antibiotics.

6. Prophylactic antibiotics should be used in most human, dog, and cat bites, intraoral lacerations, open fractures, and exposed joints or tendons.

K. Compromised skin grafts and flaps (Figures 6.11a and 6.11b)

   1. With HBOT:

      a) Improved survival of split thickness skin grafts

      b) Reversal of distal flap ischemia

      c) Decreased ischemia reperfusion injury

L. Thermal injury (Figure 6.12)

   1. Can evolve for 24 hours

   2. Initially treated with cold water

   3. Blisters may be unroofed or left intact, depending on size and location.

   4. Burns on the face and hands or affecting children may require admission to a burn center (refer to Chapter 17, page 143).

RESOURCES

1. Dissemond J, Witthoff M, Brauns TC, Haberer D, Goos M. [pH values in chronic wounds. Evaluation during modern wound therapy.] [Article in German] *Hautarzt.* 2003; 54(10):959-65.

2. Leveen HH, Falk G, Borek B, et al. Chemical acidification of wounds. An adjuvant to healing and the unfavorable action of alkalinity and ammonia. *Ann Surg.* 1973; 178(6):745-53.

3. Monaco JL, Lawrence TL. Acute wound healing: an overview. *Clinics in Plastic Surgery.* 2003; 30: 1-12.

4. Lazarus GS, Cooper DM, Knighton DR, et al. Definitions and guidelines for assessment of wounds and evaluation of healing. *Arch Dermatol.* 1994; 130:489-93.

5. Martin P. Wound healing: aiming for perfect skin regeneration. *Science.* 1997; 276:75-81.

6. Falanga V. Growth factors and wound healing. *Dermatologic Clinics.* 1993; 11(4):667-75.

7. Hunt TK, Zabel DD. Critical care of wounds and wounded patients. In: Ayres SM, Grenvik A, Holbrook PR, et al., editors. *Textbook of Critical Care.* 3rd ed. Philadelphia: WB Saunders Co; 1995: 1475-86.

8. Witte MB, Barbul A. General principles of wound healing. *Surg Clin North Am.* 1997; 77:509-28.

9. Stanley A, Osler T. Senescence and the healing rates of venous ulcers. *J Vasc Surg.* 2001; 33(6):1206-11.

10. Mulder OD, Vande Berg JS. Cellular senescence and matrix metalloproteinase activity in chronic wounds. *J Am Podiatr Med Assoc.* 2002; 92(1):34-7.

11. Perrins DJD. Influence of hyperbaric oxygen on the survival of split skin grafts. *Lancet.* 1967; 1:868-71.

12. Bowersox JC, et al. Clinical experience with hyperbaric oxygen therapy in the salvage of ischemic skin flaps and grafts. *J Hyperb Med.* 1986; 1:141-9.

13. Zamboni WA, et al. Morphologic analysis of the microcirculation during reperfusion of ischemic skeletal muscle and the effect of hyperbaric oxygen. *Plastic Reconstr Surg.* 1993; 91:1110-23.

14. American Orthopaedic Foot and Ankle Society. Diabetic foot ulcer [Internet]. Accessed at: https://www.aofas.org/education/OrthopaedicArticles/Diabetic-foot-ulcer.pdf.

15. Kruse I, Edelman S. Evaluation and treatment of diabetic foot ulcers. *Clinical Diabetes.* 2006 Apr; 24(2):91-3. Accessed at: http://clinical.diabetesjournals.org/content/24/2/91.full.

SAMPLE QUESTIONS

1. All of the following are characteristics that virtually all chronic wounds have in common except:
   a) Senescent cells
   b) High concentrations of MMPs
   c) Reduced activity of growth factors
   d) Decrease concentrations of MMPs

2. For wounds to close, angiogenesis must occur before significant epithelialization.
   a) True
   b) False

3. Most chronic wounds are likely stalled in what phase of wound healing?
   a) Proliferative phase
   b) Inflammatory phase
   c) Remodeling phase
   d) Coagulation phase

4. Chronic wounds tend to have pH in the range of:
   a) 3.5-5.5
   b) 4.5-6.5
   c) 6.5-8.5
   d) 7.5-9.5

5. Chronic wounds are stuck in inflammatory phase, which leads to all of the following except:
   a) Chronic, non-progressive inflammation and non-healing
   b) A pro-inflammatory cytokine environment
   c) Increased ratio of cytokines TNF alpha and IL-1b to their inhibitors
   d) A decrease in MMPs and increase in growth factors

6. All of the following are mechanisms of electricity-induced injury except:
   a) Electrical energy causing direct tissue damage, altering cell membrane resting potential, and eliciting muscle tetany
   b) Conversion of electrical energy to thermal energy, causing coagulative necrosis
   c) Conversion of electrical energy to mechanical energy, causing ischemic necrosis
   d) Mechanical injury from falls or violent muscle contraction

7. Factors that determine the degree of electrical injury include:
   a) Magnitude of energy delivered
   b) Resistance encountered
   c) Type of electrical current
   d) Duration of contact
   e) All of the above

8. A patient, who is a carpenter by profession, is injured while working on wood furniture and presents to the ER with pain in his left foot. The best radiological test to evaluate this patient is:
   a) X-ray
   b) Triple phase bone scan
   c) MRI
   d) None of the above

9. All of the following are characteristics of radiation wounds except:
   a) Hypoxic
   b) Hypovascular
   c) Hypocellular
   d) Hyperoxic

10. All of the following factors determine the severity of a chemical burn except:
    a) Type of chemical
    b) Chemical temperature
    c) Chemical concentration
    d) Skin pH of 4.5-5.5

See answers on page 40.

NOTES

ANSWER KEY

1. d) Virtually all chronic wounds have senescent cells, high concentrations of MMPs, and reduced activity of growth factors.

2. a) For wounds to close, angiogenesis must occur before significant epithelialization.

3. b) Most chronic wounds are stalled in the inflammatory phase of wound healing.

4. c) Chronic wounds tend to have pH in the range of 6.5-8.5.

5. d) Chronic wounds see an increase in MMPs and a decrease in growth factors.

6. c) Electrical energy can cause tissue damage, alter cell membrane resting potential, and elicit muscle tetany. It converts to thermal energy, causing coagulative necrosis or can cause mechanical injury from falls or muscle contraction.

7. e) Factors that determine the degree of electrical injury include the magnitude of energy delivered, resistance encountered, type of electrical current, and duration of contact with the electrical current.

8. c) There is really no good radiological test to identify wood as a foreign body in soft tissue. Of the tests listed, MRI would be the best option. Ultrasound might be useful but MRI is the better option. X-ray and triple phase bone scan are unable to identify wood in soft tissues.

9. d) Radiation wounds usually are hypoxic, hypocellular, and hypovascular.

10. d) The factors that determine the severity of a chemical burn include the type of chemical causing the burn, the temperature of chemical, and the concentration of chemical. A pH of 4.5-5.5 is the normal pH of skin.

PATIENT PREPARATION AND EDUCATION
7

Dianne Rudolph, RN, GNP-BC, DNP, CWOCN
Ellen T. Heiderich, RN, CWS

INTRODUCTION

The purpose of this chapter is to describe the options available to help prepare the patient for wound care, with an emphasis on maintaining patient comfort with pain management, time-outs, and positioning. The use of patient education to increase compliance and improve desirable outcomes is discussed, as well as the active role of the patient and family in the continuation of care. A list of wound-specific instructions and considerations for the patient is reviewed.

OBJECTIVES

Participants should be able to describe three techniques to comfort patients when preparing for wound care, explain Spaulding's classification scheme for level of sterilization or disinfection, and describe the tools available for self-reporting pain existence and intensity.

I. Preparing the patient for wound care

A. Transfers (tools needed for safe transfer)
1. Chair to chair: gait belt, slide board, assisted pivot, dependent pivot
2. Chair to bed: gait belt, slide board, assisted pivot, dependent pivot (Figure 7.1)

3. Bed to stretcher: draw sheet, full-length slide board
4. Bed to chair: gait belt, slide board, assisted or dependent pivot
5. Considerations for individual patient conditions and mobility issues should be assessed (e.g., contractures, amputations, hemiparesis, or paraplegia)

B. Patient comfort
1. Positioning to achieve comfort and protection of patient
2. Allows for the best wound care
3. Considerations should be taken for the patient's size, mobility, and wound site.
4. What works best for the patient and the provider?
5. Treatment environments: instruments, supplies, and dressings should be readily available.
6. Area should be clean and private with a relaxed atmosphere.

C. Pain scales
1. Visual analog scale (VAS) (Figure 7.2a)
a) Scale: 0 = no pain, 1-3 = mild pain, 4-7 = moderate pain, 8-10 = severe pain

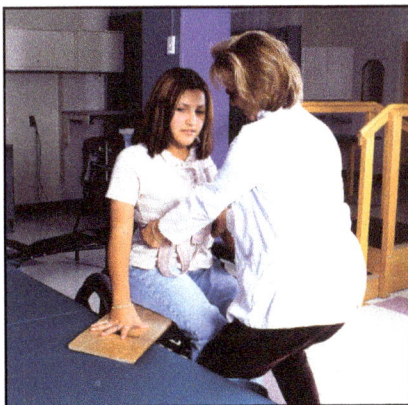

Figure 7.1: Patient transfer from chair to bed.
Courtesy of the Muscular Dystrophy Association (MDA).

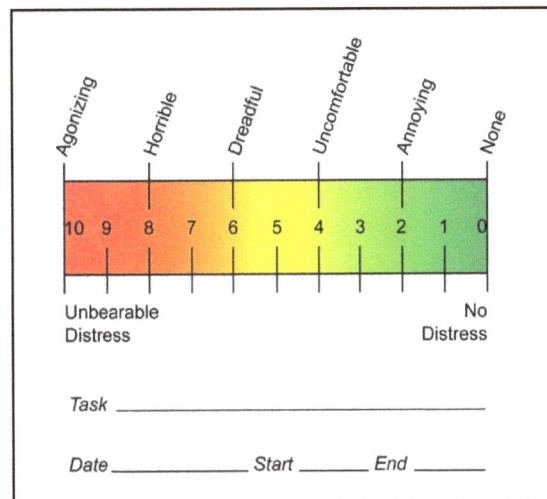

Figure 7.2a: Example of a visual analog scale.

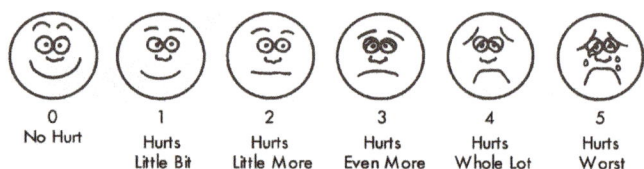

Figure 7.2b: Wong-Baker FACES Pain Rating Scale.
From Hockenberry MJ, Wilson D: *Wong's essentials of pediatric nursing*, ed. 8, St. Louis, 2009, Mosby. Used with permission. Copyright Mosby.

   2. Numeric pain intensity scale
       a) Scale is 0-10; 0 = no pain, 1-3 = mild, 4-6 = moderate, 7-9 = severe, 10 = worst possible pain
   3. Wong-Baker FACES Pain Rating Scale (for pediatric patients and patients with limited understanding) (Figure 7.2b)
       a) Happy face (no pain) to crying face (worst pain)
       b) Most reliable source: patient's self report of pain existence and intensity
       c) Monitor for signs of pain in nonverbal patients: increased agitation, crying, grimacing, acting out, pacing
D. Premedication
   1. Assess for pain prior to wound care or debridement
   2. Employ appropriate measures to eliminate or control the source of pain, e.g., cover wounds, adjust support surfaces, reposition the patient, provide analgesic as needed and when appropriate
   3. Assess for pain during and after wound care or procedure
   4. Medicate as needed: intravenous (IV), oral (PO), or sublingual (SL); allow time for the medication to take effect
E. Time-outs
   1. Dressing removal
   2. Debridement
   3. Procedures
   4. Repositioning
   5. Dressing application
F. Dressing removal/cleansing
   1. Dispose of contaminated dressings and linens in moisture-proof bags.
   2. Remove gloves and clean hands with alcohol-based sanitizer, or wash with soap and water.
   3. Clean the wound with normal saline or an approved wound cleanser.
   4. Place a clean towel or drape under the clean wound.
G. Sterile versus clean
   1. Sterile fields
       a) Free of any living organisms
       b) Use of sterile drapes, instruments, glove, gowns
   2. Clean versus sterile technique
       a) Sterile technique requires all sterile supplies and instruments, including gloves, gown, mask, drapes.
       b) Clean technique requires disinfected, clean and/or sterile instruments, sterile and non-sterile sup-

plies, and clean gloves.
H. Choice of sterilization (Spaulding's classification)
   1. Critical items that enter into tissue or vascular space: sterilization
   2. Semi-critical items that come into contact with mucus membranes or non-intact skin: high-level or intermediate disinfection
   3. Non-critical items that come into contact with intact skin: intermediate or low-level disinfection
I. Disinfecting equipment
   1. Know the organisms.
   2. Follow the recommended concentration and contact duration.
   3. Follow the recommended temperature (most are room temperature).
   4. Some disinfectants are ineffective in the presence of soap.
   5. Remove all organic material, e.g., blood, excretions.
   6. All equipment surfaces should be in contact with the solution.
J. Infection control/safety issues
   1. Always use standard precautions.
       a) Based on the principle that all blood, body fluids, secretions, excretions (except sweat), non-intact skin, and mucous membranes may contain transmissible infectious agents
       b) Include infection prevention practices that apply to all patients, regardless of suspected or confirmed infection status, in any setting where healthcare is delivered
       c) Include hand hygiene (Figure 7.3), gloves, gown, mask, eye protection, or face shield (depending on the anticipated exposure), and safe injection practices
   2. Material Safety Data Sheets (MSDS)
       a) Information on hazardous materials
       b) Instructions on how to handle exposures
       c) Contain numbers to call for help
       d) Know their location

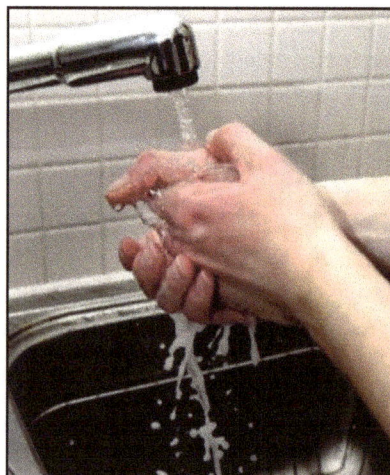

Figure 7.3: Hand washing

II. Patient education in wound care

A. Educating the patient can increase compliance and improve desirable outcomes. Empower the patient and family to take an active role in patient care. Assess the patient's healthcare literacy to appropriately plan and provide relevant education.

B. General guidance: patients need to have a basic understanding of their wounds, contributing factors, and their treatment plans.

C. Dressings: dressings should meet the needs of the wound and the patient's ability to obtain them.

D. Compression therapy: patients should have an understanding of why compression is chosen for the treatment of their wound.
   1. Compression therapy application should be by a trained professional.
   2. Potential adverse reactions should be explained to patients, such as skin reactions to the materials in bandages, pressure points, and skin injury from a slipping wrap.
   3. Proper home care: keeping wraps clean and dry, monitoring toes and edema.

E. Wound cleansing: the proper technique should be demonstrated to the patient or family with a return demonstration.
   1. Document the interaction and verbal understanding.
   2. Use positive reinforcement.

F. Reduction of pressure: the patient and family should be informed of their roles in the prevention of pressure ulcers.
   1. Turning schedule: what works best for the patient and protects the skin?
   2. Obtaining pressure reduction devices for durable medical equipment (Figure 7.4)
   3. Monitoring pressure points—how to assess, what to look for, what to report, and follow up
   4. Moisture balance, temperature
   5. Patient positioning using pillows or bolsters; no more than a 30 degree angle in a supine or prone position

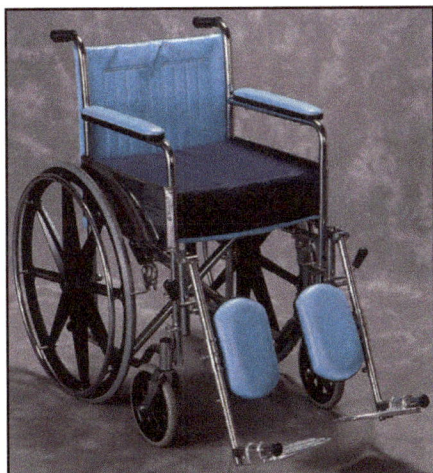

Figure 7.4: Conforma Cushion for pressure reduction.
Courtesy of Medline Industries, Inc.

G. Off-loading insensate feet
   1. Patients and family/caregivers should be taught how to properly use the device.
   2. Ability to obtain devices should be considered.
   3. Include instruction for the daily assessment of pressure points, making sure off-loading is properly applied.
   4. Careful consideration of an appropriate off-loading device can positively influence compliance.
   5. Options include rocker bottom walker, wound care shoe with custom molded inserts, total contact casting, post-op surgical shoe, etc.

H. Skin care/protection
   1. Keep moist areas dry where skin touches skin.
   2. Keep dry areas moist—no lotion between toes.
   3. Avoid hot showers and baths.
   4. Use moisturizing soap.
   5. Moisturize dry skin after bathing.
   6. Protect bony prominences, check for calluses.

I. Shoe wear
   1. Shoe wear patterns give insight to where and why a wound may occur or how one has occurred.
   2. Selection of proper fitting shoes is essential to protect from and prevent recurring wounds.
   3. Shoes should be fitted by a qualified specialist.

J. Hand washing/standard precautions
   1. Demonstrate proper hand washing and have the patients and family give a return demonstration.
   2. Instruct the patient and family to wash hands often when in contact with contaminated dressing or linens and to use alcohol-based hand sanitizer between glove changes and as needed.
   3. Explain that this will decrease the spread of microorganisms.

K. Reinforcement of smoking cessation
   1. Encourage the patient to stop smoking.
   2. Direct the patient to programs designed to help with smoking cessation.

L. Psychosocial issues
   1. Etiology—response to a wound can be closely related to how the injury occurred and associated trauma, disease processes, and infection.
   2. Preparedness—some patients and their families cannot emotionally deal with the reality of a wound. They may be dealing with something much deeper.
   3. Visibility—a wound can dramatically affect the patient's body image.
   4. The response of others can have a direct impact on the patient's self-esteem.
   5. Pain greatly affects the patient's quality of life.
   6. Odor and leakage can cause isolation from family and friends due to embarrassment.
   7. Healing outcomes—patients and family members want to know if the wound will heal, how long it will take to heal, and if the treatments cause pain.

8. Some patients consider staying wounded to be beneficial: continued nurse visits, meals on wheels, home health aides, extended time off work or unemployment, and continued attention from family and healthcare professionals.

9. All things must be considered, especially with chronic wounds. Each patient should be assessed individually.

RESOURCES

1. Coe P, Clark J. Infection control in the wound care setting. In: Sheffield PJ, Fife CE, editors. *Wound Care Practice.* 2nd ed. North Palm Beach: Best Publishing Company; 2007: 1133-45.

2. Kozier B, Erb G, Berman A, Snyder S. *Fundamentals of Nursing: Concepts, Process, and Practice.* 7th ed. Upper Saddle River: Pearson/Prentice Hall; 2004: 1092-6, 646-67.

3. Krasner DL. Wound pain management: a wound care specialist perspective. In: Sheffield PJ, Fife, CE, editors. *Wound Care Practice.* 2nd ed. North Palm Beach: Best Publishing Company; 2007: 827-44.

4. Soto LL, Sheffield KM. Comforting the patient. In: Sheffield PJ, Fife CE, editors. *Wound Care Practice.* 2nd ed. North Palm Beach: Best Publishing; 2007: 1035-54.

5. McDaniel KC, Brownin KK. Smoking, chronic wound healing and implications for evidence based practice. *J Wound Ostomy Continence Nurs.* 2014; 41(5):415-23.

6. McCarthy DM, Waite KR, Curtis LM, Engel KG, Baker DW, Wolf MS. What did the doctor say? Health literacy and recall of medical instructions. *Med Care.* Apr 2012; 50(4): 277–82. doi: 10.1097/MLR.0b013e318241e8e1.

SAMPLE QUESTIONS

1. Spaulding's classification scheme indicates the level of sterilization or disinfection required for various items. Critical items that enter tissue or vascular space require:
   a) Sterilization
   b) High-level disinfection and/or intermediate-level disinfection
   c) Intermediate or low-level disinfection
   d) Neither sterilization nor disinfection

2. The most reliable scale for the patient's self report of pain existence and intensity is the:
   a) Visual analog scale
   b) Numeric pain intensity scale
   c) Wong-Baker FACES Pain Rating Scale
   d) Verbal rating scale

3. Which tool is not required for transfer from chair to bed?
   a) Gait belt
   b) Slide board
   c) Assisted pivot
   d) Full-length slide board

4. All of the following statements about patient education are true except:
   a) It improves healing outcomes.
   b) It improves the patient's compliance.
   c) It improves the patient's literacy.
   d) It should be planned only after assessing the patient's healthcare literacy.

5. Skin care/protection education to a patient should include which of the following:
   a) Keeping moist areas moist
   b) Keeping dry areas dry
   c) Encouraging hot showers and baths
   d) Protecting bony prominences

See answers on page 47.

NOTES

ANSWER KEY

1. a) Spaulding's classification scheme indicates critical items that enter tissue or vascular space will require sterilization.

2. c) The most reliable scale for the patient's self report of pain existence and intensity is the Wong-Baker FACES Pain Rating Scale.

3. d) The tools required for a transfer from chair to bed are gait belt, slide board, and assisted pivot. The full-length slide board is used to transfer a patient from bed to stretcher.

4. c) Patient education should be planned only after assessing the patient's healthcare literacy. Patient education improves healing outcomes and compliance, but does not improve the patient's literacy.

5. d) Skin care/protection instruction should include keeping moist areas dry and dry areas moist, avoiding hot showers and baths, and protecting bony prominences.

WOUND ASSESSMENT 8

Caroline E. Fife, MD, CWSP, FAAFP, FUHM
Jayesh B. Shah, MD, CWSP, FAPWCA, FACCWS

INTRODUCTION

Proper wound assessment is the key to successful wound management. The purpose of this chapter is to identify the barriers to healing, describe the elements of wound assessment, discuss the various wound classification systems, and give examples of how to document the assessment. This chapter includes the diagnosis of ulcers/disease states and diagnostic tools such as ABI, Doppler, TCOM, and biopsy.

OBJECTIVES

Participants should be able to discuss four wound assessment methods, state the principles of wound bed preparation, identify three barriers to healing, and discuss elements of two wound documentation systems.

I. Importance of good history

A. Even with the technological innovations of the 21st century, history taking still remains the best and cheapest tool to make a good diagnosis. Recognizing clues from a patient's history can give important information about the patient's wound.
  1. The initial step in a wound assessment is obtaining the history of the initial wounding event.
  2. A chronological history of the occurrence and progression of the wound, including previous diagnostic testing and treatment interventions, should be obtained and documented. The significance of patient history is shown in Table 8.1.

Table 8.1: Significance of patient history.
From Sheffield PJ, Fife CE, editors. *Wound Care Practice*. 2nd ed. 2007:598.

IMPORTANT CLUES FOUND IN THE PATIENT'S HISTORY	SIGNIFICANCE TO THE PATIENT'S WOUND
General history	
Age and sex	Leg ulcers more common in older women; some rheumatic diseases more common in women
Duration of wound	Acute—less than one week Subacute—one week to four weeks Chronic—more than four weeks
History of recurrence	Venous ulcers likely to be recurrent
History of previous DVT	Predisposing factor to venous disease
Previous vein surgery or pelvic trauma	Indicative of venous disease
Intermittent claudication	Indicative of arterial disease
Rest pain	Indicative of arterial disease
Systemic symptoms	Indicative of a systemic disease leading to ulcers
Arthralgia	Associated with some ulcers associated with systemic disease
Social history	
Smoking	Predisposes to or worsens arterial disease
Alcohol	Vitamin deficiency
IV drug use	HIV or ulcers related to IV drug use
Past medical history	
Diabetes	Wound could be related to neuropathy or arterial disease associated with diabetes
Connective tissue disease	Wound could be related to vasculitis, pyoderma gangrenosum, cryoglobulinemia
Sickle cell disease	Increased risk of small vessel occlusion
Dietary history	Some vitamin deficiencies common in a vegetarian diet; poor nutrition and obesity influences healing
Drug history	Steroids delays healing; hydroxyurea interferes with healing
Travel history or geographic location of patient	For example, leprosy still remains a common cause for non-healing wounds in India; spider bites are only endemic in the south, western, and midwestern areas of the United States.
Allergies	Contact dressings, bandages, and ointment can add to existing skin damage

B. The following questions should be asked:
1. What caused the initial wounding event?
2. Did the wound occur suddenly (trauma, insect bite) or develop gradually over time (neuropathic foot ulcer, venous leg ulcer)?
3. Is this the first wound at this location or a recurrent wound or pattern of wounding?
4. Is the wound painful and, if so, what is the character and nature of the pain?
5. What causes the wound to get better or worse (precipitating or ameliorating factors)?
6. Has the patient had chills, fever, or night sweats?
7. Is there any history of unusual environmental or occupational exposures?
8. Does the patient have a known underlying disease (diabetes mellitus, collagen vascular disease, peripheral arterial occlusive disease, or chronic venous insufficiency), which will be evaluated in more detail during the patient assessment section?
9. What diagnostic studies have already been completed (radiographic or nuclear medicine studies, cultures, biopsies, or vascular studies)?
10. What treatments have been applied (debridements, local wound cleansing and dressings, off-loading and protection, compression wraps or devices to control edema, vascular [arterial or venous] surgical or radiographic interventions, hyperbaric oxygen therapy, electrical stimulation, topical growth factors, cellular or tissue based products, or tertiary interventions)?
11. Has reconstructive surgery been attempted? What were the results of these interventions and were there any complications?

C. Complete patient history should also include various patient factors like:
1. Mental status
2. Age
3. Pain (visual)
4. Position/mobility
5. Comorbidities
6. Ethnicity
7. Social/family support
8. Social issues/alcohol/smoking

II. Inability to heal may be due to local factors or systemic factors

A. Local factors may include:
1. Repeated external trauma because of inappropriate off-loading
2. Foot deformity causing abnormal pressure areas
3. Uncontrolled edema
4. Injury from use of toxic substances
5. Inappropriate measures for exudate control
6. Inappropriate infection control
7. Tissue oxygen tension
8. Hematoma formation
9. Undebrided wound
10. Poor blood supply
11. Hypoxia

B. Systemic factors may include:
1. Arterial insufficiency
2. Venous insufficiency
3. Systemic conditions (collagen vascular disease, sickle cell disease, hemoglobinopathies, uremia, diabetes, jaundice)
4. Immunosuppressive drugs (systemic corticosteroids, anticancer drugs, NSAIDS)
5. Immunosuppressive diseases (HIV)
6. Local or systemic malignancy
7. Exposure to radiation
8. Malnutrition
9. Old age
10. Systemic infection

III. Wound assessment

A. Perform a complete wound-focused history, a review of systems of the wound patient, and a history directed physical examination.
B. Identify comorbid conditions or contributing underlying medical conditions and other host factors that may limit an effective response to the wound or impact the choice of options for wound treatment.
C. Categorize the wound on the basis of presumed etiology.
D. Wound assessment should at least include:
1. History of wounding event
2. Wound location (useful in differential diagnosis)
3. Edge of the wound and surrounding skin
4. Undermining of the wound edge
5. Exudate quantity and quality
6. Appearance of the wound bed
7. Measurement of wound size and depth
8. Suffering (patient pain assessment)
9. Wound grading and classification
10. Re-evaluation on a periodic basis
11. Assessment of infection

IV. Clues from examination

A. Attention to clinical clues is a good start, even before touching the wound. (11)
B. General appearance
1. Cushingoid appearance—corticosteroid use, disease with excessive release of corticosteroids
2. Rheumatoid joints—pyoderma gangrenosum, rheumatoid ulcer, vasculitis
3. Cachexia—malnutrition, AIDS, cancer, other infectious etiologies (tuberculosis)
4. Scleroderma face (purse string mouth)—calcinosis, Raynaud's phenomenon
5. Abnormal affect, posture, facial expression—factitious disorder
6. Facial palsy, weakness in one or more extremities, cerebrovascular accident—more prone to pressure ulcers if bed or wheelchair bound

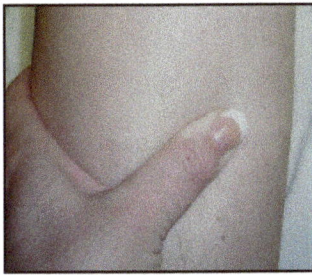

Figure 8.1a: Assessment of edema—applying pressure.

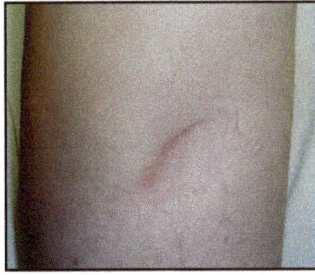

Figure 8.1b: Grade I, pits on pressure.

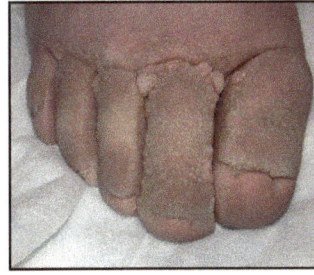

Figure 8.3a: Grade III, elephantiasis of toe.

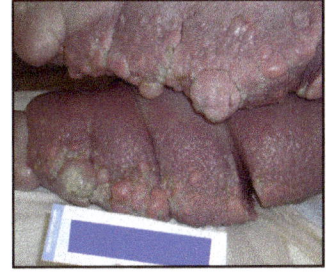

Figure 8.3b: Grade III, elephantiasis of both feet.

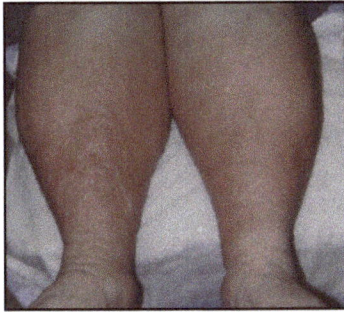

Figure 8.2: Grade II, lymphedema.

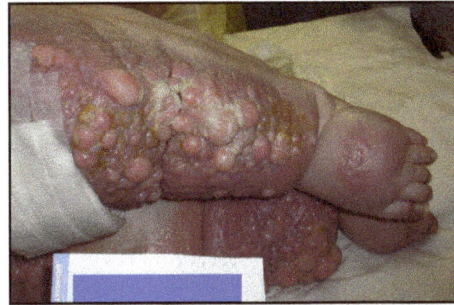

Figure 8.3c: Grade III, elephantiasis on the front of the leg.

C. Appearance of the extremity/extremities
   1. Edema—venous disease, deep vein thrombosis, lymphedema, congestive heart failure with dependent edema
       a) International Society of Lymphology (ISL) Classification of lymphedema
           i)   Grade I (Figures 8.1a and 8.1b):
                (1) Pits on pressure
                (2) Reduced on elevation
                (3) No clinical fibrosis
           ii) Grade II (Figure 8.2)
                (1) Non-pitting
                (2) Not reduced on elevation
                (3) Clinical fibrosis
           iii) Grade III (elephantiasis) (Figures 8.3a–8.3c)
                (1) Skin thick and leathery
                (2) Hypertrophy of subcutaneous tissues
                (3) Papillomas and verrucous changes
                (4) Massive localized lymphedema
   2. Foot deformities—neuropathic wounds, diabetes with autonomic neuropathy, osteomyelitis, rheumatoid arthritis
   3. Cyanosis—arterial disease, Raynaud's syndrome
   4. Dependent rubor—arterial disease
   5. Erythema—infection, contact dermatitis
   6. Livedo reticularis—cholesterol emboli, collagen vascular disease, cryoglobulinemia
   7. Sclerodactyly—scleroderma, Raynaud's disease
   8. Lipodermatosclerosis/hemosiderin pigmentation—venous disease
   9. Eczema—irritation arising from previous treatments
D. Detailed initial assessment of the wound should include
   1. Location of the wound
       a) Weight-bearing surface—neuropathic wound, pressure
       b) Digital ulcers—ischemia
       c) Gaiter area—venous disease
       d) Tibial area—arterial disease, necrobiosis lipoidica diabeticorum
       e) Vaginal ulcers—Behcet's disease
       f) Underlying internal viscera—fistula, abscess, Crohn's disease, radiation injury
   2. Physical aspects
       a) Periwound skin
       b) Painful to the touch
       c) Vasculitis and/or cellulitis
       d) Inflammation
       e) Wound odor, shape, location, duration, and quantity
       f) Tissue quality, color, and temperature
       g) Maceration
       h) Continence status
       i) Edema
       j) Exudate quality and quantity
   3. Macroscopic environment
       a) Necrosis
       b) Infection
       c) Metabolic control and nutrition
       d) Pressure
       e) Perfusion, immunity
       f) Tissue moisture balance
   4. Microscopic environment
       a) Excessive matrix metalloproteases (MMPs)
       b) Bioburden
       c) Growth factor deficiencies
       d) Proliferative capacity
       e) Abnormal microcirculation
       f) Excessive inflammatory mediators

5. Wound assessment: **MEASURE** (13)
   a) **M**easure (length, width, depth, and area)
   b) **E**xudate (quantity and quality)
   c) **A**ppearance (wound bed, including tissue type and amount)
   d) **S**uffering (pain type and level)
   e) **U**ndermining (presence or absence)
   f) **R**eevaluate (monitoring of all parameters regularly)
   g) **E**dge (condition of edge and surrounding skin)

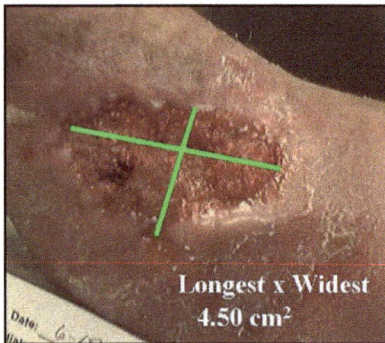

Figure 8.4: Wound measurement by ruler.

6. Wound measurement methods
   a) Wound measurement by ruler (Figure 8.4)
      i) Typically, wounds are sized according to greatest length, greatest width along the perpendicular to the length, and the greatest depth measurement. Since different techniques are used by different providers, we recommend using one method consistently to provide consistent documentation.
      ii) Other methods used include:
          (1) Greatest head-to-toe length and greatest side-to-side width perpendicular to each other
          (2) Longest length head-to-toe and the longest width side-to-side
          (3) Surface area: usually greatest length by greatest width (in centimeters)
          (4) Depth: greatest depth is measured by placing a cotton-tipped applicator into the wound at the deepest point, marking or pinching the applicator at the skin level, then comparing the applicator to a ruler; however, this two-dimensional method assumes that the wound has a geometric surface shape
              (a) Rectangle (length × width)
              (b) Circle (diameter × diameter)
              (c) Oval (maximum diameter × maximum diameter perpendicular to the first measurement)
              (d) An alternative method of calculating wound surface area is based on the formula for an ellipse (length × width × 0.785)

(5) Wound tracing: a pen is used to trace the outline of the wound directly onto sterile transparent film, which can be entered into a data processing system using a simple scanner. Can also use a "box counting" method, which estimates surface area using a grid

(6) Wound measurement by a Kundin gauge, a commercially available three-dimensional ruler used to calculate wound area and volume

(7) Wound measurement by molds: a three-dimensional cast of the wound is made using alginate filling

(8) Wound measurement by scaled photographs: uses a photograph that has been processed by a special scanner so that a scaled ruler is incorporated at the edge of the photograph

7. Exudate (Tables 8.2-8.4)

Table 8.2: Exudate quality.
From Keast DH, et al. MEASURE: A Proposed assessment framework for developing best practice recommendations for wound assessment. *Wound Rep Reg.* 2004; 12(3 Suppl):S1-S17.

EXUDATE	CONSISTENCY	COLOR	ODOR
Serous	Thin, watery	Clear to yellow	Usually odorless
Serosanguineous	Thin, watery	Pink to light red	Usually odorless
Sanguineous	Frank blood	Bright red	Usually odorless
Seropurulent	Thin, watery	White to cream	Possibly foul odor
Purulent	Thick, translucent to opaque	White to cream	Possibly foul odor

Table 8.3: Exudate quantity. (Keast DH, et al.)

	QUANTITY	CONDITION
0	None	No exudate
1	Small	Exudate fully controlled. Nonabsorptive dressing may be used. Wear time up to 7 days.
2	Moderate	Exudate controlled; absorptive dressing may be required. Wear time 2-3 days.
3	Large	Exudate uncontrolled; absorptive dressings may be required. Dressing may be overwhelmed in <1 day.

Table 8.4: Exudate odor. (Keast DH, et al.)

ODOR	CONDITION
No odor	No odor at close range
Faint odor	Faint odor at close range
Moderate odor	Moderate odor in room
Strong odor	Odor outside the room or strong odor in room

Table 8.5: Wound bed appearance. (Keast DH, et al.)

TISSUE TYPE	APPEARANCE
Granulation	Red, firm, and pebbled. Friability may indicate infection.
Fibrin	Yellow and firm. Represents collagen in the wound bed.
Slough	Yellow to gray-green and loose. May represent necrotic fascia.
Eschar	Black, soft, and wet or hard and dry. Necrotic tissue.

Table 8.6: Wound bed appearance scoring system.
(Keast DH, et al.)

APPEARANCE SCORE	GRANULATION TISSUE (RED)	FIBRINOUS TISSUE (YELLOW)	ESCHAR (BLACK)
A	100%	-	-
B	50–99%	+	+
C	< 50%	+	+
D	+/-	+/-	+

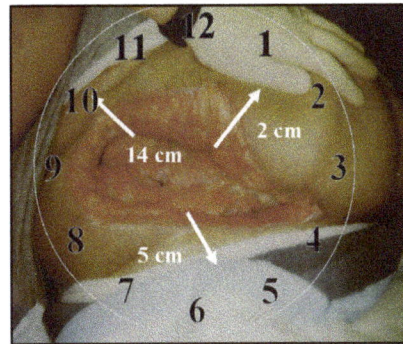

Figure 8.5: Using a clockface to document wound tunneling and undermining.

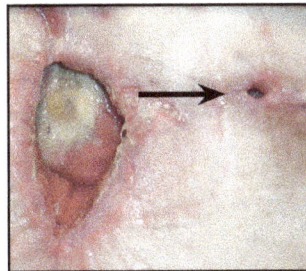

Figure 8.6a: Wound with tunnel.

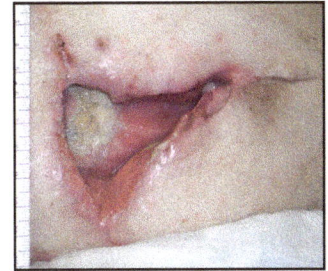

Figure 8.6b: Wound after unroofing of tunnel.

8. Appearance of wound (Tables 8.5 and 8.6)
   a) Wound base
      i) Green—*Pseudomonas* infection
      ii) Pale—pressure, ischemia
      iii) Black—arterial insufficiency
      iv) Red—good granulation/vascularity
      v) Exposed tendon—pressure, shear, tension, fistula
      vi) Exposed bone—osteomyelitis, pressure
9. Tunneling and undermining
   a) Any tunneled or undermined areas are documented according to their clockface locations
   b) The patient's head represents 12 o'clock
   c) Depth is taken in centimeters
   d) The area of additional damage extending from the wound edge, i.e., underneath intact skin
   e) For example, the wound in Figure 8.5 undermines 14 cm at 10 o'clock, 2 cm at 1 o'clock, and 5 cm at 5 o'clock
   f) Unroofing tunnels is usually necessary (Figures 8.6a and 8.6.b)
10. Tracking (Figures 8.7a and 8.7b)
    a) This trochanteric pressure ulcer tracks to bone
    b) Although small externally, it will not heal without surgical intervention
    c) Stage III and IV pressure ulcers result in significant subcutaneous tissue loss and such defects are common
11. Granulation tissue (Figures 8.8a and 8.8b)
12. Epithelialization (Figures 8.9a and 8.9b)
13. Assessing the deepest tissue exposed (Figure 8.10)
    a) Ulcers may be small or appear shallow
    b) Ulcers must be probed to determine whether an occult abscess or exposed bone or tendon is present

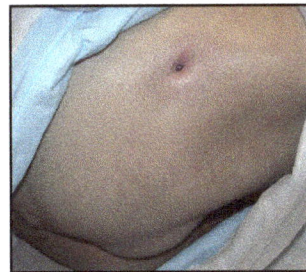

Figure 8.7a: Trochanter pressure ulcer.

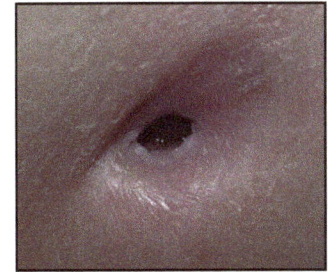

Figure 8.7b: Trochanter pressure ulcer close up.

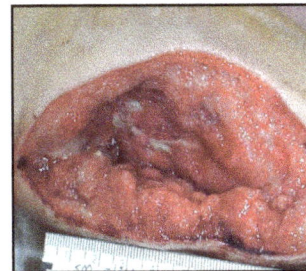

Figure 8.8a: Clean, nongranulating tissue is nongranular (deep pink or red and smooth) or striated (when muscle fibers are exposed).

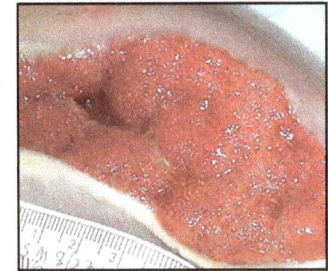

Figure 8.8b: Granulation tissue is typically deep pink or red and is characterized by an irregular, granular surface that resembles raspberries.

E. Grading and staging
   1. Diabetic foot ulcers
      a) Wagner grade classification
         i) Grade 0—callus or corn, but no ulcer (Figure 8.11a)
         ii) Grade 1—superficial ulcer, not clinically infected (Figure 8.11b)

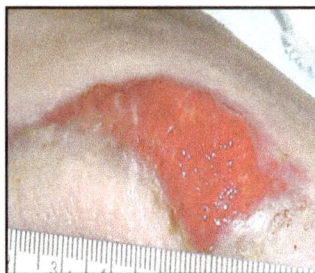

Figure 8.9a: New epithelial tissue is light pink or slightly lavender.

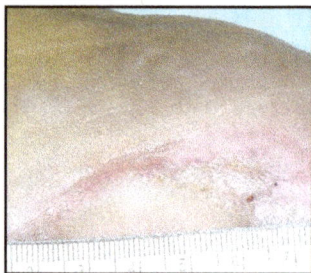

Figure 8.9b: New epithelial tissue migrates from the wound edges to gradually cover the granulation tissue.

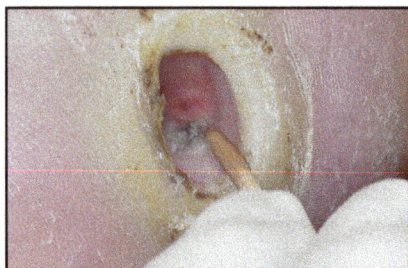

Figure 8.11a: Wagner grade 0 diabetic wound after callus removal.

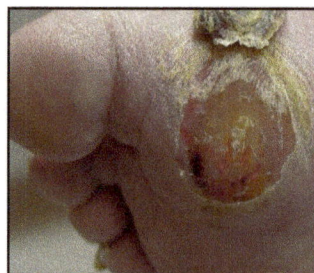

Figure 8.11b: Wagner grade 1 diabetic wound.

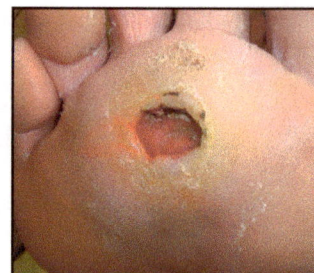

Figure 8.10: Assessing the deepest tissue exposed—probing the ulcer.

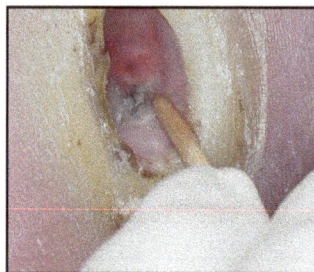

Figure 8.11c: Wagner grade 2 diabetic ulcer on the plantar foot goes up to the joint, but is not infected.

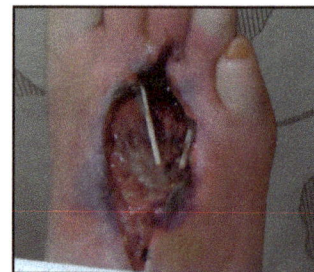

Figure 8.11d: Wagner grade 3 infected diabetic ulcer on the dorsal foot with tendon exposed, presenting with a deep abscess after debridement.

- iii) Grade 2—deep to tendon, capsule, or bone (Figure 8.11c)
- iv) Grade 3—deep with abscess, tendon, or bone infected (Figure 8.11d)
- v) Grade 4—localized gangrene of the forefoot or heel (Figure 8.11e)
- vi) Grade 5—gangrene of entire foot (Figure 8.11f)

b) University of Texas Health Science Center San Antonio (UTSA) classification system
- i) Grade 0—no open lesions, may have deformity
  - A—Without infection or ischemia
  - B—With infection
  - C—With ischemia
  - D—With infection and ischemia
- ii) Grade 1—superficial wound not involving tendon, capsule, or bone
  - A—Without infection or ischemia
  - B—With infection
  - C—With ischemia
  - D—With infection and ischemia
- iii) Grade 2—wound penetrating to tendon or capsule
  - A—Without infection or ischemia
  - B—With infection
  - C—With ischemia
  - D—With infection and ischemia
- iv) Grade 3—wound penetrating to bone or joint
  - A—Without infection or ischemia
  - B—With infection
  - C—With ischemia
  - D—With infection and ischemia

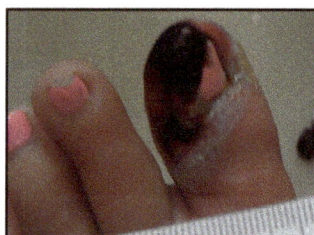

Figure 8.11e: Wagner grade 4 diabetic ulcer with a gangrenous great toe.

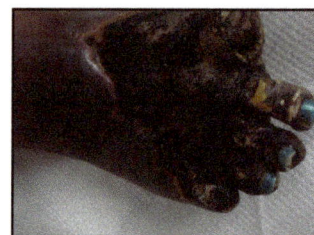

Figure 8.11f: Wagner grade 5 diabetic ulcer with extensive gangrene.

2. Pressure ulcers—NPUAP staging system
   a) Suspected deep tissue injury (Figure 8.12a). Purple or maroon localized area of discolored intact skin or blood-filled blister due to damage of underlying soft tissue from pressure and/or shear. The area may be preceded by tissue that is painful, firm, mushy, boggy, warmer, or cooler when compared to adjacent tissue.
   b) Stage I pressure ulcer (Figure 8.12b). Intact skin with non-blanchable redness of a localized area usually over a bony prominence. Darkly pigmented skin may not have visible blanching; its color may differ from the surrounding area.
   c) Stage II pressure ulcer (Figure 8.12c). Partial thickness loss of dermis presenting as a shallow open ulcer with a red-pink wound bed, without

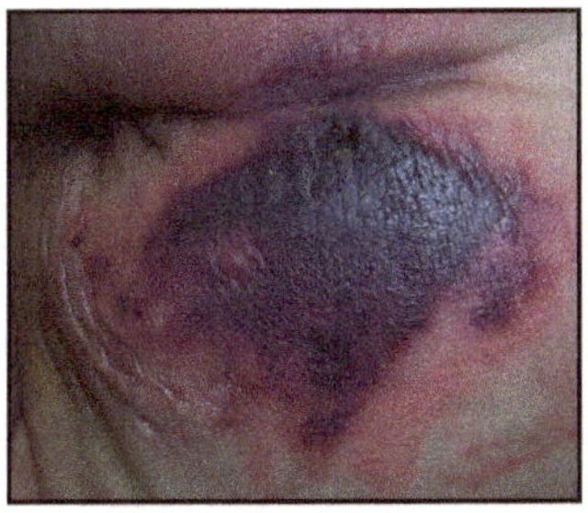

Figure 8.12a: NPUAP staging—deep tissue injury on buttocks.

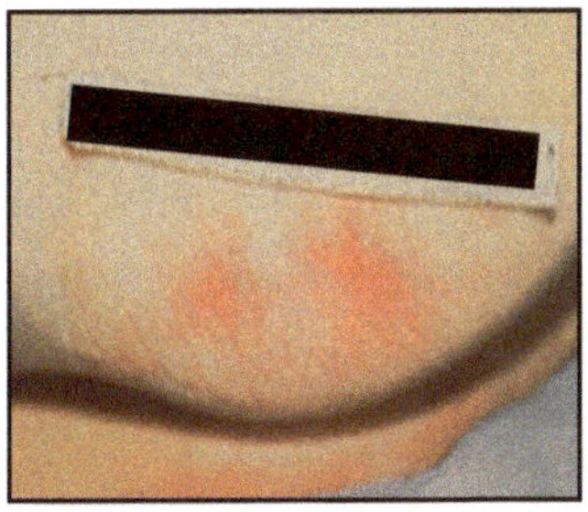

Figure 8.12b: NPUAP stage I—non-blanchable redness on buttocks.

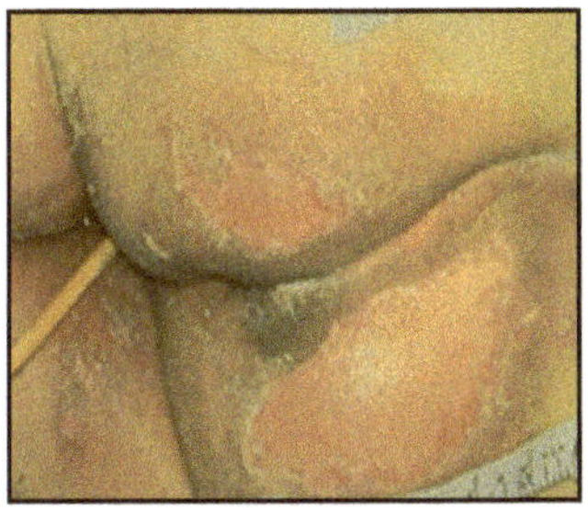

Figure 8.12c: NPUAP stage II—shallow ulcer with partial thickness loss of dermis.

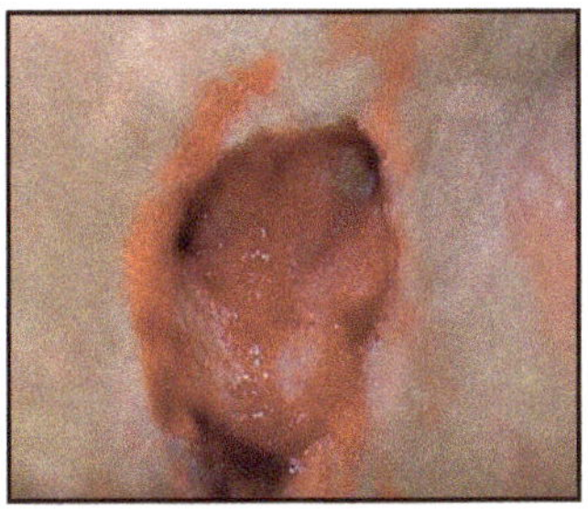

Figure 8.12d: NPUAP stage III pressure ulcer—full-thickness tissue loss on the sacrum; subcutaneous fat may be visible but bone, tendon, or muscle is not exposed.

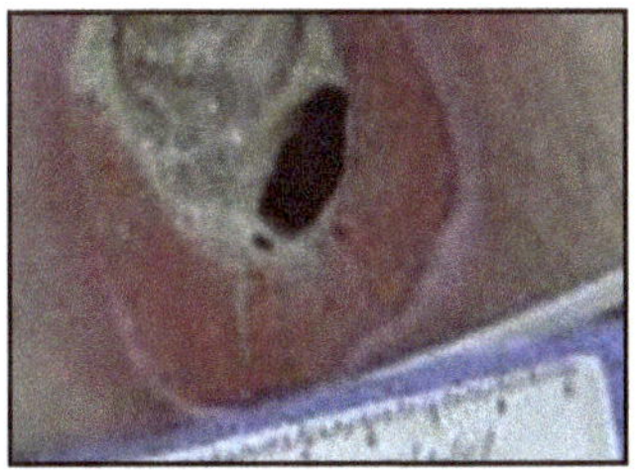

Figure 8.12e: NPUAP stage IV pressure ulcer—full-thickness tissue loss on left buttock with exposed bone, tendon, or muscle.

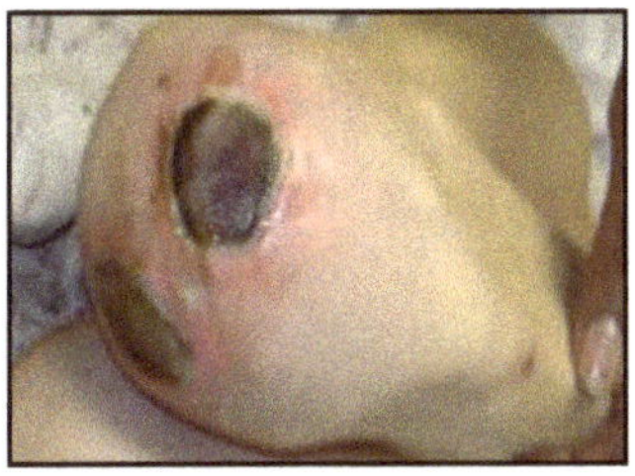

Figure 8.12f: NPUAP unstageable pressure ulcer on left knee.

slough. May also present as an intact or open/ruptured serum-filled blister.
d) Stage III pressure ulcer (Figure 8.12d). Full thickness tissue loss. Subcutaneous fat may be visible but bone, tendon, or muscle is not exposed. Slough may be present but does not obscure the depth of tissue loss. May include undermining and tunneling.
e) Stage IV pressure ulcer (Figure 8.12e). Full thickness tissue loss with exposed bone, tendon, or muscle. Slough or eschar may be present on some parts of the wound bed. Often includes undermining and tunneling.

f) Unstageable (Figure 8.12f). Full thickness tissue loss where the base of the ulcer is covered by slough (yellow, tan, gray, green, or brown) and/or eschar (tan, brown, or black) in the wound bed.
3. Classification is based on the level of tissue loss.
   a) Full thickness
   b) Partial thickness
F. Assessing pain (refer to Chapter 23)
   1. Often underestimated in the wound care population.
   2. Moderate pain was experienced 80% of the time by individuals with pressure ulcers.
   3. Pain is an issue related to patient well-being and is always subjective.
   4. Pain is whatever the patient experiencing it says it is, and it exists whenever the patient experiencing it says it does. (14)
   5. Pain assessment tools:
      a) Numeric pain intensity scale (rating of 0-10)
      b) Wong-Baker FACES Pain Rating Scale (refer to Chapter 7, page 42)
   6. All patients should be assessed for pain associated with their ulcers on an ongoing basis.
   7. Cyclic pain and non-cyclic pain, which are separate from chronic pain.
   8. Measures should be taken to eliminate or control pain caused by dressing changes, debridement, etc.

IV. Identifying barriers to healing
A. Identifying tissue viability
   1. Viable tissue (Figure 8.13a)
      a) Bright red (granulating) or pink (epithelializing) tissue represents an environment conducive to normal wound healing
   2. Nonviable tissue (Figures 8.13b and 8.13c)
      a) May be black (necrotic) or yellow (sloughy)

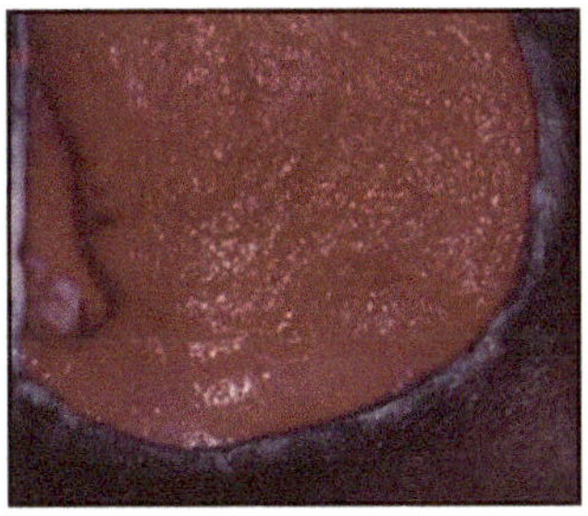

Figure 8.13a: Viable tissue is bright red (granulating) or pink (epithelializing) and represents an environment conducive to normal wound healing.

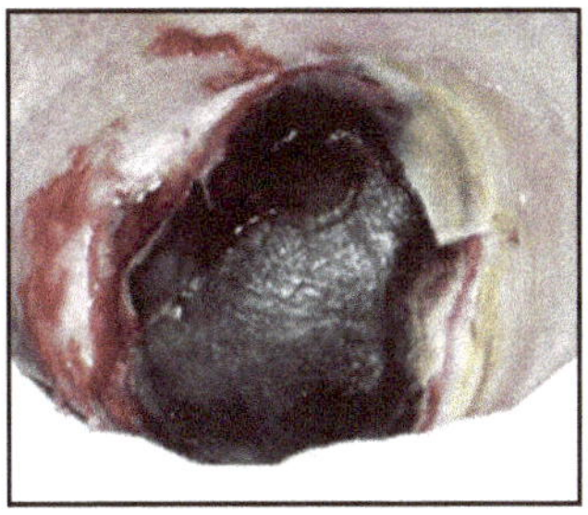

Figure 8.13b: Black (necrotic) nonviable tissue.

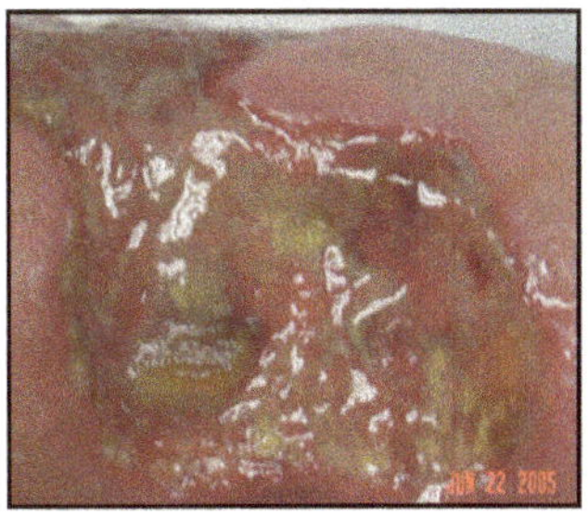

Figure 8.13c: Yellow (slough) nonviable tissue.

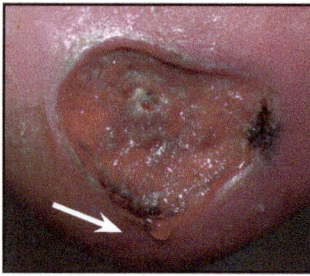

Figure 8.14a: Infected wound displaying increased exudate.

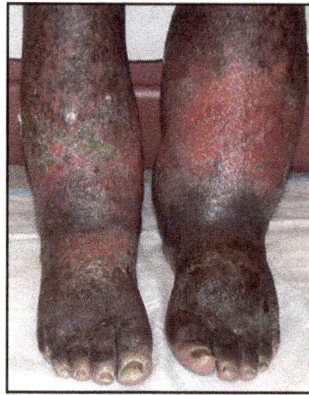

Figure 8.14b: Infected wound displaying redness and inflammation.

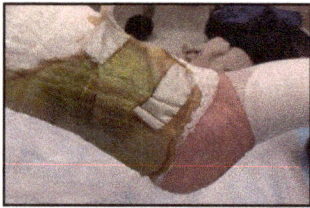

Figure 8.14c: Infected wound displaying green drainage.

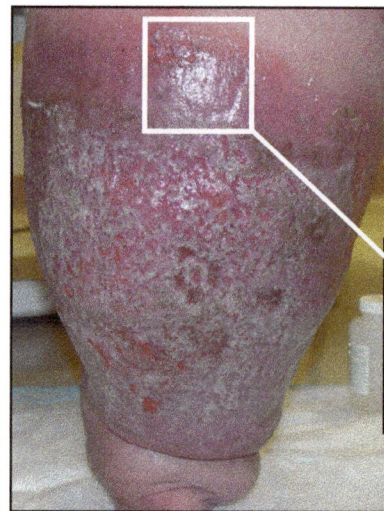

Figure 8.15a: Cellulitis patient with edema, pain, and purulent drainage.

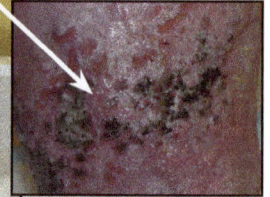

Figure 8.15b: Cellulitis (magnified).

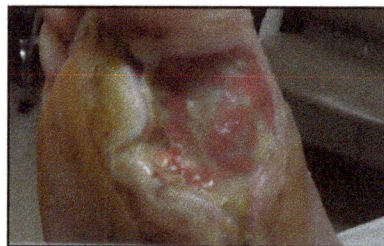

Figure 8.15c: "Slime city"—right medial foot wound on the first metatarsal head with biofilm and loose slough.

    b) If left in the wound, creates the ideal conditions for bacterial growth and infection

B. Identifying spectrum of wound infections
1. Infected wounds display particular characteristics:
   a) Increased exudates (Figure 8.14a)
   b) Redness (Figure 8.14b)
   c) Odor
   d) Green drainage (Figure 8.14c)
   e) Inflammation
   f) Tenderness
   g) Fragile or irregular tissue that bleeds easily
2. Clinical presentation of inflammation and infection
   a) Classic signs and symptoms:
      i) Acute wound infection or severe progressive or persistent chronic wound infection
         (1) Advancing erythema
         (2) Fever
         (3) Warmth
         (4) Edema/swelling
         (5) Pain
         (6) Purulence
         (7) Cellulitis (Figures 8.15a and 8.15b)
            (a) Patient with erythema, pain, and purulent drainage
   b) Signs and symptoms secondary to critically colonized bacterial bioburden causing local wound infection:
      i) Delayed healing
      ii) Change in color of wound bed
      iii) Friable granulation tissue
      iv) Absent or abnormal granulation tissue
      v) Increased or abnormal odor
      vi) Increased serous drainage
      vii) Increased pain at wound site

3. Biofilm (Figure 8.15c)
   a) A complex aggregation of bacteria that excretes a protective coating virtually impervious to topical or systemic antibiotics. Also known as a "slime city."
   b) Bacteria that secrete a glycosaminoglycan (GAG) layer, which makes them almost impervious to either topical or oral antibiotics.
   c) Must be debrided physically on a regular basis.
   d) Should be treated with topical antimicrobials.

C. Identifying moisture imbalance
1. Wounds heal better in a moist environment. Nerve endings are protected, reducing pain, and skin layers repair at a faster rate, producing less scarring than in dry wounds.
2. As part of the normal healing process, wounds exude fluid.
3. Consequence of moisture imbalance:
   a) Excess fluid causes maceration (Figure 8.16a). Maceration is white, waxy-looking tissue in the periwound area and on the wound edges.
   b) Wound dryness (dessication) leads to scabbing (Figure 8.16b).
   c) Both maceration and desiccation can interfere with wound healing.

D. Identifying edge effect (Figures 8.17a, 8.17b, 8.18, 8.19)
1. In a wound that is healing normally, epithelial cells migrate from the edge.
2. Mechanical problems at the wound edge can prevent this and include:
   a) Undermining

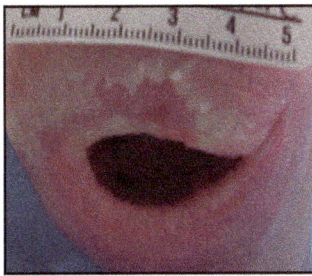

Figure 8.16a: Maceration, the white, waxy-looking tissue around the wound edges.

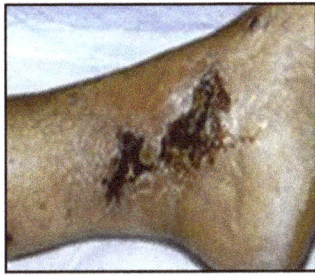

Figure 8.16b: Desiccation; note the dry eschared tissue.

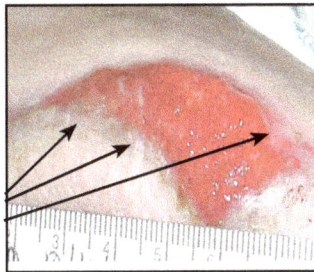

Figure 8.17a: Epithelialization.

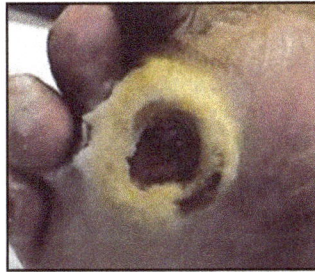

Figure 8.17b: Callus with surrounding maceration.

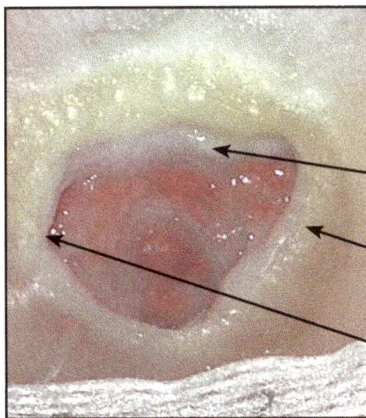

Figure 8.18: Epithelialization in a diabetic foot ulcer.

Epithelialization

Callus surrounding the wound

Undermined edges

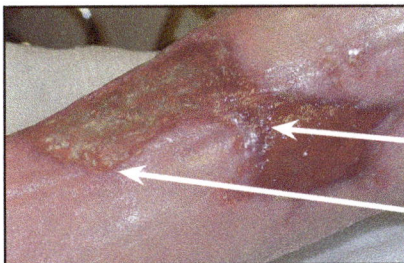

Figure 8.19: The edge effect.

Open wound edge

Closed wound edge

b) Maceration
c) Scar or other skin disease (no healthy source for epithelial cells)
3. Epithelialization in a diabetic foot ulcer (Figure 8.18).
 a) Note epithelium migrating from the top where there is no undermining.
 b) Note there is no epithelial migration from the inferior pole where there is undermining.
4. Open wound edges are characterized by a narrow border of flat, moist, red tissue that separates the surrounding skin; this represents the reproductive epithelium (Figure 8.19).
5. Closed wound edges are characterized by dry, normally pigmented skin that extends to the junction with the wound bed. In some situations, closed wound edges are also thickened and rolled.
6. No edge effect (Figure 8.20).

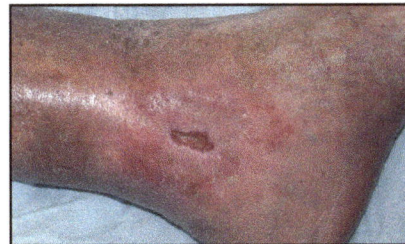

Figure 8.20: No edge effect; note the dry, thick, rolled edge in a stalled wound.

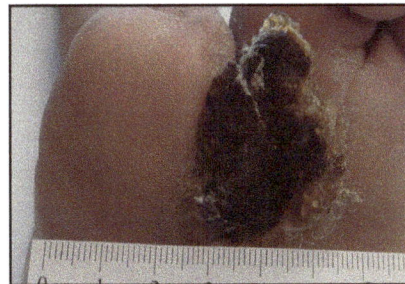

Figure 8.21: Diabetic plantar foot wound covered with callus.

7. Presence of callus (Figure 8.21)
 a) Debridement may be necessary to determine the extent of the ulcer as well as to prepare the wound bed.
E. Presence of foreign bodies
 1. Foreign bodies in a wound can prevent or slow healing and foster infection. These include:
 a) Hardware (Figure 8.22)
 b) Retained suture material
 c) Clothing, wood, glass, metal objects, etc.

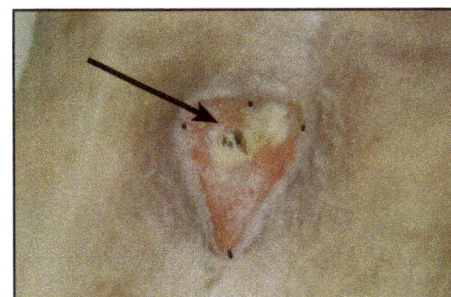

Figure 8.22: Presence of a foreign body (hardware).

V. Assessment techniques for various confounding factors related to wound healing

A. Vascular supply
1. Introduction
   a) A palpable pulse indicates a blood supply of 80 mmHg in the foot.
   b) If a regional pulse is not palpable, Doppler (Figure 8.23) or other vascular assessments (e.g., toe pressures or transcutaneous oxygen pressure, or $TcPO_2$, studies) are necessary to determine healing ability.
   c) Hypoxic conditions cause cell death and tissue necrosis, creating ideal growing conditions for microorganism contaminants that can lead to colonization.
2. Noninvasive vascular testing (refer to Chapter 16, pages 133-135)
   a) Doppler waveform analysis
   b) Ankle-brachial index (ABI)
      i) Obtaining ABI
         (1) BP cuff and handheld Doppler required.
         (2) Bilateral brachial Doppler pressures are obtained while the patient is supine. The higher of the two Doppler pressures is used as the brachial pressure in the ratio.
         (3) The blood pressure cuff is placed on the leg just above the malleoli. The Doppler probe is placed at a 45 degree angle to the dorsalis pedis or the posterior tibial artery.
         (4) The cuff is inflated until the Doppler signal is obliterated. With the Doppler probe over the artery, the cuff is slowly deflated until the Doppler signal returns. Ankle systolic pressure for that leg is recorded. A similar procedure is repeated on the other leg.
         (5) Each ankle pressure is divided by the higher of the systolic brachial pressures. This ratio is obtained for each leg, which is the ABI for each leg.

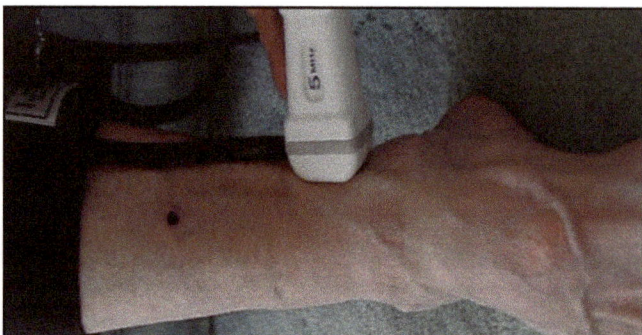

Figure 8.23: Use of Doppler

Table 8.7: Comparison of preoperative $TcPO_2$ associated with successful healing.

From Steenfos HH, Baumbach P. Transcutaneous pO_2 in Peripheral Vascular Disease. Radiometer A/S, Copenhagen; TC105: 1-18.

	# LIMBS	$TcPO_2$ WITH HEALING	PROBE TEMP	ROOM TEMP
Burgess, et al. 1982; *J Bone Joint Surg* 64(3): 378-82.	37	>40 mmHg	44-45°C	NR
Franzeck, et al. 1982; *Surgery* 91(2): 156-62.	35	>20 mmHg	45°C	25°C
Dowd, et al. 1983; *J Bone Joint Surg* 65(1): 79-83.	24	>40 mmHg	44°C	22°C
Ito, et al. 1984; *Int Surg* 69(1): 59-61.	31	>30 mmHg	45°C	NR
Benscoter, et al. 1984; *J Am Osteopath Assoc* 83(8): 560-74.	14	>37 mmHg	45°C	21°C
Rhodes.1985; *Amer Surg* 51(12):701-7.	12	>25 mmHg	NR	37°C
Christensen, et al. 1986; J Bone Joint Surg 68(3): 423-6.	42	>37 mmHg	45°C	23°C

      ii) ABI interpretation
         (1) Value interpretation
            (a) >1.2 =non-compressible vessels/calcified vessels
            (b) 0.9–1.2 = normal
            (c) 0.75–0.9 = moderate disease
            (d) 0.50–0.75 or lower = severe disease
            (e) <0.5 = rest pain or gangrene
         (2) Incompressible vessels (15)
            (a) 223 consecutive arterial leg ulcer patients
            (b) Mean ankle systolic pressure (ASP) = 88 mmHg (range 18-130)
            (c) Mean ABI = 0.6 (0.15-0.86)
            (d) Most arterial leg ulcers do not meet the criteria of chronic critical limb ischemia based on ASP (ASP <50 mmHg), which is likely due to incompressible vessels
         (3) ABI and wound healing prediction (23)

(a) ABI vs. wound healing is not correlated in DM and CRF patients
(b) ABI (macro) vs. $TcPO_2$ (microcirculation) does not correlate with wound healing
(c) $TcPO_2$ is a better indicator for healing failure compared to ABI
(d) TCOM and wound healing predictions (23) (Table 8.7)

c) Segmental pressures
d) Toe pressure
e) Color duplex imaging
f) Transcutaneous oxygen monitoring
g) Skin perfusion pressure

B. Neurological assessment
1. Sensory neuropathy involves the loss of protective sensation.
2. Sensation should be checked using a 10 g Semmes-Weinstein monofilament; the 5.07 monofilament is the limit of protective sensation (Figure 8.24).
3. Autonomic neuropathy involves poor temperature regulation. Assess for temperature, dry skin, and loss of hair on the lower limbs.
4. Motor neuropathy involves damage to nerves in the muscles of the foot. Assess motor strength and range of motion in the ankle, foot, and toes.
5. Neuropathy is diagnosed if the patient is unable to feel the 5.07 monofilament.
6. All newly diagnosed diabetics should be screened for risk factors, including:
   a) Loss of protective sensation
   b) Absent pedal pulses
   c) Severe foot deformity/abnormal biomechanics (Figure 8.25)
   d) History of foot ulcer
   e) Prior amputation
   f) Visual foot inspection EVERY visit
   g) Annual evaluations for all of the issues above

C. Biopsy
1. Indications
   a) Wounds in patients with autoimmune disease
   b) Wounds with unusual clinical presentation
   c.) Wounds that fail to respond to conventional care
   d) Wounds in which pain is out of proportion to clinical appearance
   e) Wounds for quantitative culture
2. Tissue biopsy procedure (Figures 8.26a–8.26d)
   a) Administer local anesthesia (1% lidocaine injection)
   b) Punch biopsy (0.4 mm)
   c) Wedge biopsy
   d) Place in biopsy specimen container

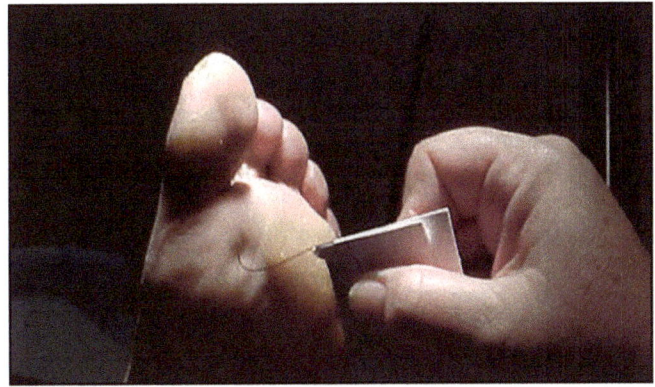

Figure 8.24: Semmes-Weinstein monofilament used for neurological assessment.

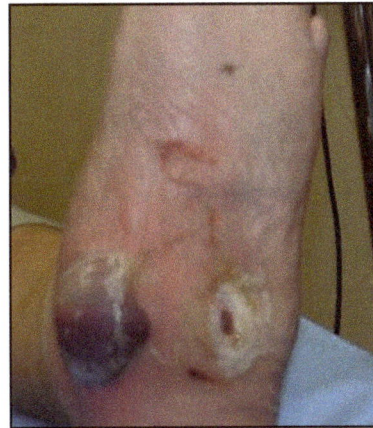

Figure 8.25: Patient with Charcot foot deformity and ulceration undermining to bullae on medial side with underlying osteomyelitis.

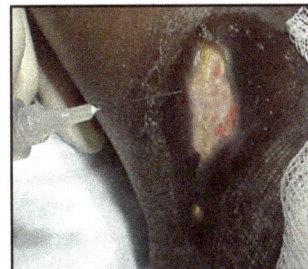

Figure 8.26a: Tissue biopsy and administration of local anesthesia with injectable lidocaine.

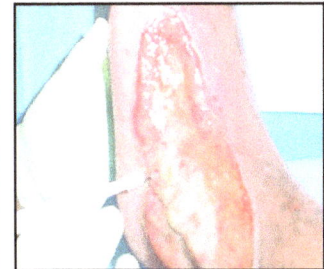

Figure 8.26b: Punch biopsy using a 0.4 mm punch to take tissue from the edge of an ulcer.

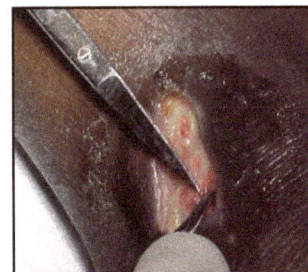

Figure 8.26c: Wedge biopsy; taking a larger tissue sample with a sharp instrument.

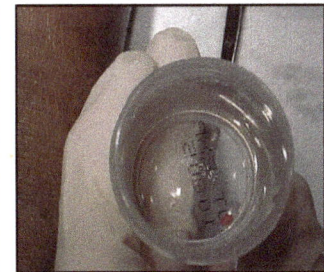

Figure 8.26d: Biopsy specimen container.

D. Techniques for assessing infection
  1. Qualitative
     a) Defines presence of bacteria, minimal inhibitory concentrations (MICs) for tested antibiotics
  2. Semi-quantitative
     a) The swab is inoculated onto a Petri dish, then streaked into four quadrants
     b) The number of quadrants in which bacteria is recovered correlates with log differences in quantitative cultures
  3. Quantitative
     a) Defines quality and quantity
     b) 10^5 CFU/gm of tissue defined as clinically infected
     c) Gram stain
        i) Initial description of components of cultured material
  4. Methods of culturing
     a) Thoroughly rinse the wound surface
     b) Don't swab through dressing residue, old exudate, necrotic tissue, or blood
     c) Choose an area that is free of nonviable tissue.
     d) Roll the end of the swab(s) over the wound surface, pressing gently to elicit fresh exudates.
     e) Don't bother swabbing dry surfaces
     f) Place the swab in the carrier and transport immediately
     g) Levine technique (swab technique)
        i) Surface swab of a 1 cm² area of healthy tissue in the wound.
        ii) Press the area with swab to extract fluid.

RESOURCES

1. Cooper D. Assessment, measurement, and evaluation: their pivotal roles in wound healing. In: Bryant R, editor. *Acute and Chronic Wounds: Nursing Management.* 2nd ed. St. Louis: Mosby; 2000: 51-84.
2. Baranoski S, Ayello EA. Wound assessment. In: Baranoski S, Ayello EA, editors. *Wound Care Essentials: Practice Principles.* Philadelphia: Lippincott Williams & Wilkins; 2004: 79-90.
3. Sibbald G, Williamson D, Orsted H, et al. Preparing the wound bed-debridement, bacterial balance, and moisture balance. *Ostomy Wound Manage.* 2000; 46(11):14-35.
4. West J, Gimbel M. Acute surgical and traumatic wound healing. In: Bryant R, editor. *Acute and Chronic Wounds: Nursing Management.* 2nd ed. St. Louis: Mosby; 2000: 189-96.
5. WOCN Society. Guidance Statement on OASIS Skin and Wound Status M0 Items. Laguna Beach, FL: WOCN; 2001.
6. Bates-Jensen B. Indices to include in wound healing assessment. *Adv Wound Care.* 1995; 8(4):25-33.
7. Bryant J, Brooks T, Schmidt B, Mostow E. Reliability of wound measuring techniques in an outpatient wound center. *Ostomy Wound Manage.* 2001; 47(4):44-51.
8. Waldrop J, Doughty D. Wound healing physiology. In: Bryant R, editor. *Acute and Chronic Wounds: Nursing Management.* 2nd ed. St. Louis: Mosby; 2000: 17-40.
9. Kerstein MD. The scientific basis of healing. *Adv Wound Care.* 1997; 10(3):30-6.
10. Black SB. Venous stasis ulcers: a review. *Ostomy Wound Manage.* 1995; 41(8):20-2, 24-6,2 8-30, 32.
11. Falanga V, Eaglstein WH. Management of venous ulcers. *Am Fam Physician.* 1986; 33:274-81.
12. Sheffield PJ, Fife CE, editors. *Wound Care Practice.* 2nd ed. North Palm Beach: Best Publishing Company; 2007.
13. Keast DH, et al. MEASURE: A Proposed assessment framework for developing best practice recommendations for wound assessment. *Wound Rep Reg.* 2004; 12(3 Suppl):S1-S17.
14. McCaffery M. *Nursing Practice Theories Related to Cognition, Bodily Pain, and Man-Environment Interactions.* Los Angeles: University of California at Los Angeles Students' Store; 1968.
15. Hafner J, Schaad I, Schneider E, et al. Leg ulcers in peripheral arterial disease (arterial leg ulcers): Impaired wound healing above the threshold of chronic critical limb ischemia. *J Am Acad Dermatol.* 2000; 43(6):1001-8.

TCOM Resources

16. Burgess EM, Matsen III FA, Wyss CR, et al. Segmental transcutaneous measurements of PO$_2$ in peripheral vascular insufficiency. *J Bone Joint Surg Am.* 1982; 64(3):378-82.
17. Franzeck UK, Talke P, Berstein EF, et al. Transcutaneous PO$_2$ measurements in health and peripheral arterial occlusive disease. *Surgery.* 1982; 9(2)1:156-62.
18. Dowd GSE, Linge K, Bently G. Measurement of transcutaneous oxygen pressure in normal and ischaemic skin. *J Bone Joint Surg Br.* 1983; 65(1):79-83.
19. Ito K, Ohgi S, Mori T, et al. Determination of amputation level in ischemic legs. *Int Surg.* 1984; 69(1):59-61.
20. Benscoter JL, Gerber A, Friedberg J. Transcutaneous oxygen measurement as a noninvasive indicator of level of tissue healing in patients with peripheral vascular disease and projected amputations. *J Am Osteopath Assoc.* 1984; 83(8):560-74.
21. Rhodes GR. Uses of transcutaneous oxygen monitoring in the management of below-knee amputations and skin envelope injuries (SKI). *Am Surg.* 1985; 51(12):701-7.
22. Christensen KS, Klarke M. Transcutaneous oxygen measurement in peripheral occlusive disease: An indicator of wound healing in leg amputation. *J Bone Joint Surg.* 1986; 68(3):423-6.
23. Padberg FT, et al. Transcutaneous oxygen (TcPO$_2$) estimates probability of healing in the ischemic extremity. *J Surg Res.* 1996; 60(2):365-9.
24. Baranoski S, Ayello EA, editors. *Wound Care Essentials: Practice Principles.* 3rd ed. Philadelphia: Lippincott Williams & Wilkins; 2012.
25. Steenfos HH, Baumbach P. Transcutaneous pO$_2$ in Peripheral Vascular Disease. Radiometer A/S, Copenhagen; TC105:1-18.

SAMPLE QUESTIONS

1. A 50-year-old female with type 2 diabetes mellitus has a long standing ulcer on her pretibial region. On examination the patient's dressings are stained green, and the wound bed of the 3 cm ulcer has friable granulation tissue. The patient is not feverish or experiencing chills. Lab values include a normal white blood cell count and an albumin level of 3.2. What would be the most probable result of a wound culture?
   a) *Proteus mirabilis*
   b) *Pseudomonas aeruginosa*
   c) *Serratia marceus*
   d) *E. coli*

2. In order to document a patient's wound exudate, the physician needs to assess the:
   a) Type of wound dressing that was applied to wound
   b) Duration of dressing on the wound
   c.) State of dressing at the time of examination
   d) All of the above

3. Which of the following is not part of wound bed preparation?
   a) Maintaining moisture balance
   b) Debridement of necrotic material
   c) Assessment of the wound edges
   d) Assessment of neuropathy with monofilament testing

4. Which of the following is not normal skin flora?
   a) *Staphylococcus epidermidis*
   b) *Staphylococcus aureus*
   c) *Escherichia coli*
   d) *Corynebacterium*

5. All of the following statements about ABI are true except:
   a) ABI is more accurate than $TcPO_2$ in predicting healing after amputation.
   b) ABI can be used as a guide in deciding whether to apply compression bandaging.
   c) Diabetic vascular calcifications can result in a falsely high ABI.

6. A 50-year-old diabetic male presents to a wound center with a 2 × 3 cm wound. The wound has good 100% granulation tissue and is on the plantar aspect of his right foot. No tendon, joint, or bone is exposed. There is no sign of infection, and the patient has a good bounding pulse. What is the UTSA grade of this wound?
   a) Grade 0D
   b) Grade 1A
   c) Grade 2C
   d) Grade 3A

7. What is the Wagner grade of the wound described in question 6?
   a) Grade 1
   b) Grade 2
   c) Grade 3
   d) Grade 4

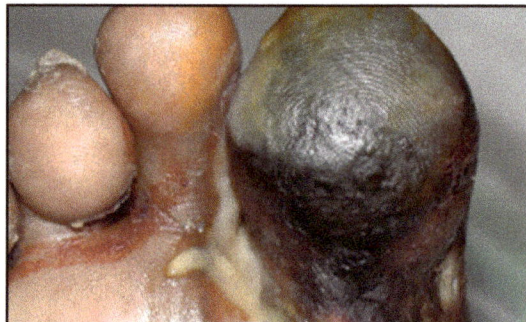

8. A 63-year-old diabetic male presents to the ER with the diabetic foot wound pictured above. What is the UTSA grade of this wound?
   a) Grade 0C
   b) Grade 1D
   c) Grade 2C
   d) Grade 3D

9. What is the Wagner grade of the wound shown in question 8?
   a) Grade 4
   b) Grade 3
   c) Grade 2
   d) Grade 1

10. An ABI greater than 1.4 in diabetics indicates:
    a) Falsely elevated ABI
    b) Non-compressible vessels
    c) Calcified arteries
    d) All of the above

See answers on page 64.

NOTES

ANSWER KEY

1. b) This 50-year-old patient has a wound infection secondary to *Pseudomonas*. Dried exudate or a green stain (caused by pyoverdin) may be found on dressings. Certain microorganisms have distinct odors; for example, *Proteus* is reminiscent of ammonia, while *Pseudomonas* is often described as "sickly sweet."

2. d) In order to document wound exudate, the physician should assess the type of dressing that was applied to the wound, the state of the dressing during the visit, and the duration the dressing was on the wound.

3. d) Wound bed preparation includes debridement, infection management, moisture balance, and monitoring wound edges. Neuropathy assessment is part of the initial assessment of the diabetic wound patient, but not part of wound bed preparation protocol.

4. c) *Escherichia coli* is usually not a skin flora; all other organisms—*Staphylococcus epidermidis, Staphylococcus aureus,* and *Corynebacterium*—are part of normal skin flora.

5. a) $TcPO_2$ is better than ABI at predicting healing failure for amputation sites. ABI is useful in non-diabetic venous stasis ulcer patients to decide on compression therapy. ABIs are falsely elevated in diabetics because of calcified vessels.

6. b) The proper UTSA grade for a superficial wound with good granulation tissue and no signs of infection or ischemia is 1A.

7. a) According to the Wagner grading system, the same wound is a grade 1.

8. d) According to the UTSA classification system, the wound in the photo, showing infected gangrene, is a grade 3D.

9. a) According to Wagner grading system, the wound in the photo is a grade 4.

10. d) An ABI greater than 1.4 indicates non-compressible vessels, calcified vessels, and falsely elevated ABI.

MICROBIOLOGY REVIEW 9

Gregory Anstead, MD, PhD
Jayesh B. Shah, MD, CWSP, FAPWCA, FACCWS

INTRODUCTION

The purpose of this chapter is to describe the classes of microorganisms and methods of bacteria classification, including gram-positive and gram-negative organisms. The process of infection will be discussed along with the concepts of contamination, colonization, critical colonization, and bioburden.

OBJECTIVES

Participants should be able to list four methods of bacteria classification, name the factors on which antibiotic selection depends, and differentiate between the concepts of contamination, colonization, and critical colonization.

I. Basic microbiology

A. Four classes of microorganisms
   1. Bacteria
   2. Viruses
   3. Fungi
   4. Parasites: protozoa (one-celled organisms) and helminths (worms)

II. Bacteria

A. Principal wound colonizers and pathogens
B. Unicellular organisms that have a cytoplasmic membrane surrounded by a cell wall; they lack a nuclear membrane and reproduce by binary fission
C. Bacteria lack many of the familiar organelles of eukaryotic cells; they possess no mitochondria, Golgi apparatus, lysozymes, or endoplasmic reticulum, but they do possess ribosomes
D. They range in size from 0.1 to 10 microns
E. Bacteria classification by morphology
   1. Spherical bacteria are called cocci
   2. Rod-shaped bacteria are called bacilli
   3. Rigid spiral bacteria are called spirilla, or spirochetes if they are more flexible
   4. Variations on these basic morphologies include coccobacilli (very short rods), curved rods, and helical rods

5. After binary fission, some bacteria aggregate into specific arrays. For the cocci there can be:
   a) Diplococci (e.g., *Streptococcus pneumoniae*)
   b) Chains (other Streptococci)
   c) Clusters (e.g., *Staphylococcus aureus*)
F. Bacteria classification based on Gram stain
   1. Gram positive
      a) Bacteria stained by crystal violet are gram positive (they appear violet on staining)
   2. Gram negative
      a) Bacteria that do not stain with crystal violet, but do stain with safranin, are termed gram negative (they appear pinkish)
   3. Gram staining characteristics reflect the differences in cell wall structure between bacteria
G. Bacteria classification by physical requirements
   1. Aerobic bacteria require an oxygen-rich environment to survive
   2. Anaerobic bacteria survive in a low-oxygen setting
      a) May be gram positive or gram negative and may have rod or coccal morphology
   3. Facultative anaerobic bacteria can adjust their metabolism to survive in a low-oxygen environment, if necessary
H. Mycobacteria
   1. Require special staining and culture techniques; an example is acid-fast bacilli (AFB) staining
   2. Infections may require specialized antibiotics for treatment
I. Bacteria are identified by
   1. Colony appearance
   2. Morphology and Gram staining characteristics
   3. AFB staining characteristics
   4. Growth on certain media and various biochemical and molecular techniques
   5. For example, an opaque gray, white, or light yellow colony on blood agar media with a Gram stain that shows gram-positive cocci in clusters that are coagulase positive is *Staphylococcus aureus*

J. Bacteria and antimicrobial agents
1. Bactericidal refers to agents that cause irreparable harm to the organism that results in bacterial death.
2. Bacteriostatic refers to the inhibition of bacterial cell growth.
3. Antibiotic selection depends on:
a) The organism involved
b) Specific susceptibility patterns
c) Safety considerations, e.g., allergies, renal and hepatic function
d) Desired route of administration, e.g., oral versus parenteral (intravenous or intramuscular)
K. Antibiotic resistance
1. An organism is resistant if it continues to grow in the presence of the agent.
2. Resistance occurs when the bacteria produce enzymes that deactivate the antimicrobial agent, alter cell metabolism, or alter permeability to prevent antimicrobial entry into the cell.
3. Resistance occurs by a Darwinian selection process whereby specific mutations or genetic changes produce subpopulations of bacteria that survive the antibiotic exposure, replicate, and then expand to become the dominant population.
L. Susceptibility testing
1. The minimal inhibitory concentration (MIC) is the lowest concentration of an antimicrobial agent that will inhibit the visible growth of a microorganism after a standard incubation period.
2. The MIC value is a standard quantitative measure of the activity of an antimicrobial agent against a particular organism.
3. Disk diffusion assay (Kirby-Bauer procedure)
a) Most commonly used test
b) Provides a qualitative result (susceptible, intermediate, or resistant)
c) A small paper disk impregnated with a specific antibiotic is placed on a lawn of bacteria or media on a culture plate, and the plate is incubated for 16-18 hours
d) A zone of inhibition develops around the antibiotic disk and the diameter of the zone is measured and compared to previously determined standards

III. The process of infection due to bacteria

A. To cause infection, a microbial pathogen must find a host niche and replicate there.
B. The microbe gains access to the host niche by a number of attributes including motility; chemotaxis, the directed movement toward specific chemical cues in the environment; and adhesive molecules (adhesins), which mediate the adherence of the microbe to eukaryotic cell surfaces.
C. Host defenses must be circumvented by the microbe to allow continued infection.

D. Methods by which bacteria cause disease:
1. Adhesion—some bacteria can bind to host cell surfaces at host cell receptor sites.
2. Colonization—some virulent bacteria produce special proteins that allow them to colonize parts of the host body.
3. Invasion—some virulent bacteria produce proteins that disrupt host cell membranes and allow the bacteria to enter host cells. Tissue invasion may be facilitated by secreted microbial enzymes that break down anatomic tissue barriers.
4. Immune response inhibitors—some bacteria produce virulence factors that inhibit the host's immune system defenses. Some bacteria have anti-phagocytic capsules, while others produce elaborate toxins that act on host immune cells or proteases that degrade immunoglobulins as a means to resist the host immune system.
5. Toxins—many virulence factors are proteins made by bacteria that poison host cells and cause tissue damage.
E. Virulence
1. Virulence is the ability of a microorganism to cause disease.
2. Virulence factors are those attributes of the organism that enhance its ability to cause disease. For example, *Staphylococcus aureus* is more virulent than *Staphylococcus epidermidis*.
3. Even within a species, different strains of bacteria may be more virulent due to the elaboration of a specific virulence factor.
4. An example is Panton-Valentine leukocidin (PVL), a pore-forming toxin produced by specific strains of *Staphylococcus aureus* that destroys leukocytes and causes tissue necrosis.
F. Contamination
1. Presence of bacteria on wound surfaces with no multiplication of bacteria.
2. The normal microflora on the skin and the mucosal surfaces of the gastrointestinal tract play an important role in protection against pathogenic organisms.
G. Colonization
1. Characterized by replication of microorganisms on the wound surface without invasion of wound tissue and no host immune response, e.g., bacteria are in the wound but are not causing tissue damage or delaying healing.
2. Intact skin can be colonized with up to 10^3 organisms per gram of tissue without adverse effects.
H. Critical colonization
1. Microbes in the wound are growing faster than they are dying, delaying healing.
2. The first sign of critical colonization may be delayed wound healing, as evidenced by no change in wound size (l × w) or increasing exudates.

I. Wound infection
    1. When host response fails to control growth of micro-organisms, localized wound infection occurs.
    2. Uncontrolled localized infection of a wound can lead to deeper, more severe infections, such as extensive cellulitis, osteomyelitis, bacteremia, and sepsis.
    3. Wound infection prolongs the inflammatory phase and disrupts the proliferative phase of wound healing.
    4. It occurs in viable wound tissue and not on the surface of the wound bed.
    5. It is manifested by the host reaction or tissue injury.
    6. Delayed healing may be the only sign of infection in some wounds.
J. Healthy skin
    1. Skin is naturally populated with microorganisms, including *Staphylococcus aureus, Staphylococcus epidermis*, some forms of *Streptococcus*.
    2. Substances in sweat, sebum, and the acid pH of the skin, which is between 4.5–5.5, help prevent these organisms from becoming pathogenic.

IV. Viral infections of the skin

A. Rashes (exanthems) are common in many viral infections, but these are usually self-limited and resolve during the course of the infection.
B. Viruses do not typically cause infection of traumatic or surgical wounds. A few viral pathogens, such as herpes simplex, varicella (chickenpox/shingles), and cytomegalovirus (CMV), cause ulcerative lesions that may heal slowly (especially in immunocompromised patients) or become secondarily infected by bacteria.
    1. Herpes simplex, varicella, and cytomegalovirus infections can be treated by antiviral agents.

V. Fungi

A. Fungi are infrequent pathogens in traumatic or surgical wounds. Some of the endemic fungal pathogens can cause primary ulcerative lesions of the skin and oral mucosa in the course of disseminated disease (which is more common in immunocompromised patients).
    1. These fungal pathogens include *Histoplasma capsulatum* (the causative organism for histoplasmosis) and *Coccidioides immitis* (the causative organism of coccidioidomycosis).
    2. Burn wounds may become infected with the yeast *Candida* species and molds of various species, especially *Aspergillus* species.
    3. Chronic wounds may also be colonized or infected with *Candida* species (*Candida albicans* in the most common species).
    4. Occasionally both traumatic and surgical wounds may become infected with a group of aggressive fungal pathogens called zygomycetes (major genera include *Rhizopus, Mucor*, and *Rhizomucor*).
B. Wound infection by zygomycetes requires aggressive debridement and long courses of antifungal treatment.

VI. Parasites

A. Parasites do not cause infections of traumatic and surgical wounds.
B. A few parasitic protozoans do cause ulcerative lesions during the course of their infections, such as *Leishmania* species (causative organism of cutaneous leishmaniasis) and *Entamoeba histolytica* (the causative organism of amebiasis).

RESOURCES

1. Le Frock JL, Mader JT. Skin, skin structure, and muscle infections. In: Sheffield PJ, Fife CE, editors. *Wound Care Practice*. 2nd ed. North Palm Beach: Best Publishing Company; 2007: 747-66.
2. Gardner SE, Frantz RA. Wound bioburden and infecton. In: Baranoski S, Ayello E, editors. *Wound Care Essentials: Practice Principles*. 3rd ed. Philadelphia: Lippincott Williams & Wilkins; 2013: 126-56.
3. Woo KY, Sibbald RG. A cross-sectional validation study of using NERDS and STONES to assess bacterial burden. *Ostomy Wound Manage*. 2009; 55(8):40-8.

SAMPLE QUESTIONS

1. Bacteria classification can be based on all of the following except:
   a) Gram stain
   b) Survival of hypoxia
   c) Acid-fast bacilli (AFB) staining
   d) Colony appearance
   e) KOH staining

2. The selection of an antibiotic is dependent on all of the following except:
   a) The organism involved
   b) Specific susceptibility pattern
   c) Allergies
   d) Renal/hepatic function
   e) The patient taking probiotics

3. The presence of microorganisms on wound surface with no multiplication of bacteria is called:
   a) Colonization
   b) Contamination
   c) Infection
   d) Critical colonization

4. The first sign of critical colonization may be:
   a) Delayed wound healing as evidenced by no change in wound size
   b) Delayed wound healing as evidenced by increasing exudate
   c) Delayed wound healing as evidence by increasing necrotic tissue
   d) Both a and b
   e) All of the above

5. All of the following statements about wound infection are true except:
   a) Wound infection occurs in viable wound tissue.
   b) Wound infection occurs on the surface of the wound tissue.
   c) Wound infection is caused by the invasion and multiplication of microbes in the wound.
   d) Wound infection is manifested by a host reaction or tissue injury.
   e) Wound infection prolongs the inflammatory phase and disrupts the proliferative phase of wound healing.

6. The classic sign of infection that is first reported by the patient is:
   a) Increasing erythema
   b Increasing warmth
   c) Increasing pain
   d) Increasing purulent exudate

7. All of the following are methods by which bacteria cause disease except:
   a) Binding to host cell surfaces at host cell receptor sites
   b) Contaminating parts of the host's body
   c) Producing proteins that disrupt host cell membranes
   d) Producing virulence factors that inhibit the host's immune system defenses
   e) Producing virulence factors that poison host cells and cause tissue damage

8. The minimal inhibitory concentration (MIC) is:
   a) The lowest concentration of an antimicrobial agent that will inhibit the visible growth of a microorganism after a standard incubation period
   b) The lowest concentration of an antimicrobial agent that will kill the microorganism after a standard incubation period
   c) The highest concentration of an antimicrobial agent that will inhibit the visible growth of a microorganism after a standard incubation period
   d) The highest concentration of an antimicrobial agent that will kill the microorganism after a standard incubation period

9. The normal pH of skin is:
   a) 3.5-4.5
   b) 4.5-5.5
   c) 5.5-6.5
   d) 6.5-7.5

10. All of the following are diseases caused by fungi except:
    a) Histoplasmosis
    b) Coccidioidomycosis
    c) Actinomycosis
    d) Sporotrichosis

See answers on page 70.

NOTES

ANSWER KEY

1. e) Bacterial classification is based on Gram stain,
        survival of hypoxia, AFB staining, and colony appear-
        ance. KOH staining is used to identify fungi.

2. e) The selection of an antibiotic is dependent on the or-
        ganisms involved, susceptibility pattern, allergies, and
        renal and hepatic function. While it is recommended
        to prescribe probiotics to patients on antibiotics to
        decrease certain side effects, the selection of an anti-
        biotic is not dependent on that factor.

3. b) Contamination is the presence of microorganisms on
        a wound surface with no multiplication.

4. d) The first sign of critical colonization is delayed
        wound healing as evidenced by no change in wound
        size and increasing exudate.

5. b) Wound infection occurs in viable wound tissue. It is
        caused by the invasion and multiplication of microbes
        in the wound, and it is manifested by a host reaction
        or tissue injury. It prolongs the inflammatory phase
        and disrupts the proliferative phase of wound healing.

6. c) The classic sign of infection that is first reported by
        the patient is increasing pain. Other signs of infec-
        tion, like increasing erythema, increasing warmth and
        increasing purulent exudate, are usually noted by a
        care provider.

7. b) Bacteria cause disease by binding to host cell surfaces
        at host cell receptor sites, producing proteins that
        disrupt host cell membranes, producing virulence fac-
        tors that inhibit the host's immune system defenses,
        and producing virulence factors that poison host cells
        and cause tissue damage. Bacteria does not cause
        disease by contaminating parts of the host's body.

8. a) The minimal inhibitory concentration (MIC) is the
        lowest concentration of an antimicrobial agent that
        will inhibit the visible growth of a microorganism
        after a standard incubation period.

9. b) The normal pH of skin is 4.5-5.5.

10. c) Histoplasmosis, coccidioidomycosis, and sporotricho-
        sis are caused by fungi. Actinomycosis is caused by
        bacteria.

INFECTION CONTROL 10

Dianne Rudolph, RN, GNP-BC, DNP, CWOCN
Ellen T. Heiderich, RN, CWS

INTRODUCTION

Healthcare providers are responsible for implementing infection control practices along the continuum of the healthcare delivery system, and adherence to these practices is essential for decreasing rates of infection. Evidence supports the consistent implementation of standard and transmission-based precautions indicated by the specific disease process to decrease the frequency of healthcare-acquired infections.

Infection control practices are required in wound care practice. Types of infections include contact, airborne, blood-borne, and special respiratory and resistant organisms. The discussion will focus on important concepts for controlling spread of infection through aseptic technique, hand hygiene, personal protective equipment, and waste management.

OBJECTIVES

Participants should be able to explain the universal precautions for infection control, discuss hand cleansing methods for infection control, and describe transmission-based contact precautions for wound infection control.

I. Regulating authorities

A. OSHA (Occupational Safety and Health Administration)—Develops standards for protection from blood-borne pathogens and respiratory pathogens (*M. tuberculosis)* and creates and enforces safety standards for the workplace.
B. CDC (Centers for Disease Control)—A major component of the Department of Health that develops standards for disease prevention.
C. NIOSH (National Institute for Occupational Safety and Health)—Conducts research and makes recommendations for the prevention of workplace diseases.
D. JCAHO (Joint Commission)—Sets the standards by which healthcare is measured.
E. APIC (Association for Professionals in Infection Control and Epidemiology)—Influences, supports, and improves the quality of healthcare through the practice and management of infection control and epidemiology.

F. State health departments—Following CDC guidelines, states have individual requirements by which healthcare institutions must abide.

II. MDROs (multidrug-resistant organisms)

A. MDROs are defined as microorganisms, predominantly bacteria, that are resistant to one or more classes of antimicrobial agents. Although the names of certain MDROs describe resistance to only one agent (e.g., MRSA, VRE), these pathogens are frequently resistant to most available antimicrobial agents. These highly resistant organisms deserve special attention in healthcare facilities. In addition to MRSA and VRE, certain GNBs, including those producing extended spectrum beta-lactamases (ESBLs) and others that are resistant to multiple classes of antimicrobial agents, are of particular concern.
B. MRSA (methicillin-resistant *Staphylococcus aureus*) infection—everyone's nemesis
   1. *S. aureus* colonizes the skin, nares, and perineum; some strains have become resistant to beta-lactam inhibitors such as methicillin
   2. 126,000 infections annually with >5,000 deaths
   3. Typically treated with vancomycin, but now there is also VISA or VRSA (vancomycin-intermediate or vancomycin-resistant *Staphylococcus aureus*)
   4. Two types of MRSA:
      a) Community acquired (CA-MRSA): soft tissue infections, boils/carbuncles, folliculitis, abscesses appearing as "spider bites." Transmitted via contact with personal items. Susceptible to ciprofloxacin, gentamicin, bactrim, and clindamycin.
      b) Healthcare associated (HA-MRSA): surgical site infections, osteomyelitis, bacteremia, pneumonia. Transmitted by contaminated environment surfaces and healthcare workers. Usually affects those already compromised. Risk factors include surgical wounds or pressure ulcers, invasive catheters or tubes, prolonged or repeat hospitalizations, immunocompromised status, end-stage renal disease on hemodialysis, burns, dermatitis, intravenous drug abuse, type 2 diabetes mel-

litus, close proximity to colonized patient, broad spectrum antibiotic use, multidrug resistance, etc.

C. VRE (vancomycin-resistant enterococci) infection
  1. Infection with VRE typically follows vancomycin-resistant enterococcal colonization, predominantly of the gastrointestinal tract. Colonization, which does not result in symptoms, may last for long periods of time and serve as a reservoir for the transmission of VRE to other patients. Within hospitals, widespread colonization with VRE may occur with a comparatively small number of documented infections. Therefore, tracking colonization with VRE through active surveillance in high-risk units is an important component of preventing further transmission.

D. ESBL (extended spectrum beta-lactamase) infection
  1. Gram-negative Enterobacteriaceae expressing ESBL are among the most multidrug-resistant pathogens in hospitals and are spreading worldwide. Infections caused by ESBL–producing organisms have resulted in poor outcomes, reduced rates of clinical and microbiological responses, longer hospital stays, and greater hospital expenses. Multiple outbreaks of ESBL-producing Enterobacteriaceae in intensive care units (ICUs) and increased rates of illness and death, especially in neonatal ICUs, have been reported. Physical contact is the most likely mode of transmission, with the gastrointestinal tract of colonized or infected patients the most frequent reservoir. Several studies indicate that transient carriage of bacteria on the hands of healthcare workers may lead to transmission to patients.

III. Current concepts in infection control practices

A. How microorganisms spread: through direct or indirect contact, droplet, vector, airborne
B. Controlling spread of infection: hand washing, wearing proper personal protective equipment (PPE), proper disposal of contaminated dressings, proper handling of contaminated equipment
C. Aseptic technique: use of dressings and equipment that have been disinfected or sterilized

IV. Standard precautions

A. Hand hygiene: hand washing with either soap and water or 70-95% alcohol products is considered the most effective method of preventing the spread of infection.
B. Use of PPE: wearing gloves, gown, eye/face protection, and respiratory mask.
C. Waste management: dispose of contaminated waste in moisture-proof bags; deposit contaminated linens in the proper containers.

V. Transmission-based precautions

A. Contact precautions
  1. Private room; if not available, cohort with another patient with the same microorganism.
  2. Wear gloves, wash hands with an antimicrobial agent after glove removal, remove gloves while inside the patient's room.
  3. Wear a gown if there may be possible contact with infectious surfaces. Protect uniform/clothing from contact with infectious surfaces.
  4. Limit patient movement outside of his or her room, and dedicate noncritical equipment to a single patient or patients with same microorganism.
  5. Clean the room thoroughly between patients. Patients with the same organism (e.g., MRSA) may be cohorted.
B. Airborne precautions
  1. Standard precautions apply, plus private room with negative pressure and air changes 6-12 times per hour.
  2. Wear a respiratory mask.
  3. Limit patient movement outside of his or her room.
  4. Susceptible persons should not enter the room.
C. Blood-borne precautions
  1. Standard precautions apply.
  2. Wash hands after contact with contaminated objects, removing gloves and gowns when entering and leaving the room.
  3. Wear a gown and/or face shield if splash is possible.
  4. Dispose of contaminated linens, dressings, and single use equipment properly.
  5. Avoid injury with sharp objects by placing them in puncture-resistant containers.
  6. Handle blood, secretions, and excretions carefully.
D. Family and visitors
  1. Educate and enforce precautions.

VI. Adverse effects of isolation

A. Decreased patient contact
B. Decreased satisfaction with patient care
C. Increased depression/isolation
D. Delays in transfer and increased length of stay (LOS)

RESOURCES

1. Coe P, Clark J. Infection control in the wound care setting. In: Sheffield PJ, Fife CE, editors. *Wound Care Practice*. 2nd ed. North Palm Beach: Best Publishing Company; 2007: 1133-46.

2. Kozier B, Erb G, Berman A, Snyder S. *Fundamentals of Nursing: Concepts, Process, and Practice.* 7th ed. Upper Saddle River: Pearson/Prentice Hall; 2004: 640-55.

3. Gudnadottir U, Fritz J, Zerbel S, Bernardo A, Sethi AK, Safdar N. Reducing health care-associated infections: patients want to be engaged and learn about infection prevention. *Am J Infect Control.* 2013; 41(11):955-8.

4. Jessee MA, Mion LC. Is evidence guiding practice? Reported versus observed adherence to contact precautions: a pilot study. *Am J Infect Control.* 2013; 41(11):965-70.

5. Bessessen MT, Lopez K, Guerin K, Hendrickson K, Williams S, O'Connor-Wright S, Granger D. Comparison of control strategies for methicillin-resistant *Staphylococcus aureus. Am J Infect Control.* 2013; 41(11):1048-52.

6. Zirakzadeh A, Patel R. Vancomycin-resistant enterococci: colonization, infection, detection, and treatment. *Mayo Clin Proc.* 2006; 81(4):529–36.

7. Centers for Disease Control and Prevention. Healthcare Infection Control Practices Advisory Committee (HICPAC). MultiDrug Resistant Organisms [Internet]. 2009 [updated 2009 Dec 29]. Accessed at: http://www.cdc.gov/hicpac/mdro/mdro_2.html.

SAMPLE QUESTIONS

1. The single most effective method for preventing the spread of infection is:
   a) Washing hands with triclosan products
   b) Washing hands with 100% alcohol products
   c) Washing hands with 70-95% alcohol products
   d) Washing hands with 50% alcohol products

2. Those with the highest risk for developing MRSA colonization and infection are patients with:
   a) Prolonged stay in a healthcare facility
   b) Invasive catheters or tubes
   c) Repeat hospitalizations
   d) Multidrug resistance
   e) All of the above

3. Contact transmission precautions require all of the following except:
   a) Assigning a private room; the patient must not occupy a room with another patient, even when that patient has the same microorganism
   b) Wearing gloves, removing them while in the patient's room, and washing hands with an antimicrobial agent after glove removal
   c) Wearing a gown to protect uniform/clothing from contact with infectious surfaces
   d) Dedicating noncritical equipment to a single patient or patients with the same microorganism
   e) Cleaning the room thoroughly between patients

4. All of the following are adverse effects of isolation except:
   a) Depression
   b) Poor patient satisfaction score
   c) Increased patient contact
   d) Increased length of stay because of delays in transfer

5. Which of the following infection control measures are recommended to prevent spread of infection?
   a) Hand washing
   b) Wearing proper PPE
   c) Proper disposal of contaminated dressings
   d) Proper handling of contaminated equipment
   e) All of the above

See answers on page 76.

NOTES

ANSWER KEY

1. c) The single most effective method for preventing the spread of infection is washing hands with 70-95% alcohol products.

2. e) Those with the highest risk for developing MRSA colonization and infection are patients with a prolonged stay in a health care facility, invasive catheters or tubes, repeat hospitalizations, and multidrug resistance.

3. a) Contact transmission precautions include assigning a private room; however, the patient can be cohorted with another patient with the same microorganism.

4. c) The adverse effects of isolation stem from decreased patient contact, which can cause depression and poor patient satisfaction. It also causes an increase in length of stay because of delays in transfer.

5. e) All of the listed infection control measures are recommended to prevent the spread of infection.

WOUND INFECTIONS 11

Gregory Anstead, MD, PhD
Jayesh B. Shah, MD, CWSP, FAPWCA, FACCWS

INTRODUCTION

The purpose of this chapter is to describe the concepts of critical colonization, bioburden, and infection. The microbiology of severe wound infections will be discussed, including gram-positive organisms, gram-negative organisms, necrotizing fasciitis, and gas gangrene.

OBJECTIVES

Participants should be able to list three primary factors in assessing infected wounds, contrast gram-positive and gram-negative organisms, and discuss necrotizing infections of skin and subcutaneous tissues.

I. Wound infection

A. The spectrum of infection range by increasing severity: contamination, colonization, critical colonization, and infection.
B. Definitions:
1. Contamination is the presence of bacteria on the wound surface with no multiplication.
2. Colonization is characterized by the replication of bacteria on wound surface without invasion of wound tissue and no host immune response.
3. Critical colonization is characterized by the replication of bacteria on the wound surface with invasion of wound edges; wound shows signs of delayed healing.
4. Infection is characterized by the replication of bacteria on the wound surface with 10^5 organisms per 1 gram of tissue with host immune response.
   a) Infection = bacterial burden × (virulence/host resistance)
C. Host resistance depends on local and systemic factors.
1. Local factors include size; foreign bodies such as bone (viable, less viable, or necrotic) suture, or metal; inciting event; and perfusion.
2. Systemic factors include behavioral (alcohol use, smoking, compliance), diabetes, immune defects (corticosteroids, chemotherapy, autoimmune illnesses), and edema-forming states.

   a) Even with 10^3 organisms, infection is possible if a highly virulent organism is in an immunocompromised host.
   b) Beta-hemolytic *Streptococcus* is considered a notable threat in wounds, regardless of the number of these microorganisms present.
D. Clinical signs of infection include erythema (redness) of skin around the wound, pus, crepitus (crackling sound upon palpation of the tissue resulting from gas in the tissue), fever with chills, tachycardia (increased pulse rate); however, all signs may not always be present.
1. Wound infection clues (Figure 11.1)
   a) Disappearance or sudden change in granulation tissue within wound
   b) Edematous, boggy, friable gray to maroon colored granulation tissue; hemorrhage
   c) Poor wound healing despite ideal care
   d) Increased wound pain
2. In an immunocompromised patient
   a) Unable to mount an appropriate immune response
   b) Infection may be clinically silent and the patient does not manifest these cardinal signs of infection
   c) Pain may be the only classic sign of wound infection present in immunocompromised patients

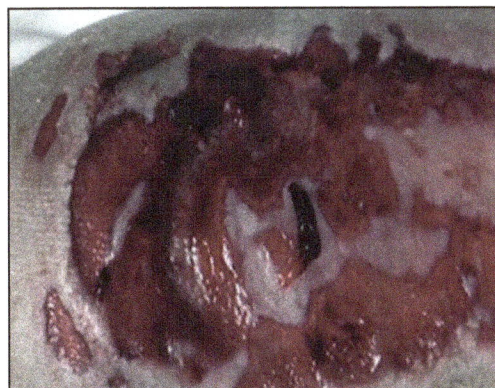

Figure 11.1: Wound infection on right lower leg, pretibial area. Clues include boggy, friable gray to maroon colored granulation tissue.

Table 11.1: Markers for identification of biofilm in a wound.
Adapted from Percival SL, Hill KE, Williams DW, et al. A review of the scientific evidence for biofilms in wounds. *Wound Repair Regen*. 2012; 20(5):647-57.

CLINICAL SIGN	MARKER	IDENTIFICATION METHOD
Non-healing wound	Slough	Visual exam
	Shiny	Visual exam
Malodor	Smell	Smell
Necrotic tissue	Necrotic tissue	Visual exam
Unresponsive to Rx	Lack of change to antimicrobial effect/ recurring	Visual exam
Polymicrobial microbiology	Cultural and molecular identification	Standard culture techniques Molecular techniques-PCR
Isolated bacteria showed a high biofilm-forming potential	Biofilm-forming potential	Use microtiter assay with crystal violet
Biopsy-visualization	Evidence of microcolonies	Gram stain Scanning electron microscopy Light microscopy
	Evidence of extracellular polymeric substances	H & E stain, Calcofluor white/ ethidium bromide, Congo red/Ziehl carbol fuchsin, Safranin/FITC-conA/ DAPI/PAS
	Evidence of an inflammatory response	H & E stain

3. Patients with wound infections usually have
   a) High bacterial counts or prolonged inflammation
   b) Increased inflammatory cytokines
   c) Increased protease activity
   d) Decreased growth factor activity
   e) Alkaline pH
4. Biofilm: bacteria with a biofilm phenotype are thought to predominate on the wound surface and have been implicated in the failure of many wounds to heal. (11)
   a) Features of chronic wound infections (biofilm)
      i) Pale wound bed
      ii) Yellow discharge
      iii) Necrotic tissue
      iv) Clear slime
      v) Putrid smell
      vi) Friable granulation tissue
      vii) Red spongy granulation tissue
   b) Biofilm in chronic wounds (Table 11.1)
      i) Causes delayed healing
      ii) Causes chronic inflammation

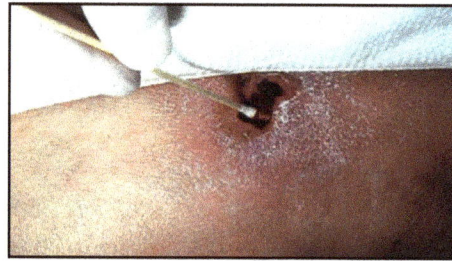

Figure 11.2a: Taking a swab culture.

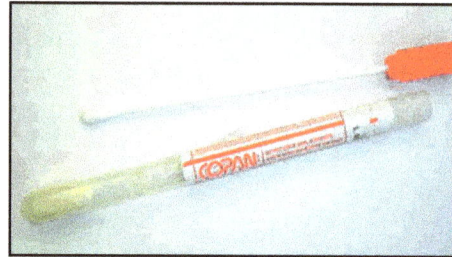

Figure 11.2b: Swab and culture medium.

E. Wound culture technique (Figures 11.2a and 11.2b)
   1. Quantitative wound culture: obtain a biopsy and send 1 gram of tissue for culture.
   2. Swab cultures
      a) Z-technique: wound cleansing is advocated before the culture. Swab using the broad Z-stroke entails rotating the swabs between the fingers as the wound is swabbed from margin to margin in a 10-point zigzag fashion.
      b) Levine technique: wound cleansing in advocated before the culture. The Levine technique consists of rotating a swab over a 1 cm² area with sufficient pressure to express fluid from within the wound tissue.
      c) Culture findings based on swab specimens obtained using Levine's technique were more accurate and concordant with culture findings based on tissue specimens than swabs taken with either wound exudate or the Z-technique.
      d) The Levine technique was the most appropriate for obtaining swab specimens of the wound.
   3. Needle aspiration (Figure 11.3)
      a) 22 G needle attached to a 10 cc syringe—obtain fluid through multiple insertions into the tissue surrounding the wound.

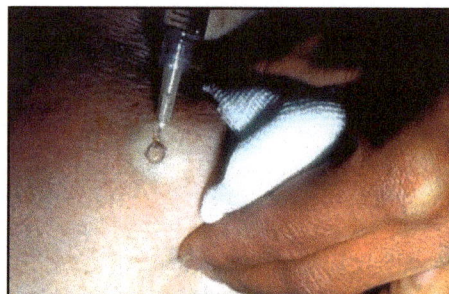

Figure 11.3: Needle aspiration.

F. NERDS and STONES (7)
1. A practical clinical approach using the mnemonics NERDS and STONES can help identify superficial and deep infection.
2. Increasing pain and wound breakdown are sufficient signs of wound infection.
3. Any three NERDS signs are indicative of critical colonization (superficial infection).
4. Any three STONES signs are indicative of deep infection.
5. Superficial infection (critical colonization) mnemonic NERDS:
    a) **N**on-healing wounds
    b) **E**xudative wounds
    c) **R**ed and bleeding wound surface granulation tissue
    d) **D**ebris (yellow or black necrotic tissue on the wound surface)
    e) **S**mell or unpleasant odor from the wound
6. Deep infection mnemonic STONES:
    a) **S**ize bigger
    b) **T**emperature increased
    c) **O**s (probes to or exposed bone)
    d) **N**ew or satellite areas of breakdown
    e) **E**xudate, Erythema, Edema
    f) **S**mell
G. Topical versus systemic therapy
1. Colonization—no treatment is indicated.
2. Critical colonization (superficial wound infections)—topical therapy is appropriate.
    a) The decision to initiate antimicrobial therapy is best guided by the failure of the wound to make progress towards healing despite the absence of devitalized tissue.
    b) Limiting the use of effective topical antibiotics to short durations with high doses can minimize the potential for the selection or development of more resistant bacteria.
    c) While treating superficial or deep infections, attention should be given to supporting or restoring host defenses to microorganism invasion, such as adequate blood supply, tissue oxygen, nutrition, management of blood sugar levels, and control of edema.
3. Infection (deep wound infections)—treatment through systemic antibiotic therapy.
    a) Parenteral therapy may be indicated when the infection involves deeper tissue and is accompanied by systemic signs such as fever, chills, and elevated WBC count.
    b) The effectiveness of systemic antibiotics is dependent on an adequate blood supply to the wound.

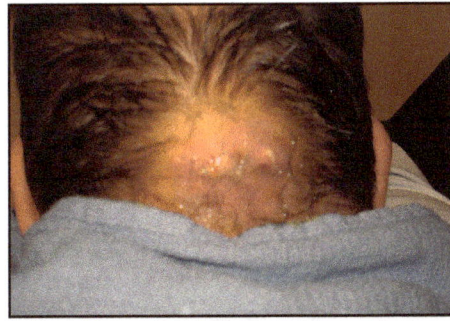

Figure 11.4a: Cellulitis of the scalp.

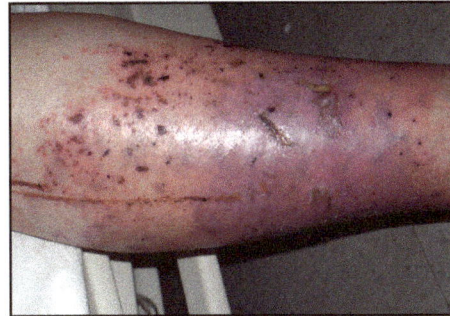

Figure 11.4b: Cellulitis of the leg.

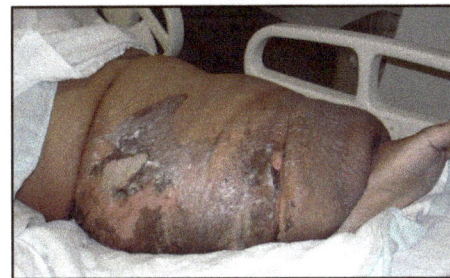

Figure 11.4c: Cellulitis in a lymphedema patient.

II. Infections/disorders

A. Cellulitis (Figures 11.4a-c)
1. An acute inflammatory condition of the skin caused either by indigenous flora colonizing the skin or by a wide variety of exogenous bacteria
2. Characterized by localized pain, erythema, swelling, and heat

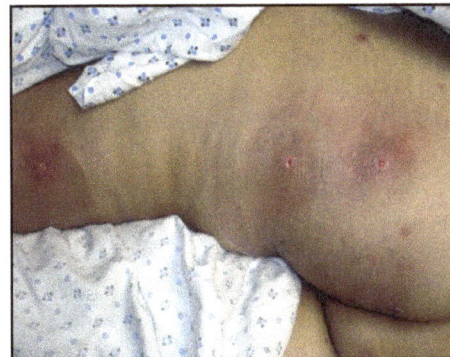

Figure 11.5: Multiple boils.

B. Boils/abscess (Figure 11.5)
1. Deep-seated infection of a hair follicle; most often located on the buttocks, face, or neck
C. Carbuncle (Figures 11.6a and 11.6b)
1. Deep infection of a group of contiguous follicles
2. Painful necrotic lesions often accompanied by high fever and malaise

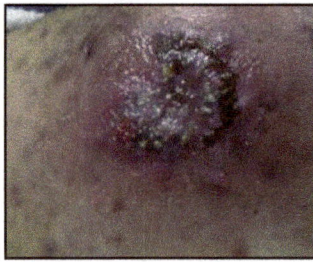

Figure 11.6a: Carbuncle before surgery.

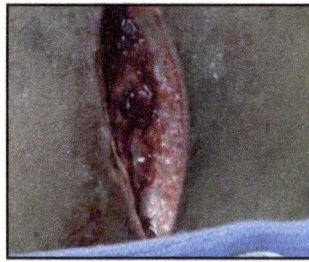

Figure 11.6b: Carbuncle after surgery.

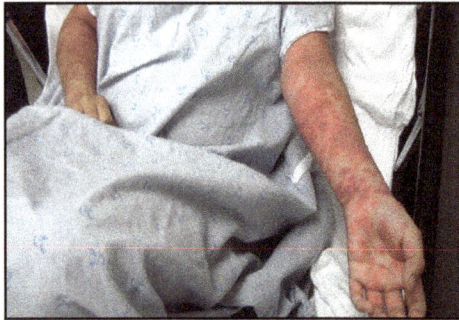

Figure 11.7: Impetigo.

  3. Occurs most often on back of the neck, shoulders, hips, and thighs

D. Impetigo (Figure 11.7)

  1. A superficial infection of skin secondary to either *Staphylococcus aureus* or group A beta-hemolytic streptococci

  2. The primary lesion is a superficial pustule that ruptures to form a "honey-colored" crust

E. Erysipelas

  1. Superficial cellulitis, most commonly on the face

  2. Characterized by a bright red, sharply demarcated, intensely painful warm plaque

  3. Most commonly due to infection with a group A beta-hemolytic streptococci occurring at sites of trauma or other breaks in skin

F. Surgical site infections (SSI) (Figure 11.8)

  1. Infections are considered SSIs if they:

   a) Occur within 30 days of surgery on that tissue layer

   b) Involve only skin or subcutaneous tissue of the incision and at least one of the following:

    i) Purulent drainage from the superficial incision

    ii) Organisms isolated from aseptically obtained culture of fluid or tissue from the incision

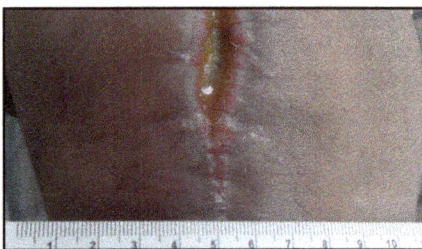

Figure 11.8: A 65-year-old diabetic male patient's surgical site infection after total knee replacement with a prosthetic.

    iii) At least one of the following, unless negative culture:

     (1) Pain or tenderness

     (2) Localized swelling

     (3) Redness or heat

     (4) Incision opened by surgeon

    iv) Diagnosis of SSI by the surgeon or attending physician

  2. Deep incisional SSIs or organ space SSIs

   a) Occur within 30 days of surgery

   b) Involve deep soft tissues (such as fascia and muscle layers) of the incision and at least one of the following:

    i) Purulent drainage from the deep incision but not organ/space

    ii) A deep incision spontaneously dehisces or is deliberately opened by the surgeon with one of the following symptoms, unless the culture is negative:

     (1) Fever greater than 100.4°F (38°C)

     (2) Localized pain

    iii) An abscess

    iv) Diagnosis of deep SSI by the surgeon or attending physician

  3. Organ/space SSI

   a) Occurs within 30 days of surgery

   b) Involves any part of the anatomy (other than the incision) opened or manipulated during the operation and at least one of the following:

    i) Purulent drainage from a drain placed in an organ/space

    ii) Organisms isolated from aseptically obtained culture of fluid or tissue in organ/space

    iii) An abscess or other evidence of infection

    iv) Diagnosis of an organ/space SSI by a surgeon or attending physician

G. Animal bites

  1. Bacterial pathogens in animal bites

   a) *Staphylococcus* and streptococci (especially *Streptococcus viridans*) are the most common pathogens found with animal bites.

   b) *Pasteurella multocida* is associated with dog and cat bites.

   c) *Eikenella corrodens* is associated with human bites.

    i) Gram-negative anaerobes are found in 11% of animal bites and 5% of human bites.

H. Diabetic wound infections

  1. Ulcers that have been infected for a short time tend to be mono-microbial and are usually caused by gram-positive pathogens.

  2. Chronic diabetic ulcers develop complex flora with gram-positive aerobes, aerobic gram-negative rods, anaerobes (gram positive and negative), and enterococci; fungi (*Candida)* and mold species also appear to disproportionately colonize the skin of diabetic patients.

Table 11.2: Suggested empiric treatment of diabetic foot infections.
Adapted from Lipsky BA. Infectious problems of the foot in diabetic patients. In: *Levin and O'Neal's The Diabetic Foot*; 2008: 305-18).

SEVERITY OF INFECTION	RECOMMENDED	ALTERNATIVES
Mild/moderate (oral for entire course)	Cephalexin (500 mg qid) or amoxicillin/clavulanate (875/125 mg bid) or clindamycin (300 mg tid)	Levofloxacin (500 mg po qd) + clindamycin (300 mg po tid) or TMP/SMX (2 ds po bid)
Moderate/severe (IV then switch to PO)	Ampicillin/sulbactam (2.1 gm IV qid) or clindamycin (450 mg po qid) + ciprofloxacin (750 mg po bid)	Linezolid (600 mg po bid) + aztreonam (2 gm tid)
Life threatening (prolonged IV)	Imipenem/cilastatin (500 mg IV qid) or clindamycin (900 mg IV tid) + tobramycin IV (5.1 mg/kg/day) + ampicillin (50 mg/kg IV qid)	Vancomycin (15 mg/kg bid) + ceftazidime (1 gm tid) + metronidazole (7.5 mg/kg IV qid)

3. Mild infections occurring in patients not previously on antibiotic therapy is usually caused by one or two species of bacteria, almost invariably aerobic gram-positive cocci (*Staphylococcus aureus* is the most common pathogen and usually part of a mixed infection).

4. Serious infections in hospitalized patients are usually caused by three to five bacterial species, including both aerobes and anaerobes.

5. Gram–negative bacilli, mainly of the family Enterobacteriaceae, are found in many patients with chronic or previously treated wounds.

6. *Pseudomonas* species are often isolated from wounds that have been soaked in water or treated with wet dressings.

7. Enterococci are commonly cultured from patients who have previously received cephalosporin.

8. Obligate anaerobic species are most frequently found in ischemic wounds with necrosis or that involve deep tissues. They are rarely the sole pathogens and are usually part of mixed infections.

9. Antibiotic–resistant organisms, especially MRSA, frequently occur in patients who have previously received antibiotic therapy.

10. Suggested empiric treatment of diabetic foot infections (Table 11.2)
   a) Case study: Charcot foot/osteomyelitis
      i) A 70-year-old female with a history of type 2 DM, coronary artery disease, and severe aortic stenosis presented with a diabetic foot infection and osteomyelitis of the cuboid bone. The bone culture was positive for MRSA. Treatment required local wound care and IV antibiotics (Figures 11.9a–11.9f).

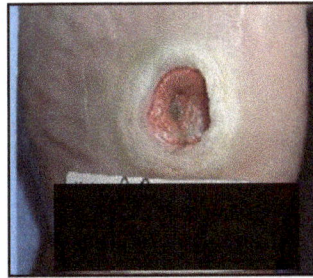

Figure 11.9a: Initial presentation of Charcot foot with plantar wound undermining down to bone.

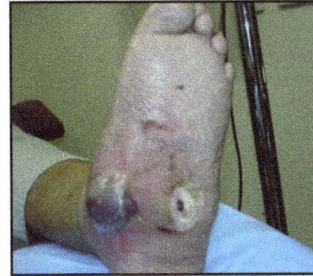

Figure 11.9b: Patient with new bullae on left medial side connected to original wound in plantar foot. Persistent infection after six weeks.

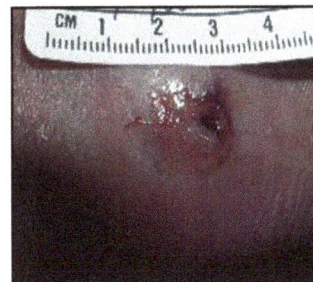

Figure 11.9c: After debridement of the bullae on left medial side and removal of sequestrum.

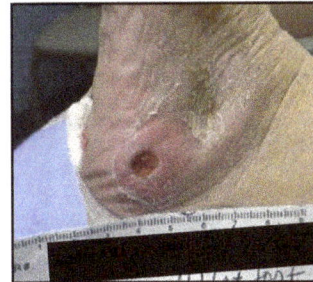

Figure 11.9d: Wound after three months of local care and continued antibiotics. Plantar wound has healed and the wound on the lateral side has almost epithelized.

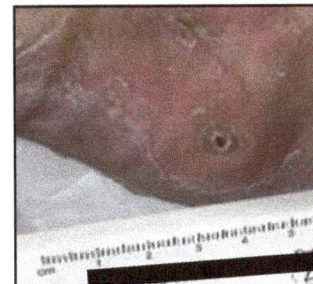

Figure 11.9e: Healed wound on medial side of left foot.

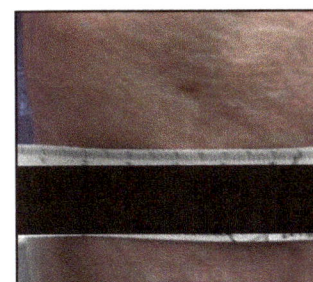

Figure 11.9f: Healed wound on plantar side of left foot.

I. Pressure ulcers

    1. Common pathogens found in infected pressure ulcers are *E. coli, Proteus mirabilis, Enterococcus* species, *Bacteroides fragilis*, other members of the *B. fragilis* group, *Prevotella* species (an anaerobic gram-negative rod), and anaerobic streptococci.

J. Necrotizing fasciitis

    1. The classic microbe responsible for necrotizing fasciitis is *Streptococcus pyogenes*, although recently *Staphylococcus aureus* has also been described as a cause.

    2. Risk factors (50% mortality associated with any combination of three or more risk factors):

       a) IV drug use

       b) Diabetes

       c) Peripheral vascular disease (PVD)

       d) Obesity

       e) Malnutrition

    3. Clinical manifestations

       a) Pain—usually out of degree to proportion of physical findings

       b) Swelling—massive "sausage-like" edema

       c) Erythema—often bullous skin changes (large blisters)

       d) Fever—low grade

       e) Lack of lymphadenopathy—misses immune recognition

       f) Skin necrosis possible—may be hypesthetic/anesthetic

       g) Striking indifference to clinical state

       h) Toxic shock appearance with rapid demise

    4. Diagnosis

       a) Culture, Gram stain

       b) Bacterial antigen testing may identify *Streptococcus* but does not establish diagnosis: basic rapid strep test

       c) Polymerase chain reaction (PCR) testing identifies streptococcal pyrogenic exotoxin genes (SPE-B)

    5. MRSA linked to necrotizing fasciitis (Figure 11.10)

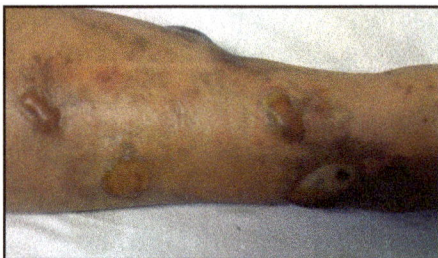

Figure 11.10: MRSA linked with necrotizing fasciitis.

       a) Necrotizing fasciitis may also be caused by community-acquired MRSA

       b) Necrotizing fasciitis case study

          i) A 61-year-old diabetic male was referred to the wound center with a large lateral and medial ulcer of the left foot (Figure 11.11a).

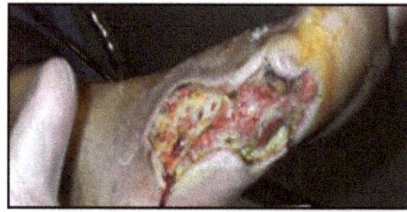

Figure 11.11a Necrotizing fasciitis of the right lateral foot before treatment.

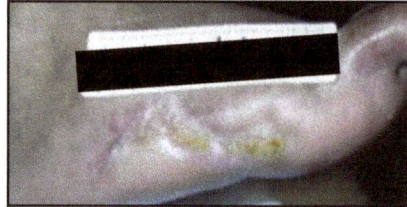

Figure 11.11b: Same wound after treatment.

          ii) He was admitted to the hospital for debridement and IV antibiotics. Cultures revealed heavy growth of group B *Streptococcus, Pseudomonas,* and *Proteus* organisms.

          iii) His transcutaneous oxygen studies revealed a very hypoxic wound.

          iv) The patient received a total of 40 hyperbaric oxygen treatments and was continued on wound care until the wound completely healed (Figure 11.11b).

K. Fournier's gangrene (Figure 11.12)

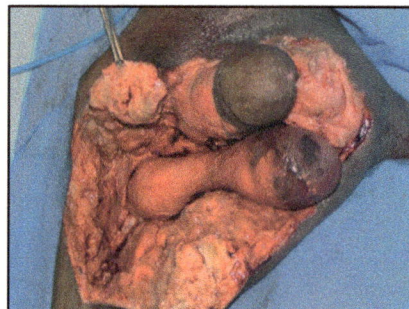

Figure 11.12: Fournier's gangrene. Courtesy of Dr. Robert Michaelson.

    1. Aggressive necrotizing infection of the perineum that may extend to the anterior abdominal wall, gluteal muscles, and in males, to the penis and scrotum.

    2. The causative organisms are a mixed collection of aerobic gram negatives, enterococci, and anaerobes, including *Bacteroides* species and peptostreptococci.

L. Clostridial cellulitis

    1. Usually occurs after trauma or surgery.

    2. The usual causative organism is the anaerobe *Clostridium perfringens.*

    3. Gas is seen in the skin, but the fascia and deeper tissues are spared.

M. Gas gangrene (Figures 11.13a–11.13c)

    1. Gas gangrene occurs after a deep penetrating injury compromises blood supply, creating the anaerobic conditions ideal for clostridial proliferation.

    2. The majority of infections are caused by *C. perfringens*, but other species of *Clostridium* have also been implicated.

    3. The patient presents with severe pain, and the skin

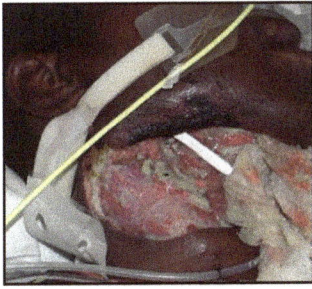

Figure 11.13a: Patient with gas gangrene of the neck.

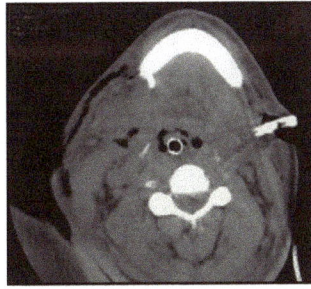

Figure 11.13b: Findings of gas on a CT scan.

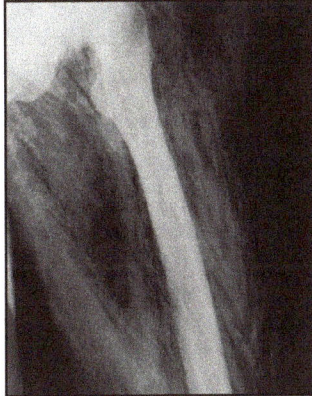

Figure 11.13c: Radiographic image of gas in a thigh muscle.

changes from pale to bronze to purplish-red with bullae formation.
4. Gas in the tissue is evident from physical exam (crepitus) or by radiography.
5. Gas gangrene—late findings
   a) Myonecrosis
   b) Hemolytic anemia
   c) Hematuria and myoglobinuria
   d) Acute renal failure
   e) Metabolic acidosis
   f) Consumptive coagulopathy
   g) Shock, seizures, and death
6. Gas gangrene—skin changes
   a) Skin in early phases appears shiny and tense
   b) Tense, bronzed, and tender
   c) Blue-black bullae
   d) Gas and crepitation may be late findings
   e) Odor
7. Earliest symptoms
   a) Fever
   b) Pain out of proportion to injury
   c) Tachycardia
   d) Diaphoresis
   e) Gray pallor
8. Earliest signs
   a) Anoxemia
   b) Apprehension, disorientation, obtundation (decreased level of alertness)
   c) Average incubation period around 48 hours
9. Other
   a) Ischemia and inoculation

   b) Bacterial proliferation
   c) Exotoxin production
   d) Tissue destruction
   e) Edema and necrosis
   f) Decreased redox potential
   g) Gangrene
   h) Hemorrhagic bullae
   i) Bronzing skin
   j) Myoglobinuria
   k) Gas in muscles (Figure 11.13c)
   l) Toxic psychosis
   m) The patient may rapidly progress to shock and multi-organ failure.
   n) Bacteremia and hemolysis may occur
   o) Renal failure may occur as a result of hemoglobinuria and myoglobinuria
N. Puncture wound
   1. It is estimated that 3-18% of puncture wounds in children become infected, resulting in cellulitis or a localized deep abscess.
   2. Osteomyelitis is the next most common complication and occurs in 0.65-1.8% of cases, with *Pseudomonas* causing the infection >90% of the time. (10)
   3. Common objects (nails, glass, plastics, rocks, sewing needles, metal wire, wood slivers, animal bites).
   4. Tetanus history
      a) Tetanus is most frequently associated with acute wounds (72%), with puncture wounds accounting for more than 50% of these.
      b) *Clostridium tetani* spores are found in soil.
      c) The leading cause of tetanus in minor wounds is *Clostridium tetani*.
O. Herpes
   1. Herpes simplex
      a) Recurrent eruption characterized by grouped vesicles on an erythematous base that progress to erosions. Often secondarily infected with *Staphylococcus* species or streptococci.
   2. Herpes zoster (Figure 11.14)

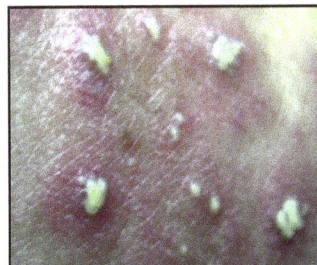

Figure 11.14: Herpes zoster with secondary bacterial infection.

      a) Eruption of grouped vesicles on an erythematous base usually limited to single dermatome.
P. Candidiasis (Figure 11.15)
   1. Fungal infection caused by a related group of yeasts.
   2. Manifestations may be localized to the skin and are rarely systemic and life threatening.
   3. Predisposing factors include type 2 diabetes mellitus, HIV, or immune deficiency.

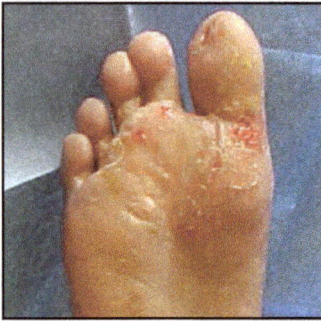

Figure 11.15: Candidiasis.

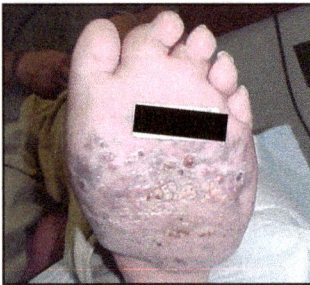

Figure 11.16a: A 32-year-old Hispanic male presents with a three-year history of multiple sinuses of the foot.

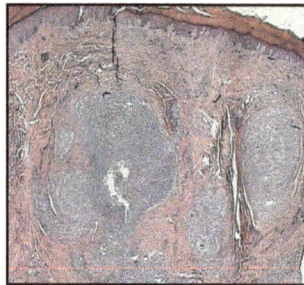

Figure 11.16b: Multiple abscesses on microscopic exam.

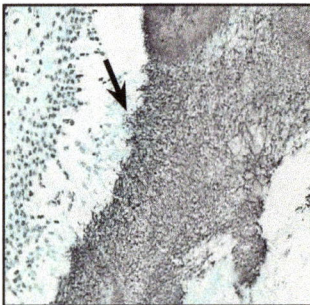

Figure 11.16c: Neutrophils and filamentous organisms (*Actinomycosis israelii*).

Q. Actinomycosis (Figures 11.16a–11.16c)
  1. It is Gram positive.
  2. It is a non-spore forming anaerobic bacilli.
  3. "Sulphur granules" (aggregates of bacteria) on Gram stain is diagnostic.
  4. *Actinomycosis israelii* is the most common species.
  5. Treatment is surgical excision and antibiotics for six months.
  6. Ampicillin is the drug of choice.
R. Mycobacteria and wounds
  1. *Mycobacterium tuberculosis* (MTB) is associated with chronic ulcers, scrofuloderma (skin involvement near an infected lymph node), lupus vulgaris (nodules or plaques), and miliary (disseminated) lesions (Figure 11.17).

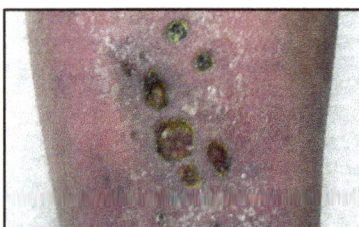

Figure 11.17: Infection from *Mycobacterium tuberculosis*.

  2. Non-tuberculous mycobacteria
    a) Swimming pool and fish tank granuloma—*M. marinum*
    b) Buruli ulcer—*M. ulcerans*
    c) Ulcer associated with *M. fortuitum*
      i) Usually isolated from nodular lesions
      ii) Usually found in diabetics and immunosuppressed patients
      iii) Usually resistant to anti-TB drugs
S. Sporotrichosis (Figure 11.18)

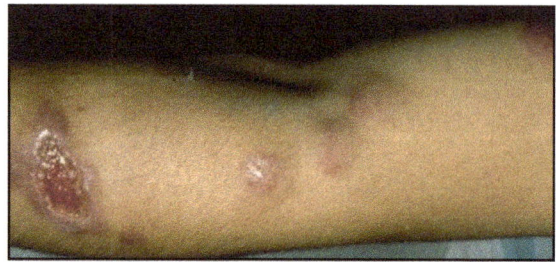

Figure 11.18. Sporotrichosis.

  1. *Sporothrix schenckii*
  2. Affects plant nursery workers, florists, gardeners
  3. Non-tender, red maculopapular granulomas that sometimes ulcerate
  4. Treatment is IV amphotericin (disseminated), oral itraconazole or posaconazole, IV potassium iodide
T. Leprosy (Figures 11.19a and 11.19b)

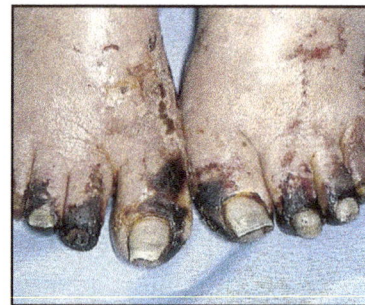

Figure 11.19a: Necrotic changes in multiple toes of a leprosy patient.

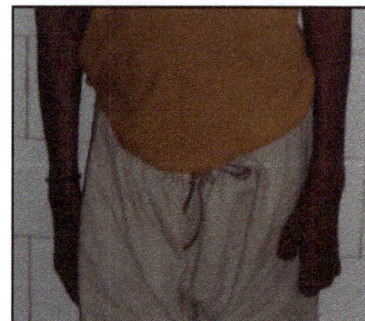

Figure 11.19b: Leprosy patient with autoamputations of the distal fingers.

  1. Chronic granulomatous disease
  2. Mainly in developing countries
  3. *M. leprae* affects skin and peripheral nerves

III. Summary
A. Treat infections seriously—they delay wound healing and can threaten life and limb.

RESOURCES

1. Le Frock JL, Mader JT. Skin, skin structure, and muscle infections. In: Sheffield PJ, Fife CE, editors. *Wound Care Practice*. 2nd ed. North Palm Beach: Best Publishing Company; 2007: 747-66.
2. Le Frock JL. Post-operative surgical site infections, non-necrotizing skin, and soft tissue infections. In: Sheffield PJ, Fife CE, editors. *Wound Care Practice*. 2nd ed. North Palm Beach: Best Publishing Company; 2007: 767-98.
3. Miller LG, Perdreau-Remington F, Rieg G, et al. Necrotizing fasciitis caused by community acquired MRSA in Los Angeles. *N Engl J Med*. 2005; 352:1445-53.
4. Horan TC, Gaynes RP, Martone WJ, et al. CDC definitions of nosocomial surgical site infections, 1992: a modification of CDC definitions of surgical wound infections. *Infect Control Hosp Epidemiol*. 1992; 13(10):606-8.
5. Mangram AJ, Horan TC, Pearson ML, et al. Guideline for prevention of surgical site infection, 1999. Hospital Infection Control Practices Advisory Committee. *Infect Control Hosp Epidemiol*. 1999; 20(4):250-78.
6. Gardner SE, Frantz RA. Wound bioburden and infection. In: Baranoski S, Ayello E, editors. *Wound Care Essentials: Practice Principles*. 3rd ed. Philadelphia: Lippincott Williams & Wilkins; 2013: 126-56.
7. Woo KY, Sibbald RG. A cross-sectional validation study of using NERDS and STONES to assess bacterial burden. *Ostomy Wound Manage*. 2009; 55(8):40-8.
8. Lipsky BA. Infectious problems of the foot in diabetic patients. In: Bowker JH, Pfeifer MA, editors. *Levin and O'Neal's The Diabetic Foot*. 7th ed. Amsterdam: Mosby Elsevier; 2008: 305-27.
9. International Working Group on the Diabetic Foot. Progress report: Wound healing and treatments for people with diabetic foot ulcers; 2003.
10. Fisher MC, Goldsmith JF, Gilligan PH. Sneakers as a source of *Pseudomonas aeruginosa* in children with osteomyelitis following puncture wounds. *J Pediatr*. 1985; 106(4):607-9.
11. Percival SL, Hill KE, Williams DW, et al. A review of the scientific evidence for biofilms in wounds. *Wound Repair Regen*. 2012; 20(5):647-57.

SAMPLE QUESTIONS

1. A wound infection in the post-operative elderly patient is a major cause of all of the following reasons except:
   a) Increased morbidity
   b) Shorter hospital stay and more outpatient visits to doctors
   c) Frequent return trips to the operating room for debridement
   d) Increased medication doses

2. Outcomes in necrotizing fasciitis are determined by all of the following except:
   a) Early recognition of tissue necrosis
   b) Prompt surgical intervention
   c) Appropriate antibiotics
   d) Adjunctive hyperbaric oxygen therapy
   e) Gender

3. Which of the following signs is not used in the differential diagnosis of necrotizing infections of skin and subcutaneous tissues?
   a) Pain
   b) Tissue gas
   c) Skin changes
   d) Odor of exudates
   e) Tissue hypoxia

4. Which of the following is the most valid indicator of a wound infection?
   a) The presence of periwound erythema and pain
   b) A quantitative culture showing 10^4 organisms per 1 gram of tissue
   c) A quantitative culture showing 10^5 organisms per 1 gram of tissue
   d) A swab culture showing large amount of methicillin-resistant *Staphylococcus aureus*

5. Topical antibiotics for the treatment of chronic wounds should be used:
   a) When there is failure of the wound to make progress towards healing despite the absence of devitalized tissue
   b) For a prolonged period until the wound has completely healed
   c) Routinely to reduce high bacterial levels even if there is no signs of infection
   d) Routinely to prevent infection

6. Which technique of swab culture is found to have more accurate results and is concordant with culture findings based on tissue specimens?
   a) Z-technique
   b) Levine technique
   c) Swab of wound exudate
   d) All of the above

7. The NERDS mnemonic for superficial wound infections includes all of the following except:
   a) Exudative wounds
   b) Debris on the wound surface
   c) Suffering (wound pain)
   d) Smell (unpleasant odor from the wound)

8. The STONES mnemonic for deep wound infections includes all of the following except:
   a) Exudate, erythema, edema
   b) Smell
   c) Os, probes to or exposed bone
   d) Excessive debris (yellow or black necrotic tissue)

9. Which of the following statements about serious, in-hospital diabetic wound infections is true?
   a) They are usually caused by three to five bacterial species, including both aerobes and anaerobes.
   b) They are usually caused by MRSA (methicillin-resistant *Staphyloccocus aureus*).
   c) They are usually caused by *Pseudomonas.*
   d) None of the above statements are true.

10. A Gram stain in patients with actinomycosis shows:
    a) Crystalline granules
    b) Sulphur granules
    c) Aerobic bacilli
    d) Aerobic cocci

See answers on page 88.

NOTES

ANSWER KEY

1. b) Wound infection in the post-operative elderly patient is a major cause of increased morbidity, prolonged hospital stay, frequent return trips to the operating room for debridement, and increased medication doses.

2. e) Outcomes in necrotizing fasciitis are determined by early recognition of tissue necrosis, prompt surgical intervention, appropriate antibiotics, and adjunctive hyperbaric oxygen therapy. Gender is not a determinant for outcome in patients with necrotizing fasciitis.

3. e) Though correction of tissue hypoxia can help in the treatment of necrotizing infections, it is not used for differential diagnosis like the clinical signs of pain, tissue gas, skin changes, and odor of exudates.

4. c) A quantitative culture taken on a wound biopsy of 1 gram of tissue showing 10^5 organisms is the most valid indicator of a wound infection.

5. a) Topical antibiotics should be used when there is failure of the wound to make progress towards healing, despite the absence of devitalized tissue. Topical antibiotics should not be used for a prolonged period. It should not be routinely used for the prevention of infection or to decrease bacterial counts.

6. b) The Levine technique of swab culture is found to have more accurate results and is concordant with culture findings based on tissue specimens.

7. c) The NERDS mnemonic for superficial wound infections includes non-healing wounds (N), exudative wounds (E), red and bleeding wound surface granulation tissue (R), debris (yellow or black necrotic tissue on the wound surface) (D), and smell or unpleasant odor from the wound (S).

8. d) The STONES mnemonic for deep infection includes size bigger (S); temperature increased (T); Os, probes to or exposed bone (O); new or satellite areas of breakdown (N); exudate, erythema, edema (E); and smell (S).

9. a) Serious, in-hospital diabetic wound infections are usually caused by three to five bacterial species, including both aerobes and anaerobes.

10. b) A Gram stain in patients with actinomycosis shows "sulphur granules" (aggregates of non spore forming anaerobic bacteria) as diagnostic.

NUTRITION AND WOUND HEALING 12

Jane Fore, MD, FAPWCA, FACCWS
Jayesh B. Shah, MD, CWSP, FAPWCA, FACCWS

INTRODUCTION

The purpose of this chapter is to describe the relationship between proper nutrition and the ability to heal. When a patient cannot ingest food orally, it may become necessary to provide either enteral or parenteral nutrition. Enteral nutrition is the delivery of nutrients directly into the stomach, duodenum, or jejunum by tube feeding. Parenteral nutrition is provided by a route other than the alimentary canal, such as subcutaneously, intravenously, intramuscularly, or intradermally, and is usually for the purpose of maintaining fluid and electrolyte balance. This chapter will focus on protein calorie malnutrition and nutritional considerations. Nutritional assessment tools and lab indicators will be discussed.

OBJECTIVES

Participants should be able to describe a nutritional status assessment, describe the physical signs of malnutrition, contrast enteral and parenteral nutrition, and discuss the role of nutrition in the enzyme systems involved in wound healing.

I. Role of nutrition
A. Nutrition and hydration are critical for tissue integrity and wound healing.
B. A strong relationship exists between pressure ulcers and nutritional status.
   1. Poor nutritional status is a major risk factor for pressure ulcer development.
   2. Weight loss is associated with poor wound healing.

II. Catabolic state stress response (Figure 12.1)

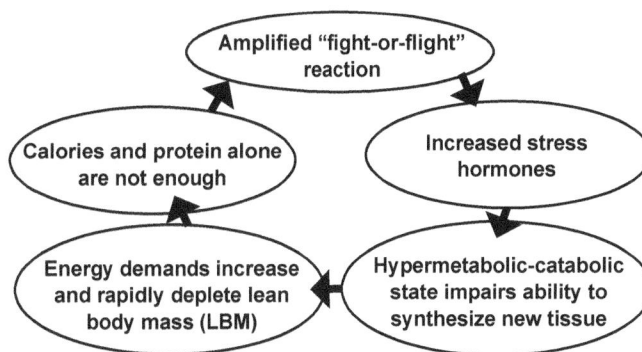

Figure 12.1: Stress response.

III. Screening for malnutrition
A. Significant weight loss
   1. 5 lbs or more in one month
   2. 5% in 30 days
   3. 10% in 180 days
B. Look for associated disease states and conditions
   1. Diabetes mellitus (DM)
   2. Dementia
   3. Malnutrition
   4. Chronic obstructive pulmonary disease (COPD)
   5. Cancer
   6. Renal disease
   7. Obesity
C. Chewing and swallowing problems
   1. Dysphagia
   2. Stroke
   3. Parkinson's disease
   4. Cerebral palsy
D. Poor food and fluid intake
E. Medication adverse events
F. Significant weight loss without any know medical condition
G. Requires help to eat or drink
H. Eats less than half of meals and snacks served
I. Has mouth pain

J. Has poorly fitting dentures
K. Has a hard time chewing or swallowing
L. Coughs or chokes while eating
M. Has sadness, crying spells, or withdrawal from others
N. Is confused, wanders, or paces
O. Other factors
    1. Medications

2. Radiation
3. Anti-inflammatory drugs
4. Immunosuppressive agents
5. Smoking
6. Mobility

IV. Physical signs of malnutrition (Table 12.1)

Table 12.1: Signs of malnutrition.

LOCATION	DEFICIENCY	DESCRIPTION
Hair	Protein energy	Dull, dry, lack of natural shine
	Zinc	Thin, sparse, loss of curl, color change
	Manganese/copper	Depigmentation and easily plucked
Eyes	Hyperlipedemia	Small, yellowish lumps around eyes, white ring around both eyes
	Riboflavin	Angular inflammation of eyelids, "grittiness" under eyelids
	Vitamin B12, folate,* and/or iron	Pale eye membranes
	Vitamin A, zinc	Night blindness, dry membranes, dull or soft cornea
	Niacin	Redness and fissures of eyelid corners
Lips	Niacin, riboflavin, iron, pyridoxine	Redness and swelling of mouth
	Niacin, riboflavin, iron, pyridoxine	Angular fissures, scars at corner of mouth
	Pyridoxine	Soreness, burning lips, pallor
Gums	Vitamin C	Spongy, swollen, bleeds easily, redness
	Folic acid, vitamin B12	Gingivitis
Mouth	Riboflavin, folic acid, pyridoxine	Cheilosis, angular scars
	Riboflavin	Soreness, burning
Tongue	Folic acid, niacin	Sores, swollen, scarlet, raw
	Riboflavin	Soreness, burning tongue, purplish color
	Riboflavin, vitamin B12, pyridoxine	Smooth with papillae (small projections)
	Iron, zinc, pyridoxine	Glossitis
	Zinc	Loss of taste
Nails	Protein	Fragility, banding
	Iron	Spoon shaped
Skin	Zinc	Slow wound healing
	Biotin	Psoriasis, scaliness
	Riboflavin	Eczema
	Vitamin C or K	Black and blue marks due to skin bleeding
	Vitamin A	Dryness, mosaic, sandpaper feel, flakiness
	Niacin	Swollen, dark, hyperpigmentation, cutaneous flushing
Gastrointestinal	Vitamin B12	Anorexia, flatulence, diarrhea
Muscular	Phosphorous or potassium	Weakness
	Protein energy, malnutrition	Wasted appearance
	Thiamin	Calf tenderness, absent knee jerks
	Magnesium or pyridoxine (excess or deficiency)	Muscle twitching
Skeletal	Vitamin D, calcium, phosphorous	Demineralization of bone, epiphyseal enlargement of leg and knee
Nervous system	Protein energy	Listlessness
	Thiamine and vitamin B12	Loss of position and vibratory sense, decrease and loss of ankle and knee reflexes, depression, inability to concentrate, defective memory, delirium
	Magnesium and zinc	Seizures, memory impairment, behavioral disturbances

*Naturally occurring form of folic acid

Table 12.2: Lab data.

TEST	NORMAL	MODERATE	DEPLETION
Albumin	3.5 g/dL or greater	2.8-3.5 g/dL	2.8 g/dL or less
Transferrin	200 mg/dL or greater	160-200 mg/dL	160 mg/dL or less
Prealbumin	14 mg/dL or greater	11-14 mg/dL	11 mg/dL or less

V. Lab data (Table 12.2)
A. TLC 1500-3000/mm^3
B. BUN/CR
C. Hemoglobin/hematocrit

VI. Starvation
A. During starvation lean body mass (LBM) will decline, resulting in complications.
B. Loss of LBM has the following effects:
1. A loss of 10% of LBM impairs immune function, resulting in increased risk of infection.
2. A loss of 15% of LBM further increases risk for infection and slows the rate of wound healing.
3. A loss of 25% of LBM results in extreme weakness, further risk of infection, and a lack of healing.
4. As loss of LBM progresses, spared protein is less available for wound healing as restoring LBM becomes the priority. When malnutrition becomes this severe, there is also a risk that new wounds will form as a result of collagen losses and a thinning of the skin.

VII. Protein—energy malnutrition
A. Marasmus
1. Chronic wasting of body tissues, especially in young children, commonly due to prolonged dietary deficiency of protein and calories
2. Impaired absorption of protein, energy, vitamins, and minerals
3. Weight loss with normal visceral protein stores (serum albumin, prealbumin, and transferrin) remaining normal. Lack of muscle and subcutaneous tissue
4. Cancer and COPD are common causes
B. Kwashiorkor
1. A form of protein-energy malnutrition produced by severe protein deficiency; caloric intake may be deficient. Protein deficit is greater than calorie deficit.
2. Muscle mass is preserved.
   a) Patient may appear well nourished
   b) Edema is present and weight may be maintained due to edema
   c) Serum albumin and cellular immunity are impaired
   d) Poor wound healing
C. Marasmic kwashiorkor
1. A condition in which there is a deficiency of both calories and protein with severe tissue wasting, loss of subcutaneous fat, and usually dehydration.

VIII. Obesity and wounds
A. Body mass index (BMI) is a weight-to-height ratio derived from body weight in kilograms divided by the square of the height in meters, or height ratio derived from body weight in pounds divided by the height in inches multiplied by 705.
B. A normally hydrated person with a BMI greater than 30 is considered obese. (5)
C. An obese patient with wounds should consume a diet adequate in protein and calories to meet wound healing needs instead of a low-calorie diet designed for weight reduction. (4)

IX. Nutrition interventions
A. Dietician consult
B. Nutritional support
1. Treatment—patients with wounds require
   a) Calories: 30-35 calories/kg/day
   b) Carbohydrates
      i) Provides 4 Kcal/gram of carbohydrates
      ii) 50-100 gm/day needed to prevent ketosis
   c) Fat
      i) Provides 9 Kcal/gram of fat
      ii) Recommended intake of total fat 20-35% of total calorie intake
   d) Proteins: 1.2-1.5 gm/kg/ day
      i) Positive nitrogen balance to promote anabolism
         (1) High loss of exudate can result in deficit of as much as 100 gm of protein in one day
C. Fluid management
D. Vitamin and mineral supplementation
1. Nutrition essentials
   a) Essential (indispensable) amino acids
      i) Isoleucine, phenylalanine, leucine, threonine, lysine, tryptophan, methionine, valine
   b) Nonessential (dispensable) amino acids
      i) Alanine, glutamine, arginine, glycine, asparagine, histidine, aspartate, proline, cysteine, serine
   c) Conditionally indispensible amino acids
      i) Arginine cysteine, glutamine, glycine, proline, tyrosine, serine
      ii) These are important to consider in wound healing and why arginine, cysteine, and glutamine are used as supplements

2. Targeted nutritional synergy (arginine and glutamine support protein synthesis; HMB increases lean mass by decreasing breakdown of protein from cells)
    a) L-arginine
        i)   Sole substrate for nitric oxide synthase
        ii) Precursor to polyamines
        iii) Regulator of nucleic acid synthesis
        iv) Stimulates IGF-1
    b) Arginine
        i)   Conditionally essential amino acid
        ii) Helps support immune function
        iii) Helps promote wound healing from help with collagen production
        iv) Enhances bacterial killing power of WBCs
        v)   By-product of nitric oxide and important for angiogenesis
    c) Glutamine
        i)   Depleted during stress
        ii)   Major component of muscle tissue
        iii) Indirect role in wound healing
        iv)   Primary fuel for lymphocytes and macrophages
        v)   Dosage is 0.57 gm/kg/day for 10 days
        vi)   Conditionally essential amino acid
        vii) Regulates cellular protein synthesis
        viii) Improves immune function
        ix)   Maintains gut integrity
        x)   Vehicle for nitrogen transfer between tissues
        xi)   Fuel for macrophages, lymphocytes, and fibroblasts
        xii) Anti-catabolic activity; positive nitrogen balance
    d) HMB (ß-hydroxy-ß-methylbutyrate)
        i) Naturally produced in humans
            (1) Metabolite of leucine
            (2) Precursor to cholesterol synthesis inside cells
            (3) Stress compromises HMB production
            (4) Anti-catabolic effect
        ii) Helps reduce muscle damage
            (1) Increased cholesterol synthesis
                (a) Protects muscle from stress-related damage
                (b) Decreases muscle breakdown in disease states
3. Omega fatty acids
    a) Alpha-linolenic acid is an omega (ω)-3 fatty acid.
        i) Found in fish oils and shellfish
        ii) Omega-3 generated eicosanoids have antiproliferative, anti-inflammatory, and antithrombotic effects
    b) Gamma-linolenic acid is an omega-6 fatty acid.
    c) Omega-6 generated eicosanoids increase cell proliferation, inflammation, and blood clotting.

4. Vitamin A
    a) Essential for epithelial cell structure and function and influences synthesis or activation of a number of proteins, hormones, and insulin
    b) Depleted during time of malnutrition, infection, and injury
5. Vitamin D
    a) Can be synthesized in the body and is considered a prohormone.
    b) 7-dehydrocholesterol is converted to D3 or cholecalciferol.
    c) Sunlight is required to produce the vitamin.
        i)   Increases with increasing pigmentation (darker skin)
        ii) Increases with age
        iii) Increases with the time of the day
        iv) Increases with season of the year
    d) Exposure to sunshine at the peak of the day for 10-15 minutes three times a week is adequate for a fair-skinned individual.
    e) Application of SPF 15 sunscreen reduces the body's ability to make vitamin D by 95%.
    f) Vitamin D regulates calcium levels.
    g) Each cell of the body has vitamin D receptors.
    h) Vitamin D is important as it acts like a hormone.
    i) Regulates cellular function to prevent cancer, mature skin, and regulate turnover of skin.
    j) Vitamin D is integral in calcium-binding proteins like calcitonin and type I collagen.
    k) Important in suppression of parathyroid hormone secretion and maintenance of good bone density (preventing or slowing osteoporosis).
    l) Rickets is due to a vitamin D deficiency.
    m) 1.25 dihydroxyvitamin D3 is the most active form.
    n) Morbidity and mortality reduction is noted with adequate vitamin D levels, as well as a reduction in cardiac disease, cancer, immune deficiency, and multiple sclerosis.
    o) Measure the 25-hydroxy D3 to judge vitamin D levels—goal is 40-50 ng/ml.
6. Vitamin E
    a) Most active form is naturally occurring D-alpha tocopherol
    b) Stored in muscle, fat, and liver
    c) Protects liposomes and mitochondria from free radical damage
    d) Increased need with consumption of polyunsaturated fats and decreased need with the intake of vitamin C and beta-carotene
    e) Acts to potentiate glutathione peroxidase
    f) Aids in the maintenance and stability of cell membranes
    g) Acts to potentiate glutathione peroxidase
    h) Aids in the maintenance and stability of cell membranes

7. Vitamin K
   a) Plant source is most active
   b) Biosynthesis in the lower GI provides the vitamin
   c) Anticoagulants, antibiotics usage, and lipid absorption impairment interferes with vitamin K activity
   d) Co-substrate for coagulation factor II, VII, IX, X
   e) Plasma proteins C and S are also vitamin K dependent
8. Nutrition and wound healing
   a) Vitamin A: 10,000-25,000 IU PO × 10 days
   b) Vitamin C: 500-1000 mg
   c) Vitamin K: 120 mcg/day
   d) Zinc sulfate: 220 mg PO × 2 weeks (required by most enzyme systems)
   e) Copper: 1.5-3.0 mg/day
   f) Iron: 45 mg/day

E. Pharmaceutical agents
   1. Appetite stimulants
      a) Megestrol acetate
      b) Dronabinol
   2. Anabolic agents
      a) Recombinant human growth hormone
      b) Oxandrolone (1)
         i) Only FDA-approved anabolic agent
         ii) Its principal clinical application in wound healing is in patients with catabolism due to injury or illness, with an accompanying LBM loss of at least 10%
         iii) Dosage 10 mg PO BID

F. Nutritional assessment and support
   1. Refer to Chapter 32, Pathway 3 for a flowchart that can be used to determine when to consider enteral and parenteral feeding.

X. Medical nutrition therapy

A. Documentation of nutrition should include: (4)
   1. Amount of food consumed in quantity and quality of type of food as related to amount needed
   2. Average fluid consumed daily as related to amount required
   3. Ability to eat—assisted, supervised, or independent
   4. Acceptance or refusal of diet, meals, or supplements
   5. Current weight and percentage gained or lost
   6. Change in medical condition affecting nutritional status
   7. New medications affecting nutritional status
   8. Current laboratory results
   9. Wound condition and stage
   10. Current caloric protein or fluid requirement

RESOURCES

1. Demling R, DeSanti L. Involuntary weight loss and the nonhealing wound: the role of anabolic agents. *Adv Wound Care*. 1999; 12(1 Suppl):1-14.
2. Dennis-Wauters A. Nutrition and hydration. In: Sheffield PJ, Fife CE, editors. *Wound Care Practice*. 2nd ed. North Palm Beach: Best Publishing; 2007: 661-96.
3. James TJ, Hughes MA, Cherry GW, et al. Simple biochemical markers to assess chronic wounds. *Wound Repair Regen*. 2000 Jul-Aug; 8(4):264-9.
4. Posthauer M et al. Nutrition and wound care. In: Baranoski S, Ayello E, editors. *Wound Care Essentials: Practice Principles*. 3rd ed. Philadelphia: Lippincott Williams & Wilkins; 2013: 245-65.
5. Centers for Disease Control and Prevention. Defining Overweight and Obesity [Internet]. 2012 [Updated 2012 Apr 27]. Accessed at: http://www.cdc.gov/obesity/adult/defining.html.
6. Barbul A, Lazarou SA, et al. Arginine enhances wound healing and lymphocyte immune responses in humans. *Surgery*. 1990; 108(2):331-7.
7. Kirk SJ, Hurson M, et al. Arginine stimulates wound healing and immune function in elderly human beings. *Surgery*. 1993; 114(2):155-60.
8. Schaffer MR, Tantry U, et al. Acute protein-calorie malnutrition impairs wound healing: a possible role of decreased wound nitric oxide synthesis. *J Am Coll Surg*. 1997; 184(1):37-43.
9. ter Riet G et al. Randomized clinical trial of ascorbic acid in the treatment of pressure ulcers. *J Clin Epidemiol*. 1995; 48(12):1452-60.
10. National Pressure Ulcer Advisory Panel and European Pressure ulcer Advisory Panel. Prevention and treatment of pressure ulcers: clinical practice guidelines. Washington, DC: National Pressure Ulcer Advisory Panel; 2009.

SAMPLE QUESTIONS

1. During starvation, wound healing slows when there is a loss of lean body mass (LBM) of more than:
   a) 5%
   b) 10%
   c) 15%
   d) 25%

2. The preferred biochemical indicator of protein status is:
   a) Albumin level
   b) Prealbumin level
   c) Transferrin level
   d) Vitamin K level

3. The supplemental metal required by most enzyme systems with regard to wound healing is:
   a) Silver
   b) Zinc
   c) Iron
   d) Copper

4. Oxandrolone is an FDA-approved drug for protein calorie malnutrition with accompanying LBM loss of at least:
   a) 5%
   b) 10%
   c) 15%
   d) 20%

5. A 50-year-old prednisone-dependent rheumatoid arthritis patient has had a refractory wound of the left leg for the past three years. Based on this evidence, which of the following vitamins would you recommend to negate the effect of the steroid?
   a) Vitamin A
   b) Vitamin C
   c) Vitamin D
   d) Vitamin E

6. Which of the following amino acids are considered conditionally indispensable during periods of stress?
   a) Lysine and valine
   b) Valine and leucine
   c) Alanine and glutamic acid
   d) Arginine and glutamine

7. According to CDC guidelines, a person is considered obese with a BMI greater than:
   a) 25
   b) 30
   c) 35
   d) 40

8. NPUAP nutrition guidelines include all of the following recommendations except:
   a) Intake of 1.2-1.5 gm protein/kg of body weight
   b) Nutritional support by enteral or parental intake if a 24-hour caloric intake is inadequate
   c) Scheduling a 24-hour caloric count and assessing a diary of 24 hours of food and fluid intake
   d) Prescribing elemental zinc and ascorbic acid twice daily

9. You are evaluating a nursing home patient with a pressure ulcer, and you find that patient is taking fat-soluble vitamins as a supplement. What will be part of your evaluation?
   a) Signs and symptoms of overdose toxicity
   b) Double the vitamin dose, as increasing supplements will help with wound healing
   c) Administer a supratherapeutic dose of vitamin C to accelerate wound healing
   d) Administer thiamine and riboflavin

10. Which of the following laboratory values is useful in evaluating a patient with dehydration?
    a) Serum sodium
    b) Albumin
    c) BUN
    d) BUN/creatinine ratio
    e) Urine-specific gravity
    f) All of the above

See answers on page 96.

NOTES

ANSWER KEY

1. c) During starvation, wound healing slows when there is a loss of lean body mass (LBM) of more than 15%.

2. b) The preferred biochemical indicator of protein status is prealbumin level.

3. b) Zinc is the supplemental metal required by most enzyme systems with regard to wound healing.

4. b) Oxandrolone is an FDA-approved drug for protein calorie malnutrition with accompanying LBM loss of at least 10%.

5. a) Vitamin A has shown evidence in negating the effects of steroids on wound healing.

6. d) Arginine and glutamine are considered conditionally indispensable amino acids during period of stress.

7. b) According to CDC guidelines, a BMI greater than 30 is considered obese.

8. d) The NPUAP nutrition guidelines (10) recommend an intake of 1.2-1.5 gm protein/kg body weight, possible nutritional support by enteral or parental intake if a 24-hour caloric intake is inadequate, and scheduling a 24-hour caloric count and assessing a diary of 24 hours of food and fluid intake. Prescribing elemental zinc and ascorbic acid is not part of the NPUAP nutrition guidelines.

9. a) A nursing home patient with a pressure ulcer taking fat-soluble vitamins as a supplement should be evaluated for signs and symptoms of vitamin toxicity, as the body does not excrete excess fat-soluble vitamins. Increasing the dose of fat soluble vitamins, administering supratherapeutic doses of vitamin C, or administering thiamin and riboflavin will not assist the patient in wound healing.

10. f) Patients with dehydration can be evaluated by several lab values. Usually patient dehydration shows hypernatremia (increased sodium), higher than normal albumin, increased BUN, increased BUN/creatinine ratio, and increased urine-specific gravity.

WOUND BED PREPARATION & ADVANCED TECHNOLOGIES FOR WOUND HEALING 13

Caroline E. Fife, MD, CWSP, FAAFP, FUHM
Jayesh B. Shah, MD, CWSP, FAPWCA, FACCWS

INTRODUCTION

This chapter describes wound bed preparation as the management of a wound to accelerate endogenous healing or to facilitate the effectiveness of other therapeutic measures. Wound bed preparation is a systematic approach to correcting molecular and cellular abnormalities, which is critical to promoting healing of chronic wounds. The TIME O_2 paradigm (tissue, infection/chronic inflammation, moisture balance, edge effect, and correction of hypoxia) is discussed. Advanced therapy options include cellular and/or tissue based products (CTPs), stem cells, and epidermal harvesting.

OBJECTIVES

Participants should be able to describe the TIME O_2 concept for wound bed preparation, discuss the modified wound bed preparation score, and contrast selective debridement versus nonselective debridement.

I. Wound bed preparation

A. Definition: wound bed preparation is a systematic approach to correcting molecular and cellular abnormalities, which is critical to promoting healing of chronic wounds.

B. Foundation for wound bed preparation
1. Includes good history taking
2. Comprehensive general examination and wound assessment
3. Debridement
4. Moist wound dressings
5. Off-loading
6. Edema control
7. Nutritional support
8. Glycemic control
9. Appropriate use of new technologies
   a) Newer debridement technologies
   b) Growth factors
   c) Cellular and/or tissue based products (CTPs)
   d) Negative pressure wound therapy (NPWT)
   e) Electrical stimulation
   f) Electromagnetic therapy
   g) Hyperbaric oxygen therapy (HBOT)
   h) Gene therapy
   i) Angiogenesis technology

C. Goal for wound bed preparation
1. Creating a well-vascularized, stable wound bed with minimal exudates (Figures 13.1a and 13.1b)

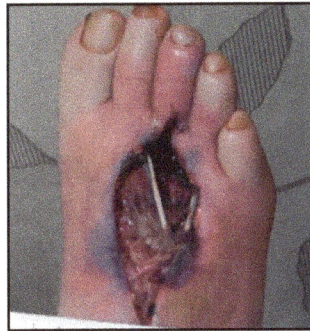

Figure 13.1a: A 50-year-old diabetic male with an infected and ischemic diabetic wound.

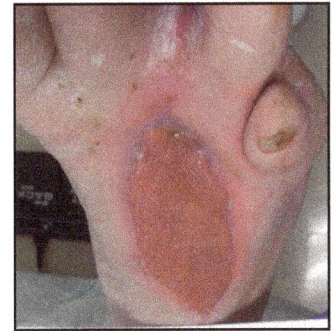

Figure 13.1b: Wound after IV antibiotics, debridement, negative pressure wound therapy, and hyperbaric oxygen therapy.

II. Determining the healing ability of a wound

Table 13.1: Factors to determine wound healing ability. Adapted from Sibbald RG, Woo KY, Ayello E. Special considerations in wound bed preparation 2011: an update. *Wound Healing Southern Africa.* 2011; 4(2):55-72.

WOUND PROGNOSIS	TREAT THE CAUSE	BLOOD SUPPLY	COEXISTING MEDICAL CONDITIONS/ DRUGS
Healable	Yes	Adequate	None that prevent healing
Maintenance	No	Adequate	+/- prevent healing
Non-healable	No	Often inadequate	May prevent healing

Table 13.2: Agents for the maintenance wound management of non-healable wounds.

AGENT	EFFECTS
Acetic acid (0.5–2%) Hydrochloric acid	Lower PH Effective against *Pseudomonas* May cause local stinging and burning May select out (*S. aureus*)
Chlorhexidine 2% alcohol solution or 0.5% aqueous solution	Active against gram-positive and gram-negative organisms Low tissue toxicity Water-based formulation
Povidone iodine 10% aqueous solution delivers 0.9% iodine at wound bed	Broad spectrum activity May be toxic to thyroid Autolytic debridement
Crystal violet Methylene blue	Broad spectrum antimicrobial Lower tissue toxicity Can be used with enzymatic debridement

A. Non-healable wound
1. Maintenance wound management preferred (Table 13.2)

B. For healable and maintenance wounds, follow the TIME O_2 protocol for wound bed preparation

III. Modified wound bed preparation score

A. Practitioners should try to achieve a wound bed score of 14 and above, as shown in Table 13.3.

Table 13.3: Modified wound bed preparation score.
Adapted from Falanga V, Saap LJ, Ozonoff A. Wound bed score and its correlation with healing of chronic wounds. *Dermatol Ther.* 2006; 19(6):383-90.

WOUND BED CHARACTERISTICS	0	1	2
Healing edges	None	25-75%	>75%
Black eschar	>25% of wound surface area	0-25%	None
Greatest wound depth/ granulation tissue	Severely depressed or raised when compared to periwound skin	Moderate	Flushed or almost even
Exudate amount	Severe	Moderate	None/mild
Edema	Severe	Moderate	None/mild
Periwound dermatitis	Severe	Moderate	None/mild
Periwound callus/ fibrosis	Severe	Moderate	None/ minimal
Pink wound bed	None	50-70%	>75%
Wound duration prior to treatment	>or equal to 1 year	—	<1 year

IV. TIME O$_2$ paradigm (tissue, infection/ inflammation, moisture balance, edge effect, correction of hypoxia)

A. TIME paradigm modified to include correction of hypoxia (refer to Chapter 32, page 287)

B. Tissue (refer to Chapter 32, page 288)
1. Assessment
   a) Color
   b) Tissue perfusion
   c) TcPO$_2$, Doppler, angiography
2. Debridement (episodic or continuous)
   a) Goals
      i) Restoration of wound base and functional extracellular matrix proteins
      ii) Viable wound base
   b) Objectives
      i) To get rid of necrotic tissue
      ii) To prevent infection
      iii) To correct abnormal wound repair
   c) Non-selective debridement
      i) Wet-to-dry dressings: wet (or moist) gauze dressing is placed on the wound and allowed to dry; wound drainage and dead tissue can be removed when the dry dressing is removed
      ii) Whirlpool (hydrotherapy): formerly called hydropathy; involves the use of water for pain relief and wound treatment
   d) Selective debridement
      i) Sharp
         (1) Most rapid means of debridement
         (2) Selective for nonviable tissue
         (3) May require analgesia (topical or local)
      ii) Enzymatic
         (1) Using chemical enzymes to selectively debride necrotic tissue
      iii) Autolytic
         (1) Uses the body's own enzymes and moisture to rehydrate, soften, and finally liquefy hard eschar and slough with the use of occlusive or semi-occlusive dressings
         (2) Best use is on clean wounds with slight to moderate exudate
         (3) Advantages
            (a) Very selective, with no damage to surrounding skin
            (b) Little to no pain for the patient
         (4) Disadvantages
            (a) Slow
            (b) May promote anaerobic growth
      iv) Biosurgical debridement
         (1) The use of sterile larvae or leaches for debridement
   e) Advanced debridement techniques
      i) Laser

Table 13.4: Key factors in deciding the method of debridement.
Adapted from Sibbald RG, Woo KY, Ayello E. Special considerations in wound bed preparation 2011: an update. *Wound Healing Southern Africa*. 2011; 4(2):55-72.

FACTORS	SURGICAL	ENZYMATIC	AUTOLYTIC	BIOLOGIC	MECHANICAL
Speed	1	3	5	2	4
Tissue selectivity	3	1	4	2	4
Painful wounds	5	2	1	3	4
Exudate	1	4	3	5	2
Infection	1	4	5	2	3
Cost	5	4	1	3	2

In choosing a debridement method, it is important to consider a variety of factors. A grade of 1 is the most effective choice of debridement for a given factor, while a grade of 5 is the least likely choice for effective debridement for that factor.

(1) Wound debridement in which a pulsed CO_2 laser beam is caused to impinge upon exposed tissue with individual pulses sufficiently energetic to ablate a thin layer of tissue.
(2) Each pulse has a time duration short enough to avoid deleterious heat penetration but long enough so that it does not cause atmospheric breakdown.
(3) The CO_2 laser, with a wavelength in the far infrared region, is operated to produce a pulsed beam with individual pulses having an energy of about one joule per pulse or greater.
ii) Jetox debridement system: uses saline and oxygen
iii) Versajet (hydrosurgery): specialized waterjet-powered surgical tools designed to establish new standards for patient care and procedural efficiency in wound debridement
iv) Ultrasound-assisted wound debridement: an advanced wound care technology that transmits low frequency ultrasonic energy directly to the wound surface and subsurface tissues resulting in tissue debridement and microcavitations
    (1) Debridement
    (2) Bacterial control
    (3) Vascular enhancement
v) Biosurgical debridement
    (1) Sterile larvae or leaches used for debridement, "the world's smallest surgeons"
    (2) Sterile larvae of *Lucilia sericata*
    (3) Larvae release proteolytic enzymes
    (4) Promote granulation tissue formation
C. Infection/chronic inflammation (refer to Chapter 32, page 289)
    1. Infection causes
        a) High bacterial counts or prolonged inflammation
        b) Increase inflammatory cytokines
        c) Increased protease activity
        d) Decreased growth factor activity
        e) Alkaline pH

2. Signs of heavy bioburden
    a) Sudden deterioration in quantity or quality of granulation tissue such as granulation tissue that is edematous, pale, friable, and nongranular
    b) Persistent high volume wound exudates
    c) Increased wound pain
3. Treatment for infection (refer to Chapter 11, page 79)
    a) Any three NERDS, treat topically: non-healing, exudate, red-friable tissue, debris, smell
    b) Any three STONES, treat systemically: size, temperature, os, new breakdown, exudate, erythema/edema (cellulitis), smell
    c) Persistent inflammation (non-infectious): topical or systemic anti-inflammatory drugs (26)
D. Moisture balance (refer to Chapter 32, page 290)
    1. Clinical clues of inadequate moisture control
        a) Examine color of surrounding skin to evaluate moisture
        b) Examine surrounding skin for transepidermal water loss
        c) Maceration of wound margin
        d) Desiccation slows epithelial cell migration
    2. Management of moisture (30)
        a) Apply moisture balance dressings (refer also to Chapter 24)
            i) Healable wounds: autolytic debridement: alginates, hydro-gels, hydrocolloids, acrylics
                (1) Critical colonization: silver, iodides, PHMB (polyhexamethylene biguanidine), honey
                (2) Persistent inflammation: anti-inflammatory dressings
                (3) Moisture balance: foams, hydrofibers, alginates, hydrocolloids, films, acrylics
        b) Compression (refer to Chapter 14, pages 116-117)
        c) Negative pressure wound therapy (NPWT) (Figure 13.2)
            i) All existing negative pressure systems have regulated suction and tubing but differ in type of dressing used and amount of suction delivered.
            ii) Mechanisms of action of NPWT:
                (1) Provides moist healing environment
                (2) Clears matrix metalloproteases (MMPs)

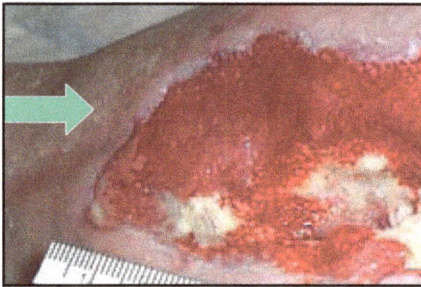

Figure 13.2: Granulation tissue in response to NPWT.

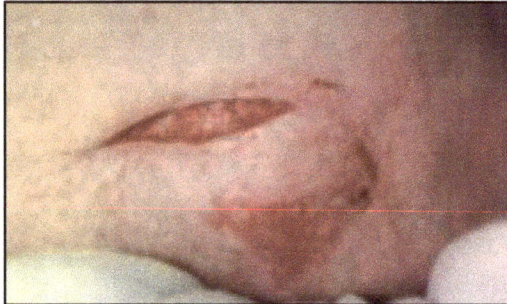

Figure 13.3a: Original left shoulder wound.

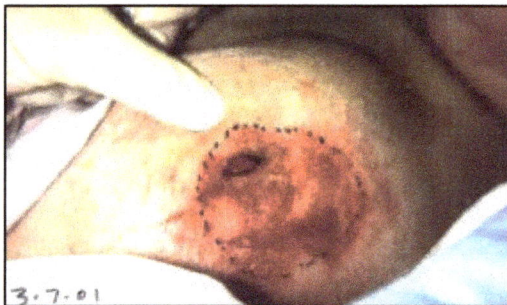

Figure 13.3b: Granulation tissue growing through skin from improperly applied NPWT sponge (note smaller original wound). This demonstrates the powerful effect of NPWT to stimulate angiogenesis.

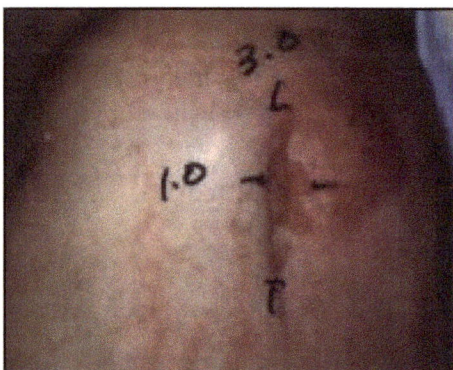

Figure 13.3c: Periwound skin healing after NPWT sponge was discontinued.

(3) Mechanical distraction stimulates mitosis

(4) Converts an uncontrolled open wound to a controlled closed wound

(5) Controls edema

(6) Removes excess interstitial fluid to decrease the intercellular diffusion distance

(7) Improves blood flow

(8) May reduce bacterial colonization (conflicting data)

(9) Sequestration of excess MMPs and wound exudation

(10) Augments local functional blood perfusion

(11) Causes microstrain (releases growth factors) and macrostrain (helps with wound contraction)

iii) General contraindications for NPWT

(1) Malignancy in the wound

(2) Untreated osteomyelitis

(3) Non-enteric and unexplored fistula

(4) Necrotic tissue with eschar

(5) Exposed blood vessels and organs

iv) Case study 1 for NPWT (Figures 13.3a-13.3c)

v) Case study 2 for NPWT (Figures 13.4a-13.4d)

vi) Case study 3 for NPWT (Figures 13.5a-13.5e)

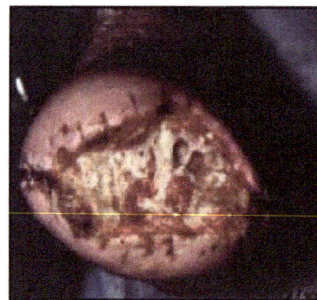

Figure 13.4a: Failed transmetatarsal amputation.

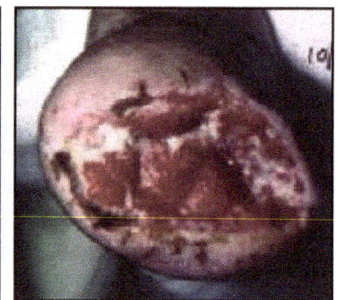

Figure 13.4b: Wound after two weeks of NPWT.

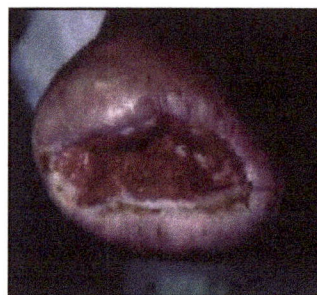

Figure 13.4c: Wound after four weeks of NPWT.

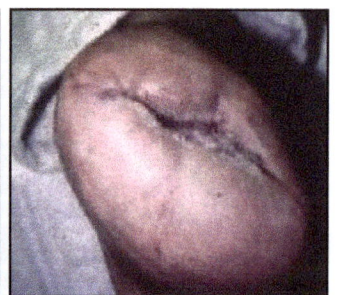

Figure 13.4d: Wound after eight weeks of NPWT.

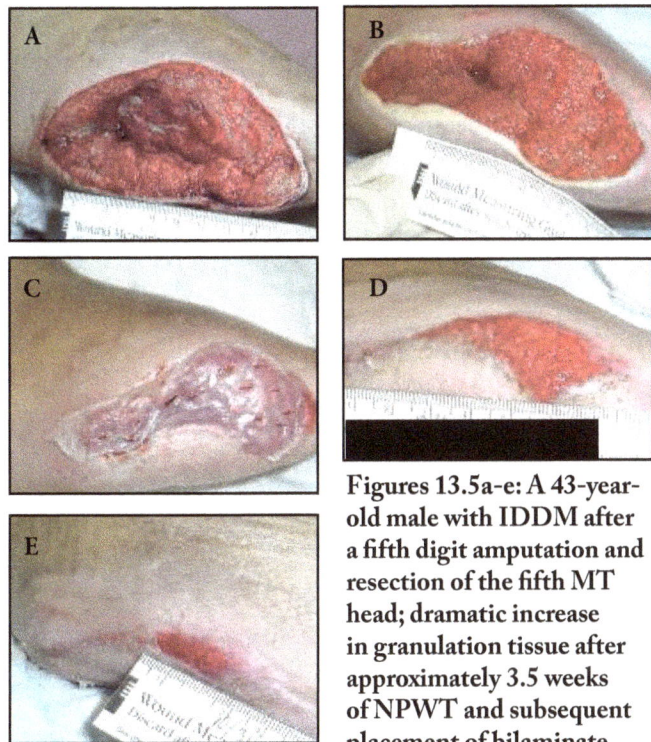

Figures 13.5a-e: A 43-year-old male with IDDM after a fifth digit amputation and resection of the fifth MT head; dramatic increase in granulation tissue after approximately 3.5 weeks of NPWT and subsequent placement of bilaminate skin.

Table 13.5: Cells and PDGF.

CELLS THAT PRODUCE PDGF	CELLS THAT PDGF ACT ON	CELLULAR RESPONSE TO PDGF
Fibroblasts, keratinocytes, smooth muscle cells, macrophages, platelets, endothelial cells	Neutrophils	Stimulates chemotaxis
	Macrophages	Stimulates chemotaxis, induces release of other GFs
	Fibroblasts	Stimulates proliferation and chemotaxis, stimulates production of matrix molecules (collagen, fibronectin, proteoglycans, etc.)
	Endothelial cells	Stimulates proliferation and new blood vessel formation
	Smooth muscle cells	Stimulates proliferation and chemotaxis, recruits smooth muscle cells to site of new blood vessel formation

E. Edge effect (refer to Chapter 32, page 291)
   1. Characteristics of edge effect in chronic wounds
      a) Edge of wound: nonadvancing or undermined
      b) Nonmigrating keratinocytes, nonresponsive wound cells, and abnormal protease activity
   2. Advanced wound care technology to help with edge effect
      a) Growth factor therapy: GFs are subgroups of cytokines that are biologically active polypeptides recognized for their contributions to the cell activation during wound healing
         i) Platelet-derived growth factor BB
            (1) The first FDA-approved recombinant human growth factor was Regranex® Gel (becaplermin) 0.01% (rhPDGF-BB)
            (2) Synthesized by recombinant biotechnology using yeast cells genetically engineered to secrete rhPDGF-BB into medium
            (3) Prescription form is active rhPDGF-BB
            (4) Activates endothelial cells and fibroblasts
            (5) Stimulates vascular proliferation, migration, new blood vessel formation
            (6) Recruits smooth muscle cells and pericytes to stabilize newly formed vessels
            (7) rhPDGF-BB (Regranex® or becaplermin) gel is indicated for the treatment of lower extremity diabetic neuropathic ulcers that extend into the subcutaneous tissue of beyond and have an adequate blood supply
            (8) Black box warning for Regranex®: increased risk of cancer mortality in patients who use three or more tubes of the product
            (9) Cells and PDGF (Table 13.5)
            (10) Case study: ischemic diabetic foot after debridement. Patient was treated with growth factor and hyperbaric oxygen therapy (Figures 13.6a-13.6d)

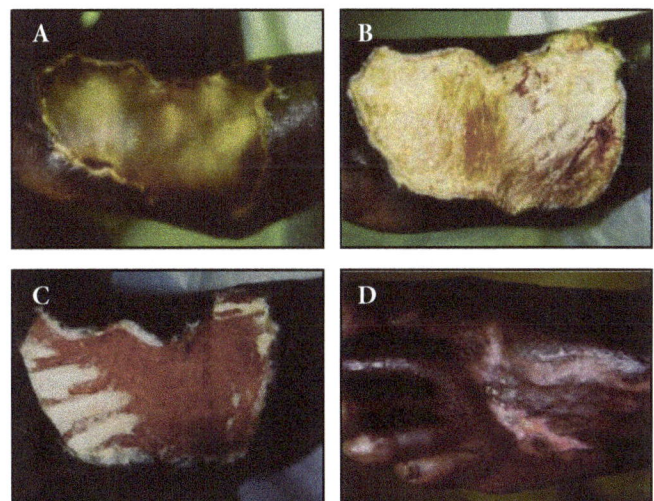

Figures 13.6a-d: Diabetic foot wound treated with Regranex® and HBOT.

Table 13.6: Wound healing growth factors.

GROWTH FACTORS	MAJOR SOURCES	FUNCTIONS
Fibroblast GFs	• Fibroblasts • Endothelial Cells	Mitogenic for endothelial cells, fibroblasts and keratinocytes Stimulates angiogenesis
Keratinocyte GFs	• Fibroblasts	Mitogenic and chemotactic for keratinocyte and epithelial cells
Epidermal GFs	• Platelet • Macrophage • Keratinocyte	Mitogenic for fibroblasts, epithelial cells, endothelial cells and smooth muscles Stimulates keratinocyte differentiation, proliferation and migration
Transforming GFs	• Platelets • Macrophages • Lymphocytes • Keratinocytes • Fibroblasts	Stimulates fibroblasts and angiogenesis Induces extracellular matrix production
Vascular endothelial GFs	• Neutrophils • Platelets	Stimulates endothelial cells and neoangiogenesis
Granulocyte colony stimulating factors	• Monocytes • Fibroblasts • Lymphocytes	Stimulates production and function of neutrophils

ii) Other growth factors used in wound healing (Table 13.6)
iii) Autologous platelet gel
   (1) Platelet gels or releasates are prepared from platelet-rich plasma obtained by differential centrifugation of whole blood.
   (2) Other components are added to platelet rich plasma:
     (a) Cryoprecipitate gives a firmer consistency to gel
     (b) Other components (Figure 13.7)

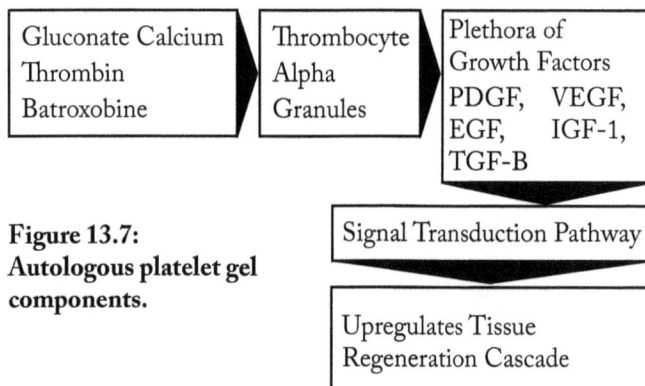

Figure 13.7: Autologous platelet gel components.

Table 13.7: Autologous grafts.

AUTOLOGOUS GRAFTS	GRAFT COMPOSITE
Epicel®	Keratinocytes
EpiDex®	Keratinocytes
TransCell®	Keratinocytes in fibrin sealant

b) Cellular and/or tissue based products (CTPs)
  i) Characteristics of ideal CTPs
   (1) Be able to develop rapid sustained adherence to wound surface
   (2) Allow water vapor transmission
   (3) Resist friction and shear stresses
   (4) Prevent proliferation of bacteria
   (5) Contain low antigenicity
   (6) Be free of local and systemic toxicity
  ii) Autologous grafts (autografts)
   (1) Cultivated from patient's own skin cells.
   (2) The cells are then separated and cultured for expansion and placed on the wounds.
   (3) As these are the patient's own cells, there is less likelihood of rejection.
  (iii) Epidermal cellular autologous grafts (Table 13.7)
  (iv) Dermal acellular grafts (Table 13.8)
   (1) OASIS®
    (a) Porcine small intestinal submucosa
    (b) Single layer sheet
    (c) Acellular/non-living
    (d) Freeze-dried sheet
    (e) Fenestrated
    (f) Contains no cells
   (2) Integra™
    (a) Bilayer silicone and glycosaminoglycan layer
    (b) Useful in wounds with tendon and bone exposed

Table 13.8: Dermal acellular grafts.

DERMAL ACELLULAR GRAFTS	DERIVED FROM
AlloDerm®	Human cadaveric dermis
Biobrane®	Porcine dermal template bonded to nylon mesh and silicone membrane
EZ Derm®	Porcine collagen cross-linked with an aldehyde
Graftjacket®	Cadaveric human skin with epidermis and dermal cells removed
Integra™	Matrix containing bovine tendon collagen, glycosaminoglycans, and a silicone layer
OASIS®	Porcine collagen matrix

Table 13.9: Dermal cellular composite grafts.

DERMAL CELLULAR-COMPOSITE GRAFTS	DERIVED FROM
Apligraf® Graftskin®	Bilayer bovine collagen matrix containing allogenic human fibroblasts and keratinocytes isolated from human infant foreskin
GammaGraft®	Gamma irradiated cadaveric allograft
OrCel®	Bilayer matrix of epidermal keratinocytes and dermal fibroblasts embedded into bovine collagen sponge

(3) Graftjacket® scaffold repair
   (a) Replacement of authentic human dermal matrix in deficient skin wounds
   (b) Intact vascular channels for rapid revascularization
   (c) Cryogenically preserved extracellular matrix for rapid cell repopulation
(v) Dermal cellular composite grafts (Table 13.9)
  (1) Apligraf®
    (a) Epidermis/dermis
    (b) Derived from human infant foreskin
    (c) Fresh culture has a 10-day shelf life
    (d) FDA approved (May 1998/June 2000)
      ((i)) Venous leg ulcers
      ((ii)) Diabetic foot ulcers
    (e) 7.5 cm single use round
    (f) Clinical observations of Apligraf® appearances as it progresses toward wound healing (Figures 13.8a–13.8f)
  (2) TheraSkin® is a biologically active, cryopreserved human skin allograft composed of living cells, fibroblasts and keratinocytes, with a fully developed extra cellular matrix (ECM) in its epidermis and dermis layers

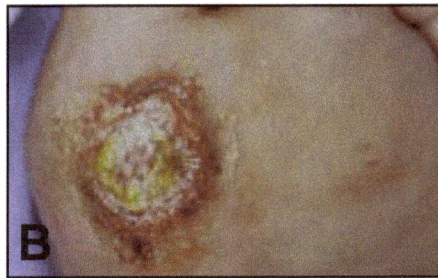

Figure 13.8a: The sheer cellophane-like appearance of Apligraf®.

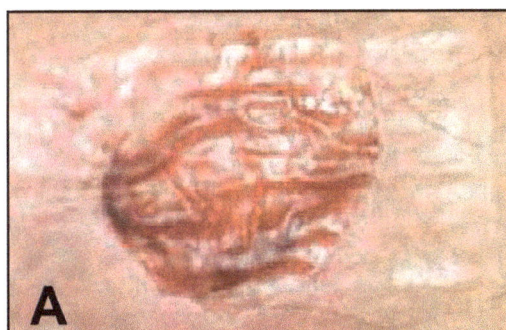

Figure 13.8b: Yellowish-white, gelatinous appearance.

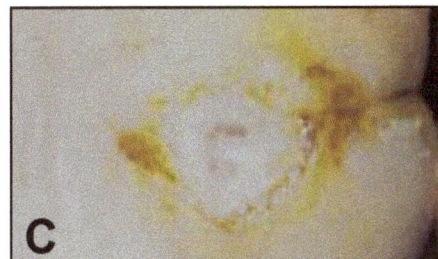

Figure 13.8c: Rapid epithelialization.

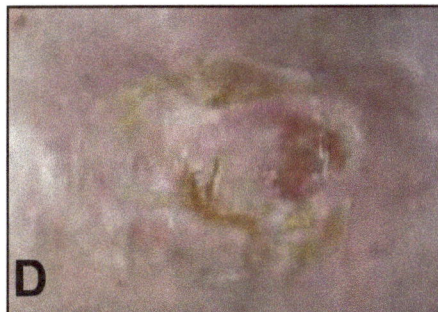

Figure 13.8d: Thin epithelial covering.

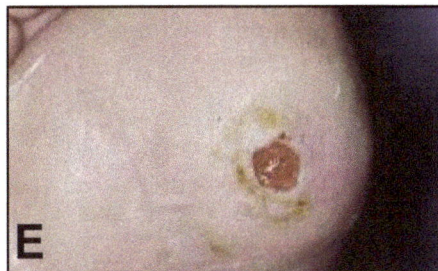

Figure 13.8e: Wound contraction, epidermal edge effect.

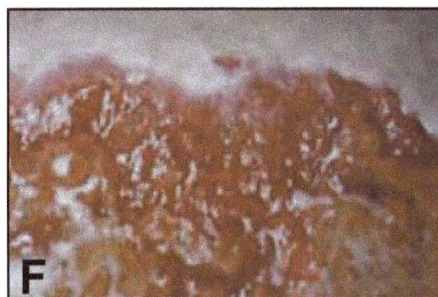

Figure 13.8f: Granulation tissue; wound bed flush with surrounding skin. Figures 13.8a–13.8f courtesy of Vincent Falanga, MD, Boston University School of Medicine, Boston, MA, and Roger Williams Medical Center, Providence, RI.

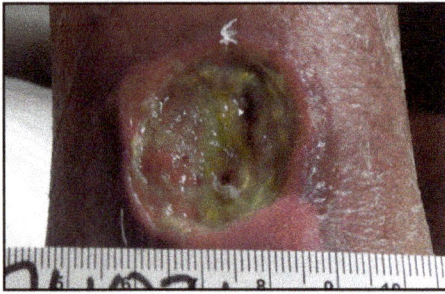

Figure 13.9a: A 52-year-old female with a history of lupus on immunosuppressants with a vasculitic ulcer.

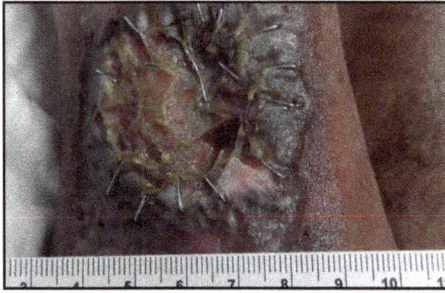

Figure 13.9b: Lupus vasculitis after debridement and STSG with non-take.

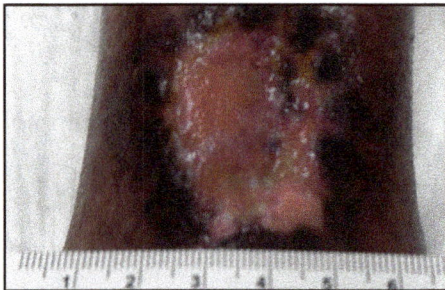

Figure 13.9c: Lupus vasculitis ulcer after application of TheraSkin®.

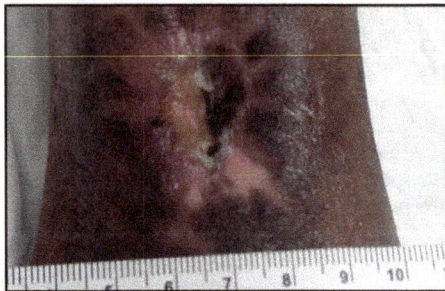

Figure 13.9d: Lupus vasculitis ulcer patient epithelized after eight weeks of TheraSkin® application.

Table 13.10: Dermal cellular dermal grafts.

DERMAL CELLULAR-DERMAL	DERIVED FROM
Dermagraft®	Human fibroblast and extra cellular matrix in a polyglactin mesh
TransCyte®	Fibroblast from human new born foreskin covered by outer layer of non-permeable silicone

100% DENSITY (PER MM³)	COMPONENT	Dermagraft®	Apligraf®
	Neonatal fibroblasts	8,000 cells	500 cells
	TGF-B	0.4 pg	4 pg
	PDGF	1 pg	1 pg
	Collagen	18.75 µg	2 µg
	Hyaluronan	80 µg	7.45 µg

Table 13.11: Comparison of the dermal components in Dermagraft® and Apligraf®.
From Waugh HV, Sherratt JA. Modeling the effects of treating diabetic wounds with engineered skin substitutes. *Wound Repair Regen.* 2007;15(4):556–65.

(a) TheraSkin® case study (Figures 13.9a–13.9d)
(vi) Dermal cellular dermal grafts (Table 13.10)
(1) Dermagraft®
(a) Dermis with matrix
(b) Derived from foreskin
(c) Cryopreserved for six-month shelf life
(d) FDA approved for diabetic foot ulcers (October 2001)
(e) 5 × 7.5 cm single use
(f) Comparison of the dermal components in Dermagraft® and Apligraf® (Table 13.11)
vii) Other newer CTPs
(1) Cryopreserved placental membrane (Grafix®) is an alternative to autologous skin graft shown to be beneficial in supporting natural wound repair.
(2) Cryopreserved amniotic membrane allograft (AmnioGraft®) is also used as an alternative to autologuous skin graft for wound healing.
(3) Wound care products composed of naturally occurring urinary bladder matrix (MatriStem®) maintain an intact epithelial basement membrane.
(4) Epidermal harvesting system (CelluTome™) is intended to harvest a thin skin graft for autologous skin grafting. It produces an array of epidermal micrografts ready for immediate transfer onto a recipient site.
(a) Epidermal bubble skin graft case study (Figures 13.10a–13.10f)
viii) Things to remember before the application of CTPs
(1) Topical agents, such as antibiotic ointments, must be safe to use with CTPs. These prescriptions include, but are not limited to:
(a) Bacitracin zinc

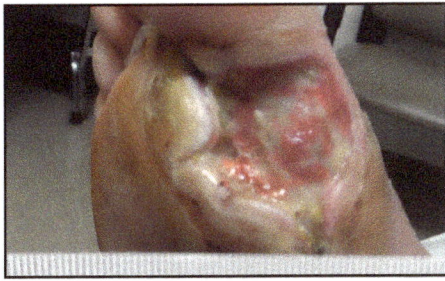

Figure 13.10a: Initial presentation of a 60-year-old diabetic male with an infected neuroischemic diabetic foot ulcer.

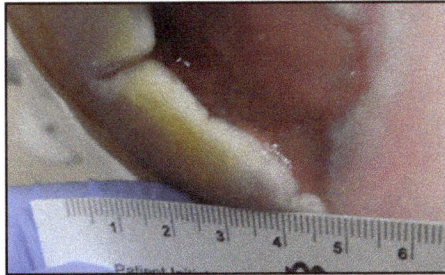

Figure 13.10b: Wound after debridement, antibiotics, and HBOT—six weeks after initial presentation.

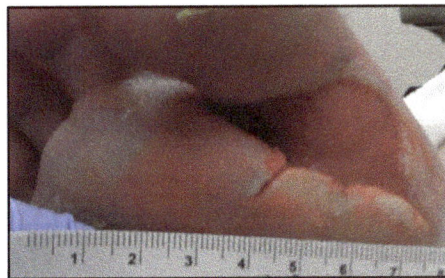

Figure 13.10c: Acticoat® applied for two weeks to decrease bacterial bioburden.

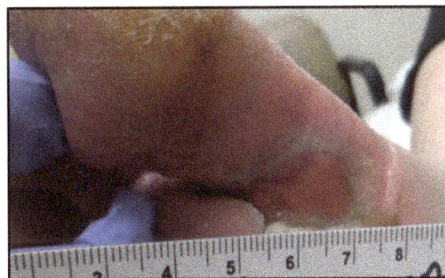

Figure 13.10d: One week after the epidermal bubble skin grafting application.

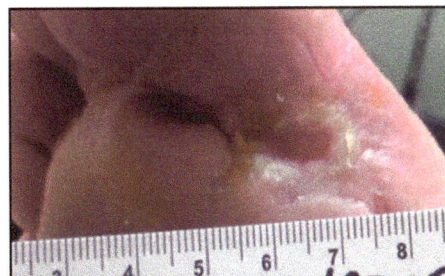

Figure 13.10e: Three weeks after the epidermal bubble skin grafting application.

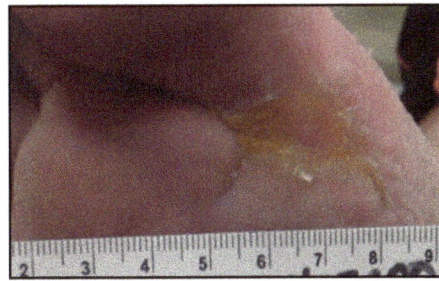

Figure 13.10f: Four weeks after the epidermal bubble skin grafting application.

(b) Gentamicin sulfate
(c) Neomycin sulfate
(d) Bactroban
(e) Silver sulfadiazine
(2) Avoid using cytotoxic topical agents immediately before or after the application of CTPs. These prescriptions include, but are not limited to:
(a) Chlorhexidine gluconate
(b) Dakin's solution
(c) Polymyxin/nystatin
(d) Mafenide acetate
(e) Povidone iodine solution
(f) Scarlet red dressing
(g) Tincoban
(h) Zinc sulfate
(3) If cytotoxic agents are used prior to CTP application, the wound bed must be thoroughly cleaned with saline before applying the CTPs.
ix) CTPs are not recommended in cases of:
(1) Patients with severe, uncontrolled diabetes mellitus or arterial disease
(2) Patients with known sensitivity to the components of CTPs
(3) Clinically infected wounds
(4) Wound with severe dermatitis
(5) Wounds with unprepared wound beds
c) Stem cells
i) Definition: a cell that can self-replicate and give rise to more than one type of mature daughter cell
ii) Characteristics
(1) Unlimited self-renewal capacity
(2) Long term viability
(3) Multi-lineage potential
(4) Participation in tissue repair
(5) Preservation of somatic homeostasis
(6) Replication of a single cell can potentially result in whole populations of cells and cause tissue regeneration
iii) Types
(1) Embryonic stem cells
(2) Stem cells harvested from adult tissue

d) Electrical stimulation
   i) High-voltage pulsed current (HVPC) 75-150 V, 60-120 pps
   ii) Pulsed low-frequency stimulation
   iii) Both have proven to accelerate healing

F. Correction of hypoxia with hyperbaric oxygen therapy (refer to Chapter 32, page 292)
   1. Definition: the administration of 100% oxygen under increased atmospheric pressure of at least 1.4 ATA and above
   2. Oxygen transport by two mechanisms
      a) Chemical binding to hemoglobin
      b) Physical dissolution in plasma
   3. Once Hb is saturated, increases in FiO_2 can affect only the plasma dissolved oxygen fraction
   4. As the PO_2 increases, the amount of O_2 physically dissolved in plasma increases in a linear fashion (22)
   5. Physiological effects of increased oxygen partial pressure (Figure 13.11)
   6. Wound healing impairment with decreasing $TcPO_2$ (or $PtcO_2$) (Figure 13.12)
   7. Defining hypoxia (9)
      a) Hypoxia is defined as a $TcPO_2$ <40 mmHg (respiring air).
      b) Normal extremities reach $TcPO_2$ >100 mmHg (respiring O_2).

Physiological Effects of Increased Oxygen Partial Pressure

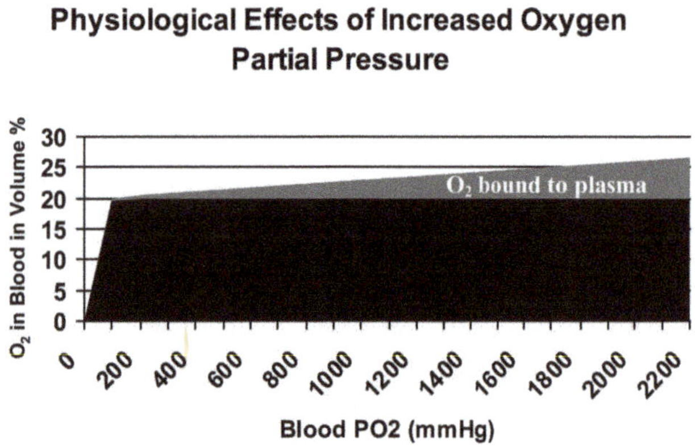

Figure 13.11: Physiological effects of increased oxygen partial pressure.

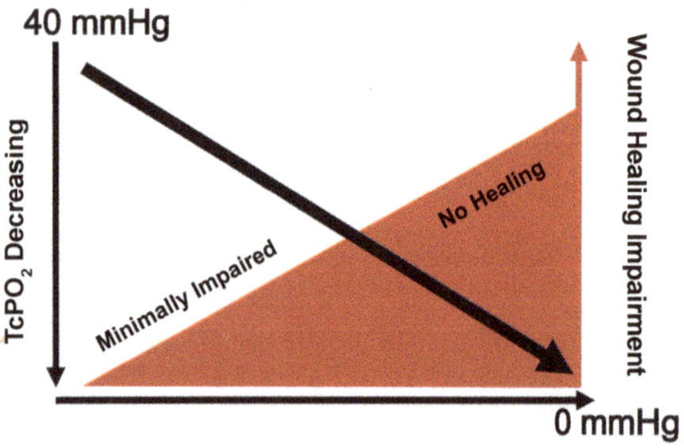

Figure 13.12: Wound healing impairment with decreasing $TcPO_2$.

   c) Critical limb ischemia usually has a $TcPO_2$ <30 mmHg.
   d) Amputation healing is unlikely at a $TcPO_2$ <40 mmHg, or if the $TcPO_2$ rise on O_2 is <10 mmHg.
   e) After revascularization, healing usually occurs if $TcPO_2$ increases to >40 mmHg (increase may be delayed).
   f) $TcPO_2$ obtained while breathing normobaric air can identify patients who will not heal spontaneously.

8. $TcPO_2$ as a predictor of wound healing in diabetic foot wounds
   a) $TcPO_2$ <20 mmHg indicated a 39-fold increased risk of early healing failure. (20)
   b) Multicenter study of diabetic wounds showed relationship between in-chamber TCOM and HBOT success. (8)
      i) As in-chamber transcutaneous oxygen measurements (TCOM) increase, the likelihood of success from HBOT increases (Figure 13.13).
      ii) Overall, 75.6% of diabetic foot ulcers improved after HBOT.
      iii) Best indicator of success or failure was $TcPO_2$ >200 mmHg during HBOT. (8)
   c) A cohort study showed that a reliable test is a combination of 1 ATA air and oxygen $TcPO_2$. Mean values simultaneously taken at the same anatomic level (TC-air >0 mmHg; TC-O_2 >35 mmHg; TC % rise >50 %) were more reliable than single air values in predicting healing outcome. (25)

9. The role of oxygen in wound healing
   a) Enhanced WBC killing
   b) Inhibition of toxin formation
   c) Inactivation of toxins (*Clostridium perfringens*)
   d) Bacteriostasis
   e) Antibiotic transport across cell wall (11,17)
   f) Collagen cross-linking (13)
   g) Angiogenesis

10. HBOT in diabetic wounds of the lower extremity (evidence-based studies)

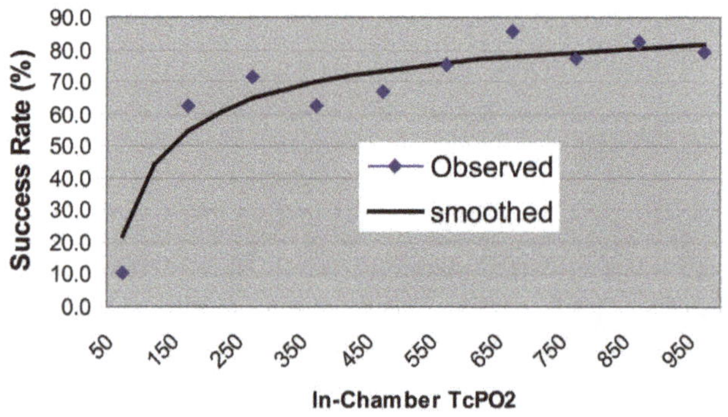

Figure 13.13: In-chamber $TcPO_2$ vs. success rate.

a) Six randomized controlled clinical trials on HBOT in diabetic foot ulcers

b) Two randomized controlled trials on non-diabetic leg ulcers or wound healing, not outcome indicator

c) Two controlled trials on HBOT in diabetic foot ulcers

d) One prospective case series on HBOT and infrapopliteal angioplasty in diabetic foot ulcers

e) Eight prospective or retrospective uncontrolled case series on HBOT in diabetic foot ulcers

f) Medicare coverage indication: HBOT for diabetic foot ulcers
   i)   Lower extremity wound due to type 1 or 2 diabetes mellitus
   ii) Wagner grade 3 or higher
   iii) Failed standard wound care, i.e., no measurable signs of healing for 30 days
   iv) Wound must be re-evaluated every 30 days during the course of HBOT
   v)   Continued HBOT will not be covered if there are no measurable signs of healing during the 30 day period

g) Case study for hyperbaric oxygen therapy (Figures 13.14a–13.14c)

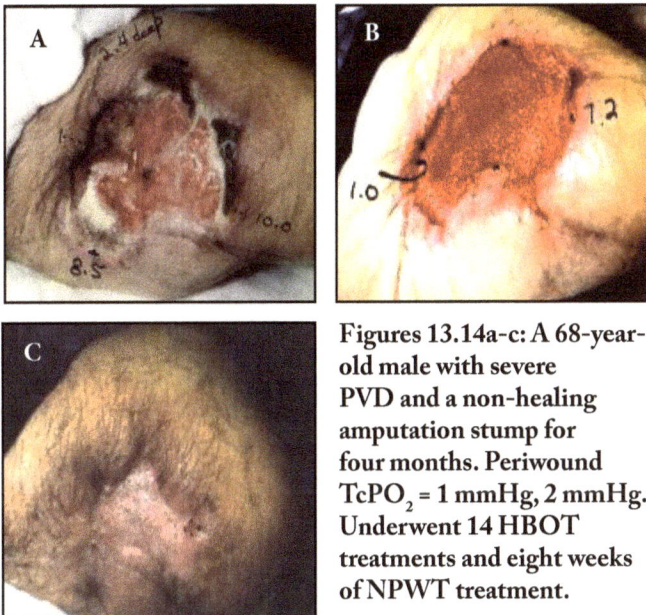

Figures 13.14a-c: A 68-year-old male with severe PVD and a non-healing amputation stump for four months. Periwound $TcPO_2$ = 1 mmHg, 2 mmHg. Underwent 14 HBOT treatments and eight weeks of NPWT treatment.

V. Guidance on when to use advanced therapy (refer also to Chapter 32)

A. If conventional therapy has not been successful within four weeks, alternative therapies should be considered.

B. The initial rate of healing during the first four weeks can predict whether ulcers are likely to heal by 24 weeks. If the initial healing rate is <0.1 cm/wk at the four week interval, advanced therapy should be considered.

C. Ulcers with a poor prognosis should be treated with a more advanced therapy.

D. Rapid identification of patients who are unlikely to respond to conventional care will allow for earlier interventions with advanced therapies.

VI. Conclusion

A. In chronic wounds, the orderly sequence of events seen in acute wounds becomes disrupted or stuck at one or more of the different stages of wound healing. For the normal repair process to resume, the barrier to healing must be identified and removed through application of the correct techniques.

B. It is important to understand the molecular events that are involved in the wound healing process in order to select the most appropriate intervention.

C. Wound bed preparation is the management of a wound in order to accelerate endogenous healing or to facilitate the effectiveness of other therapeutic measures.

RESOURCES

1. APHA drug treatment protocols: management of foot ulcers in patients with diabetes. *J Am Pharm Assoc.* 2000; 40(4):467–74.
2. Attinger CE, Janis JE, Steinberg J, Schwartz J, Al-Attar A, Couch K. Clinical approach to wounds: debridement and wound bed preparation including the use of dressings and wound-healing adjuvants. *Plast Reconstr Surg.* 2006 Jun; 117(7 Suppl):72S-109S.
3. Brem H, Young J, Tomic-Canic M, et al. Clinical efficacy and mechanism of bilayered living human skin equivalent (HSE) in treatment of diabetic foot ulcers. *Surg Technol Int.* 2003; 11:23-31.
4. Dowsett C. Using the TIME framework in wound bed preparation. *Br J Community Nurs.* 2008 Jun; 13(6):S15-6, S18, S20
5. Falanga V, Sabolinski M. A bilayered living skin construct (Apligraf®) accelerates complete closure of hard-to-heal venous ulcers. *Wound Repair Regen.* 1999; 7:201-7.
6. Falanga V, Sabolinski ML. Prognostic factors for healing of venous ulcers. *WOUNDS.* 2000; 12(5 Suppl A):42A–46A.
7. Fife CE. Hyperbaric oxygen therapy applications in wound care. In: Sheffield PJ, Fife CE, editors. *Wound Care Practice.* 2nd ed. North Palm Beach: Best Publishing Company; 2007: 947-80.
8. Fife CE, Buyukcakir C, Otto GH, et al. The predictive value of transcutaneous oxygen tension measurement in diabetic lower extremity ulcers treated with hyperbaric oxygen therapy: a retrospective analysis of 1144 patients. *Wound Repair Regen.* 2002; 10:198-207.
9. Fife CE, Smart DR, Sheffield PJ, et al. Transcutaneous oximetry in clinical practice: consensus statements from an expert panel based on evidence. *Undersea Hyperb Med.* 2009; 36(1):43-53.
10. Gilman TH. Parameter for measurement of wound closure. *WOUNDS.* 1990; 2(3):95-101.
11. Hart GB, Lamb RC, Strauss MB. Gas gangrene. *J Trauma.* 1983 Nov; 23(11):991-1000.
12. Heldin CH, Westermark B. Mechanism of action and *in vivo* role of platelet-derived growth factor. *Physiol Rev.* October 1999; 79(4):1283-316.
13. Hunt TK, Pai MP. The effect of varying ambient oxygen tensions on wound metabolism and collagen synthesis. *Surg Gynecol Obstet.* 1972; 135:561-7.
14. Joseph E, et al. A prospective randomized trial of vacuum assisted closure versus standard therapy of chronic non-healing wounds. *WOUNDS.* 2000; 12(3):60-7.
15. Kantor J, Margolis DJ. Efficacy and prognostic value of simple wound measurements. *Arch Dermatol.* 1998; 134:1571-74.
16. Kantor J, Margolis DJ. A multicenter study of percentage change in venous leg ulcer area as a prognostic index of healing at 24 weeks. *Br J Dermatol.* 2000; 142:960–4.
17. Mader JT. Phagocytic killing and hyperbaric oxygen: antibacterial mechanisms. *HBO Rev.* 1981; 2:37-49.
18. Moneta G, Falanga V, Altman M, et al. Nonoperative management of venous leg ulcers: evolving role of skin substitutes. Vasc Endovascular Surg 1999; 33(2):197-210.
19. Panuncialman J, Falanga V. The science of wound bed preparation. *Surg Clin North Am.* 2009 Jun; 89(3):611-26.
20. Pecoraro RE, Ahroni J, Boyko E, et al. Chronology and determinants of tissue repair in diabetic lower-extremity ulcers. *Diabetes.* 1991; 40:1305-13.
21. Robson MC, Hill DP, Woodske ME, et al. Wound healing trajectories as predictors of effectiveness of therapeutic agents. *Arch Surg.* 2000; 135:773-7.
22. Saltzman HA. Rational normobaric and hyperbaric oxygen therapy. *Ann Intern Med.* 1967; 67:843–52.
23. Schultz GS, Sibbald RG, Falanga V, et al. Wound bed preparation: a systematic approach to wound management. *Wound Repair Regen.* 2003 Mar; 11(Suppl 1):S1-28.
24. Sheehan P, Jones P, Caselli A, et al. Percent change in wound area of diabetic foot ulcers over a 4-week period is a robust predictor of complete healing in a 12-week prospective trial. *Diabetes Care.* 2003; 26(6):1879- 82.
25. Sheffield PJ, Dietz D, Posey KI, et al. [Abstract] Mean PtcO$_2$ values as an outcome predictor in hyperbaric oxygen treatment of hypoxic wounds. *Undersea Hyperb Med.* 2008; 35(4):272.
26. Sibbald RG, Woo KY, Ayello E. Special considerations in wound bed preparation 2011: an update. *Wound Healing Southern Africa.* 2011; 4(2):55-72.
27. Smith APS, Bozzuto TM. Advanced therapeutics: the biochemistry and biophysical basis of wound products. In: Sheffield PJ, Fife CE, editors. *Wound Care Practice.* 2nd ed. North Palm Beach: Best Publishing Company; 2007: 981-1034.
28. Steed DL, the Diabetic Ulcer Study Group. Clinical evaluation of recombinant human platelet-derived growth factor for the treatment of lower extremity diabetic ulcers. *J Vasc Surg.* 1995; 21(1):71-81.
29. Thomas Hess C. Meeting the goal: wound bed preparation. *Adv Skin Wound Care.* 2008 Jul; 21(7):344.
30. Waugh HV, Sherratt JA. Modeling the effects of treating diabetic wounds with engineered skin substitutes. *Wound Repair Regen.* 2007; 15(4):556-65.
31. Woo K, Ayello EA, Sibbald RG. The edge effect: current therapeutic options to advance the wound edge. *Adv Skin Wound Care.* 2007; 20(2):99-117.

Resources for product information

1. AmnioGraft®: http://www.biotissue.com/products/amniograft.aspx
2. Apligraf®: http://www.apligraf.com
3. CelluTome™: http://www.kci1.com/KCI1/cellutome
4. Dermagraft®: http://www.dermagraft.com/portal/
5. Grafix®: http://www.osiris.com/grafix
6. Graftskin: http://www.pharmacopeia.cn/v29240/usp29nf24s0_m35846.html
7. Hydrotherapy: http://en.wikipedia.org/wiki/Hydrotherapy
8. Laser debridement: http://www.podiatrytoday.com/laser-debridement-can-it-have-impact-chronic-wounds?page=2
9. MatriStem®: https://acell.com/matristem-devices/
10. OASIS®: http://www.oasiswoundmatrix.com/aboutowm
11. Platelet rich plasma: http://en.wikipedia.org/wiki/Platelet-rich_plasma
12. Regranex®: http://www.regranex.com
13. TheraSkin®: http://www.solublesystems.com/Products/TheraSkin
14. Stem cells: http://stemcells.nih.gov/info/basics/pages/basics1.aspx
15. Ultrasound assisted wound debridement: http://www.google.com/url?sa=t&rct=j&q=&esrc=s&source=web&cd=17&ved=0CEEQFjAGOAo&url=http%3A%2F%2Fwww.moh.gov.my%2Findex.php%2Fdatabase_stores%2Fattach_download%2F347%2F165&ei=7oyEVLi5Go6hyATCwILIDA&usg=AFQjCNFLomu2Ctlkap9bYw7jNZXbMQRfDw&sig2=V0CRFoIsID7GttOW94ya7w&bvm=bv.80642063,d.aWw
16. Wet-to-dry dressing: http://www.nlm.nih.gov/medlineplus/ency/patientinstructions/000315.htm

SAMPLE QUESTIONS

1. Wound bed preparation includes all of the following except:
   a) Hydrogel dressings
   b) Negative pressure wound therapy
   c) Medihoney
   d) Flaps

2. The modified wound bed preparation score includes:
   a) Black eschar
   b) Exudate amount
   c) Edema
   d) Wound duration prior to treatment
   e) All of the above

3. Cellular and/or tissue based products (CTPs) are not indicated for:
   a) Infected wounds
   b) Wound bed with 100% granulation tissue
   c) Wounds with scant exudate
   d) A patient with well controlled diabetes mellitus

4. All of the following are composite grafts/CTPs except:
   a) Apligraf®
   b) Dermagraft®
   c) Graftskin
   d) OrCel®
   e) GammaGraft®

5. In which patient is advanced wound therapy for wound bed preparation most appropriate?
   a) A 32-year-old female who presents to a wound clinic with a non-healing surgical wound after a Cesarean section three weeks ago.
   b) A 70-year-old diabetic male with a neuropathic wound who is refractory to healing with standard wound care after four weeks.
   c) A 99-year-old nursing home resident with dementia, CVA, and contractures and an unstageable left heel wound for more than one year.
   d) A 12-year-old male who was injured while playing football and subsequently developed a large wound on the right pretibial area two days ago.

6. The mechanism of action of hyperbaric oxygen therapy includes which of the following:
   a) Increased oxygen carrying capacity via plasma dissolved oxygen
   b) Decreased collagen synthesis
   c) Decreased white cell function
   d) Topical application of oxygen causing increasing oxygenation in the wound bed

7. Which of the following is not commonly described with negative pressure wound therapy?
   a) Increased tissue oxygen
   b) Decreased tissue edema
   c) Increased granulation
   d) Change in bacterial flora colonizing the wound bed

8. Becalpermin, Apligraf®, and Dermagraft® have which of the following in common?
   a) They are believed to increase wound growth factor levels
   b) They have been shown to improve diabetic foot ulcer closure rates
   c) They are more likely to be effective in a clean wound bed
   d) All of the above

9. Which of the following products is appropriate for use in non-healable wounds?
   a) Acetic acid
   b) CTPs
   c) Growth factors
   d) Hyperbaric oxygen therapy

10. The preferred method of debriding a painful wound is:
    a) Sharp debridement
    b) Biosurgical debridement
    c) Autolytic debridement
    d) Mechanical debridement

See answers on page 112.

NOTES

ANSWER KEY

1. d) Wound bed preparation is a systematic approach to correcting molecular and cellular abnormalities and is critical to promoting healing in chronic wounds. Wound bed preparation with TIME O$_2$ principles includes controlling moisture with hydrogel, medihoney, and negative pressure wound therapy. Flap is indicated after the wound bed is prepared.

2. e) The modified wound bed preparation score, as proposed by Dr. Falanga, includes all the factors listed, i.e., black eschar, exudate amount, edema, wound duration prior to treatment, healing edges, greatest wound depth/granulation tissue, periwound dermatitis, periwound callus/fibrosis, and pink wound bed.

3. a) Cellular and/or tissue based products (CTPs) are not indicated if the wound is infected. The wound bed requires infection and exudate control as well as the debridement of necrotic tissue before CTPs can be applied.

4. b) Composite grafts have both epidermal and dermal tissue and cells. Dermagraft® has dermal matrix but does not have epidermis or epidermal cells. All other choices have both epidermal and dermal cells.

5. b) Advanced wound therapy is most appropriate in the 70-year-old diabetic male with a neuropathic wound that has not healed with standard wound management for four weeks. Advanced therapy should be considered if conventional therapy has not been successful within four weeks, as the initial rate of healing during this time can predict whether ulcers are likely to heal by 24 weeks. If the initial healing rate is <0.1 cm/wk at the four week interval, then advanced therapy should be considered.

6. a) Hyperbaric oxygen therapy is the administration of 100% oxygen with increased pressure of at least 1.4 ATA. It increases oxygen carrying capacity via plasma dissolved oxygen. It also helps with increased collagen synthesis and improves white cell function. Topical application of oxygen causing increasing oxygenation in the wound bed is not considered hyperbaric oxygen therapy.

7. a) Negative pressure wound therapy has not proven to increase tissue oxygen. It does help to decrease tissue edema and increase granulation tissue, and evidence shows there is a change in bacterial flora colonizing the wound bed, which may create a more favorable environment for wound healing.

8. d) Becalpermin, Apligraf®, and Dermagraft® are believed to increase wound growth factor levels. They all have been shown in randomized trials to improve diabetic foot ulcer closure rate. All advanced wound therapies are more likely to be effective when the wound bed is well prepared.

9. a) Acetic acid is appropriate to use in non-healable wounds, as the therapy goals in the non-healable wound bed are to control pain, odor, exudates, and bleeding. Acetic acid is cytotoxic but appropriate to use when the goal of therapy is to control infection, exudate, and odor.

10. c) The preferred method to debride a painful wound is autolytic debridement, as all other modes of debridement usually increase pain during the debridement process.

VENOUS INSUFFICIENCY ULCERS 14

Jayesh B. Shah, MD, CWSP, FAPWCA, FACCWS

INTRODUCTION

This chapter describes the anatomy of the venous system and the pathophysiology of venous insufficiency and ulceration. The CORE (compression, optimization of local wound environment, review of contributing factors, establishment of a maintenance plan) principles of venous ulcer management is discussed. Included are methods for edema management, ulcer prevention, and five "pearls" for venous ulcer management.

OBJECTIVES

Participants should be able to describe the characteristics of a venous stasis ulcer, discuss various methods of edema management, describe the management options for venous ulcers, and discuss the treatment plan for a venous ulcer that shows no signs of healing after three months.

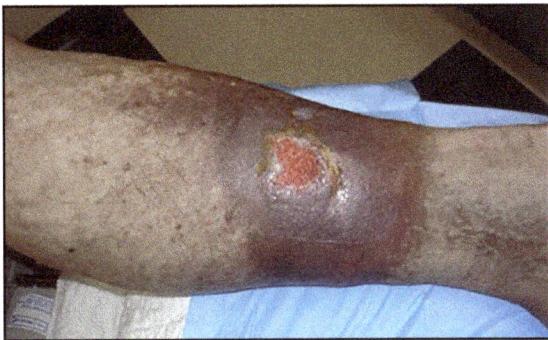

Figure 14.1: Venous insufficiency.

I. Venous insufficiency ulcers: disease impact

A. Impaired quality of life: pain, social isolation, depression, negative self-image
B. Healthcare costs
   1. Wide range, dependent on disease severity and duration
   2. Frequent office visits/hospitalizations
   3. Lost work days
   4. Between $775 million and $1 billion spent on outpatient treatments annually in the United States
   5. Total medical treatment cost per patient averages $9,685 (median $3,036) per episode
   6. Average cost per month of care ~$24,005
C. Physical impairment
   1. Decreased mobility
   2. Loss of productivity

II. Incidence and epidemiology (9-13)

A. Worldwide prevalence ~1-1.3%
B. ~500,000 treated annually in the United States
C. Equates to 80-90% of all leg ulcer cases

III. Venous system (normal anatomy and physiology)

A. Anatomy
   1. Major superficial veins: 10%
      a) Greater saphenous vein and lesser saphenous vein
      b) Found in subcutaneous tissue/outside fascia
      c) Venous return from skin and subcutaneous fat
   2. Major deep veins: 90%
      a) Femoral vein, anterior tibial vein, popliteal vein, posterior tibial vein
      b) Responsible for returning blood to the heart
      c) Lie within leg muscles/fascia
   3. Communicating venous system
      a) Perforators (communicating veins)
      b) Connects superficial veins to deep veins
      c) Allows flow from superficial veins to deep veins
   4. Valves (bicuspid)
      a) Allow blood to flow in one direction
      b) Prevent retrograde flow
      c) Leg muscles augment venous flow
B. Physiology
   1. Normal venous flow (calf muscle pump)
      a) Venous physiology during walking
         i) Calf muscle action—systolic: the calf muscle flexes, compresses deep veins, and blood flows cephalad towards the heart.

ii) Calf muscle action—diastolic: the calf muscle relaxes, perforator valves open, and blood flows from superficial to deep veins.

iii) The cycle repeats itself with each step.

b) Hemodynamics of venous flow (Figure 14.2)

IV. Pathophysiology of the venous ulcer

A. Calf muscle pump dysfunction (water hammer effect)

1. Dilated veins and incompetent valves cause blood vessel congestion resulting in fluid leakage, leading to congestion in surrounding tissue.

2. The surrounding tissue becomes poorly perfused and dies, forming an ulcer.

B. Fibrin cuff theory (14-16)

1. Dermal leakage causes fibrin formation, which leads to venous hypertension. This causes distended capillaries and fibrinogen leakage into subcutaneous tissue and results in a pericapillary fibrin cuff.

2. Pericapillary fibrin cuff results in a decreased exchange of oxygen and other vital nutrients to subcutaneous tissue and dermis, which causes anoxia and ulceration.

C. White cell trapping theory (14-16)

1. Endothelial cell damage causes neutrophil activation, which leads to adherence of neutrophils to the endothelium, causing damage to the intimal lining of vessel.

2. Damage to the intimal lining of vessel leads to the release of toxic oxygen metabolites and enzymes, which damage the capillaries and cause distended capillaries and ulceration.

V. Predisposing factors for venous stasis ulcers and edema

A. Prior pregnancy

B. Deep venous thrombosis

C. Leg trauma

D. Cardiac disease

E. Poor nutrition

F. Absence of or poor calf muscle pump

VI. Clinical features

A. Associated with insidious onset of edema

B. Edema could be pitting or non-pitting

C. Usually below the knee

D. Usually located near the ankle or lower calf

E. Usually recurrent

F. Usually patient complains of heavy, aching leg

G. Varicose veins are present in 10% of patients (Figure 14.3)

H. Surrounding skin is usually reddened or brown

I. Skin temperature is warm to the touch (normal)

J. Peripheral pulses are usually present and palpable

K. Capillary refill is usually normal

L. Hyperpigmentation is usually present (Figure 14.4)

M. Lipodermatosclerosis (indurated and fibrotic skin) may

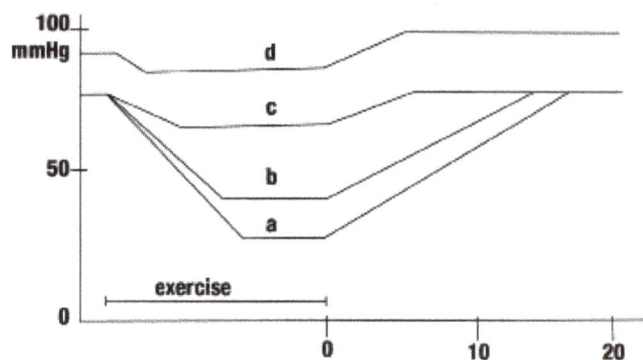

Figure 14.2: Hemodynamic charting of (a) healthy patients, (b) patients with only varicose veins, (c) patients with incompetent perforator veins, and (d) patients with deep and perforator incompetence.

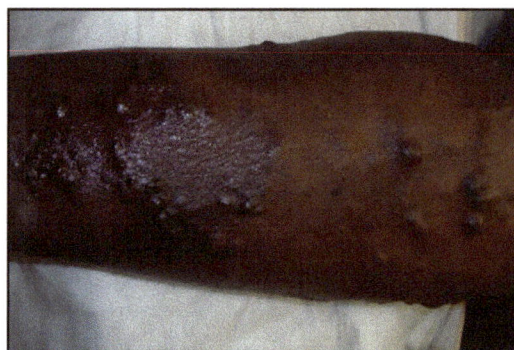

Figure 14.3: Varicose veins.

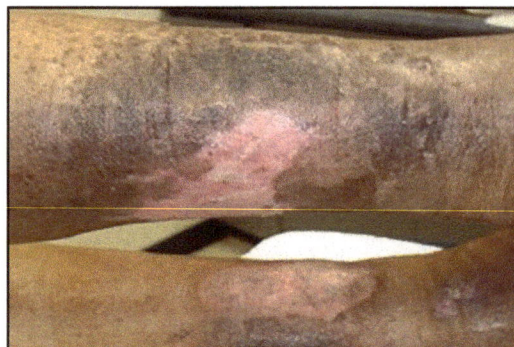

Figure 14.4: Hyperpigmentation.

be present in patients with long-standing disease (Figure 14.5)

N. Inverted champagne bottle appearance is typically seen

P. Venous dermatitis (Figure 14.6)

1. Frequent finding

2. Anterior shin/ankle

3. Often bilateral

4. Warmth and pruritus

5. Differential diagnosis (D/D) cellulitis

Q. Venous ulcer characteristics (Figure 14.7)

1. Irregular border

2. Flat, flush edges

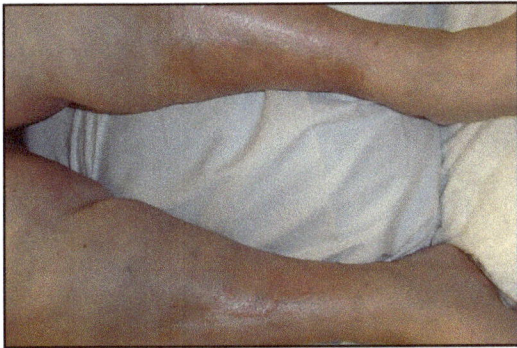

Figure 14.5: Lipodermatosclerosis.

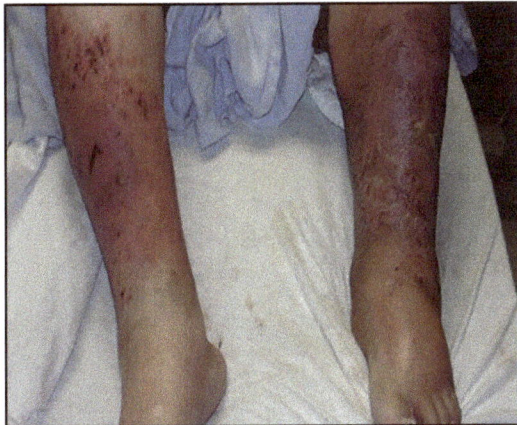

Figure 14.6: Venous dermatitis.

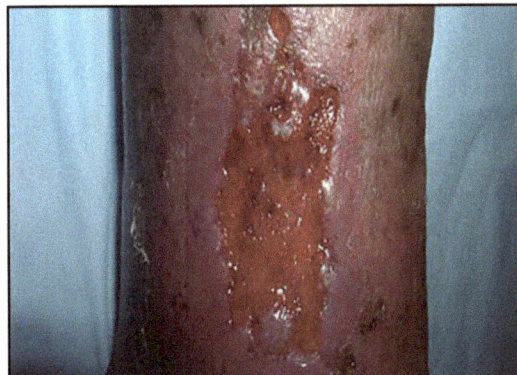

Figure 14.7: Venus ulcer characteristics.

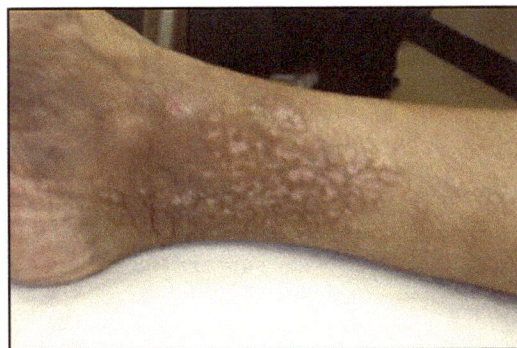

Figure 14.8: Atrophie blanche.

3. Surrounded by fibrosed skin and erythema
4. Usually develop in the malleolar area along the distribution of the saphenous vein (61%)
5. Necrotic eschar is generally not present
6. Friable, purple tissue (usually ruddy color base)
7. Ulcers are usually of shallow depth
8. Ulcers usually have moderate to heavy exudate
9. Exudate is protein rich
10. Granulation tissue is usually present
    a) Usually painless unless infected or of mixed disease

R. Atrophie blanche (Figure 14.8)
1. Type of vasculopathy (as opposed to vasculitis)
2. In vasculopathy, the primary process is occlusion of vessels leading to tissue necrosis. The inflammatory changes are secondary. The pathophysiologic process is thought to be deposition of fibrin with subsequent formation of thrombi within superficial and deep dermal vessels. These lead to infarction and ulceration of the dermis and epidermis
3. Characterized by smooth, ivory-white plaque stippled with telangectasias surrounded by hyperpigmentation
4. Often seen in association with chronic venous insufficiency, but can be a primary skin disorder
5. Alternate names include capillaritis alba, livedo vasculitis, and livedo vasculopathy
6. More common in females
7. In 30% of cases the area breaks down into an exquisitely painful ulcer
8. Divided into two categories
   a) Primary: lesions located on the lower extremity without any underlying disease
   b) Secondary: seen with other systemic or local diseases

VII. Chronic venous insufficiency (CVI) classification (CEAP)

A. C = clinical presentation (class 1-6)
1. Class 0: no signs of venous disease
2. Class 1: telangiectasia or reticular veins
3. Class 2: varicose veins
4. Class 3: edema
5. Class 4: skin changes
6. Class 5: healed ulceration
7. Class 6: active ulceration

B. E = etiologic basis: primary, secondary, congenital
C. A = anatomic distribution: superficial, deep, perforators
D. P = pathophysiologic basis: reflux, obstruction, pathophysiology

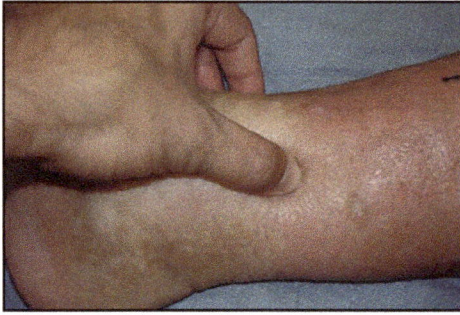

Figure 14.9: Examining for edema.

VIII. Differential diagnosis
A. Edema (Figure 14.9)
1. Venous edema
2. Lymphedema
3. Lipedema
4. Congestive heart failure (CHF)
5. Renal disease
6. Cirrhosis of liver
7. Hypothyroidism
8. Drug-induced edema (e.g., from antihypertensive medications)
B. Ulcer differential diagnosis
1. Arterial ulcer (Figure 14.10)

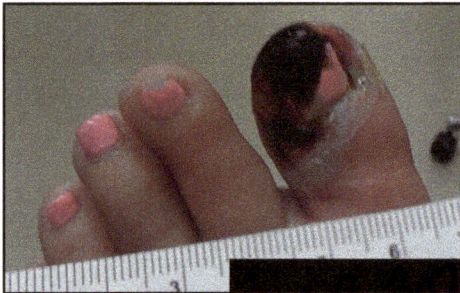

Figure 14.10: Arterial ulcer.

a) Painful
b) Punched out
c) Black eschar
d) Involves deep tissue
e) Arterial coexists in 20% of venous insufficiency patients
2. Vasculitis (Figure 14.11)

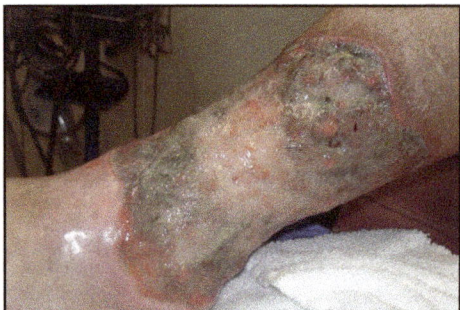

Figure 14.11: Vasculitis.

a) Usually painful
b) Associated with systemic symptoms and systemic disease
c) Biopsy is helpful
d) May need referral

IX. Diagnostic tools
A. ABI (ankle-brachial index)
B. TBI (toe-brachial index)
C. TCOM (transcutaneous oximetry)
D. Arterial Doppler
E. Photoplethysmography
F. Doppler ultrasonography
G. Hand-held Doppler system
H. Duplex ultrasonography with color flow imaging

X. Management of venous ulcers
A. CORE principles of venous ulcer management
1. C = compression
2. O = optimize the local wound environment
3. R = review contributing factors
4. E = establish a maintenance plan
B. Other
1. Control venous hypertension
2. Treat infection
3. Treat dermatitis
4. Debride ulcer
5. Prevention
6. Surgical management of varicose veins
C. Edema management
1. Compression
a) Compression dressings (Figure 14.12)

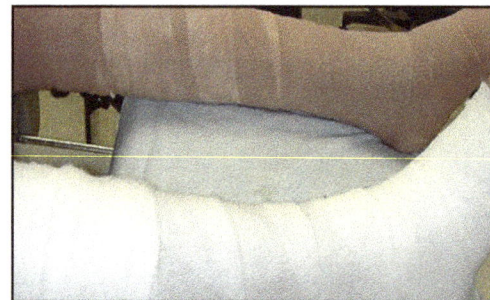

Figure 14.12: Compression dressings.

b) Unna's boot
c) Profore™
d) Profore™ light
e) SurePress®
f) ACE® bandage
g) Stretch options
i) Short stretch (Figure 14.13a)
(1) Low resting and high working pressure lowers the possibility of developing toe ischemia
(2) Less useful in non-ambulatory patient
(3) Compresses lower extremity by resisting changes in force during walking

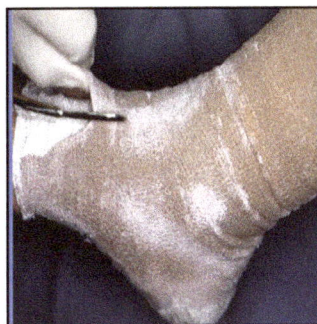

Figure 14.13a: Short stretch plus elastic bandage.

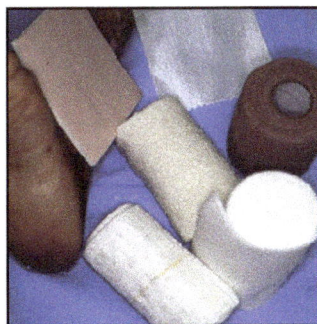

Figure 14.13b: Long stretch multilayered bandaging systems.

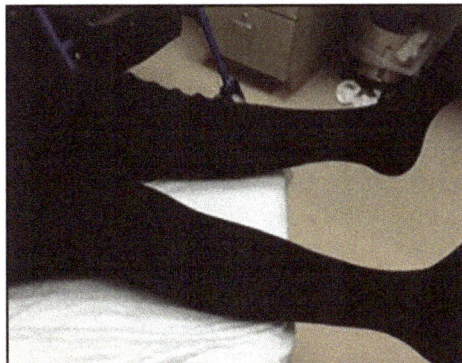

Figure 14.14a: Zipper thigh-length stockings.

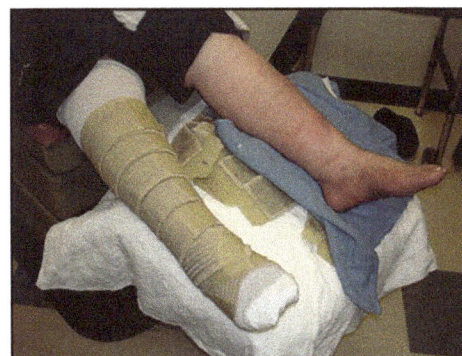

Figure 14.14b: Class 2 knee-high compression stockings.

        (4)   Examples: Unna-FLEX® (ConvaTec), Comprilan® (Beiersdorf), Unna's boot, Coban™ 2 Layer (3M)

    ii)   Long stretch (Figure 14.13b)

        (1)   Extensible bandage

        (2)   Returns to original length when force is removed

        (3)   Loses elasticity over time

        (4)   Examples: Setopress® (ACME United Co.), Profore™ (Smith & Nephew), Dyna-Flex® (Johnson & Johnson)

D. Ulcer management

    1.   DIME (debridement, infection management, moisture control and edge effect)

    2.   Split-thickness skin graft (STSG)

    3.   Cellular and/or tissue based products (CTPs)

    4.   Apligraf®

    5.   OASIS®

    6.   Advanced collagen dressings

E. Review contributing factors—surgery (32)

    1.   Chronic venous leg ulceration can be managed by compression treatment, elevation of the leg, and exercise.

    2.   The addition of ablative superficial venous surgery to this strategy has not been shown to affect ulcer healing, but it does reduce ulcer recurrence.

    3.   Venous leg ulcers are also correlated with increased ambulatory venous pressures (AVP). Patients with venous leg ulcers with increased AVP may benefit from procedures such as a venous valve transplant, which reduces the AVP to less than 30 mmHg.

XI. Ulcer prevention: compression stockings (Figures 14.14a–14.14c)

A. Over-the-counter gradient compression stockings are usually <20 mmHg.

    1.   Class 0: 15-20 mmHg; used for aching/fatigued legs, mild ankle and foot edema, mild varicosities, prophylaxis during pregnancy

    2.   Class 1: 20-30 mmHg; used for simple varicose veins, light edema, leg fatigue, DVT prevention, superficial thrombophlebitis

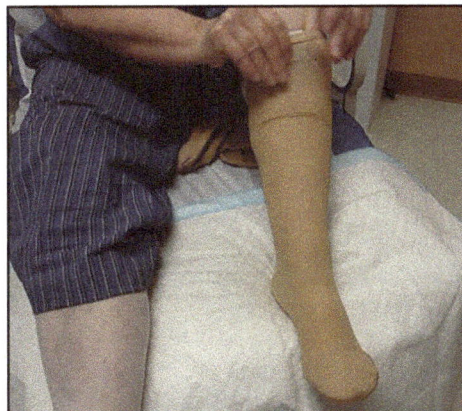

Figure 14.14c: Velcro-tabbed stockings (Farrow wrap).

    3.   Class 2: 30-40 mmHg; used for moderate edema, severe varicosities, moderate venous insufficiency, moderate and post traumatic edema, post phlebectomy, post sclerotherapy, orthostatic hypotension, moderate lymphedema, post-thrombotic syndrome

    4.   Class 3: 40-50 mmHg; used for severe tendencies towards edema, severe lymphedema, and severe chronic venous insufficiency, in conjunction with the management of open venous ulcers

    5.   Class 4: >60 mmHg; used for severe edema, venous insufficiency, post-thrombotic lymphatic edema, and elephantiasis

XII. Pearls for venous ulcer management

A. Venous ulcers can exist in the presence of mixed arterial/venous pathology; however, treatment of only the elevated venous pressure will not succeed when significant arterial disease is present. Level 1 evidence. (18-21)

B. Patients presenting with an apparent venous ulcer and are suspected of having sickle cell disease should have a sickle cell prep and hemoglobin electrophoresis. Level 2 evidence. (22-23)

C. Apparent venous ulcers that have been open continuously without signs of healing for three months or do not demonstrate any response to treatment after six weeks should be biopsied for histological diagnosis. Level 3 evidence. (24-27)

D. Apparent venous ulcers, as well as any wounds that are excessively painful and progressively increase in size after debridement and/or despite treatment, should be considered for a diagnosis of pyoderma gangrenosum. This suspicion should be especially high if the ulcer is darker in color with blue/purple borders, or if the patient has a systemic disease. Level 2 evidence. (28-31)

E. Color duplex ultrasound scanning performed with proximal compression or Valsalva maneuver is useful in providing anatomic and physiologic data to help confirm a venous etiology for the leg ulcer. Level 1 evidence. (18-21)

RESOURCES

1. McCulloch JM, Kloth LC, Feedar JA (editors). *Wound Healing Alternatives in Management*. 2nd ed. Philadelphia: F.A Davis Company; 1995.

2. Sheffield PJ, Fife CE (editors). *Wound Care Practice*. 2nd ed. North Palm Beach: Best Publishing Company; 2007.

3. Chaurasia BD. *B.D. Chaurasia's Handbook of General Anatomy*. New Delhi: CBS Publishers & Distributors; 1985.

4. Moore KL, Dalley AF. *Clinically Oriented Anatomy*. Philadelphia: Lippincott Williams & Wilkins; 1999.

5. Krasner DL, Rodeheaver GT, Sibbold RG. *Chronic Wound Care*. Malvern: HMP Communications; 2001.

6. Bowker JH, Pfeifer MA. *Levin and O'Neal's The Diabetic Foot*. St. Louis: Mosby; 2001.

7. Robson MC, et al. Guidelines for the treatment of venous ulcers. *Wound Rep Reg*. 2006; 14:649-62.

8. Wound Healing Society. Wound Care Guidelines [Internet]. Accessed at: http://www.woundheal.org.

9. Angle N, Bergan JJ. Chronic Venous Ulcer. *BMJ*. 1997; 314:1019-23.

10. Coon WW, et al. Venous thromboembolism and other venous disease in the Tecumseh community health study. *Circulation*. 1973; 48(4):839-46.

11. Mathias SD, et al. Skin replacement in venous stasis ulcer. *Adv Skin Wound Care*. 2000; 13:76-8.

12. Phillips TJ, Dover JS. Leg ulcers. *J Am Acad Dermatol*. 1991; 25:965-87.

13. Olin JW, et al. Medical costs of treating venous stasis ulcers: evidence from a retrospective cohort study. *Vasc Med*. 1999; 4(1):1-7.

14. Browse NL, et al. The cause of venous stasis ulceration. *Lancet*. July 1982; 2:243-5.

15. Falanga V, et al. The 'trap' hypothesis of venous ulceration. *Lancet*. 1993; 341:1006-8.

16. Coleridge Smith PD, et al. Causes of venous stasis ulceration. *BMJ*. 1988; 296:1726-7.

17. Robson MC, et al. Wound Healing Society guidelines for the treatment of venous ulcers. *Wound Repair Regen*. 2006; 14:649-62.

18. Porter JM, Moneta, GL. Reporting standards in venous disease: an update. International Consensus Committee on Chronic Venous Disease. *J Vasc Surg*. 1995; 21(4):635-45.

19. Beebe HG, Bergan JJ, et al. Classification and grading of chronic venous disease in lower limbs: a consensus statement. *Eur J Vasc Endovasc Surg*. 1996; 12(4):487-92.

20. Porter JM, Rutherford RB, Clagett GP, et al. Reporting standards in venous disease. *J Vasc Surg*. 1988; 8:172-81.

21. Kjaer ML, Mainz J, Soerensen LT, et al. Clinical quality indicators of venous leg ulcers: development, feasibility and reliability. *Ostomy Wound Manage*. 2005; 51(5):64-74.

22. Karayalcin G, Rosner F, Kim KY, et al. Sickle cell anemia-clinical manifestations in 100 patients and review of the literature. *Am J Med Sci*. 1975; 269(1):51-68.

23. Wolfort FG, Krizek TJ. Skin ulceration in sickle cell anemia. *Plast Reconstr Surg*. 1969; 43(1):71-7.

24. Hansson C, Andersson E. Malignant skin lesions on the legs and feet at a dermatological leg ulcer clinic during five years. *Acta Derm Venereal*. 1997; 78:147-8.

25. Synder RJ, Stillman RM, Weiss SD. Epidermoid cancers that masquerade as a venous ulcer disease. *Ostomy Wound Manage*. 2003; 49:63-6.

26. Mekkes JR, Loots MA, Vanderwal AC, et al. Causes, investigation and treatment of leg ulceration. *Brit J Dermatol*. 2003; 148:388-401.

27. Chakrabarty A, Phillips T. Leg ulcers of unusual causes. *Int J Low Extrem Wound*. 2003; 21:207-16.

28. Reichrath J, Bens G, Bonowitz A, et al. Treatment recommendations for pyoderma gangrenosum: an evidence based review of the literature based on more than 350 patients. *J Am Acad Dermatol*. 2005; 53:273-83.

29. Su WP, Schroeter AL, Perry HO, et al. Histopathologic and immuno-pathologic study of pyoderma gangrenosum. *J Cutan Patho*. 1986; 13:323-30.

30. Wines N, Wines M, Ryman W. Understanding pyoderma gangrenosum: a review. *MedGenMed*. 2001; 3:6-12.

31. Bennet ML, Jackson JM, Jorizzo JL, et al. Pyoderma gangrenosum. A comparison of typical and atypical forms with emphasis on time to remission. Case review of 86 patients from 2 institutions. *Medicine*. 2000; 79:37-46.

32. Barwell JR, et al. Comparison of surgery and compression with compression alone in chronic venous ulceration (ESCHAR study): randomized controlled trial. *Lancet*. 2004; 363:1854-59.

33. Nicholaides AN, et al. The relation of venous ulceration with ambulatory venous pressure measurements. *J Vasc Surg*. 1993; 17(2):414-9.

SAMPLE QUESTIONS

1. A typical venous stasis ulcer has all of the following characteristics except:
   a) Irregular edge
   b) Deep depth
   c) Moderate exudates
   d) Present peripheral pulses

2. A 67-year-old female with a history of type 2 DM, hypertension, and peripheral vascular disease has a non-healing wound on her right leg. The ulcer is 5 × 7 cm with an irregular edge, shallow depth, necrotic eschar, with +2 edema. The patient has an ABI of 0.6. The next step in the management of this patient is:
   a) Compression bandage
   b) Vascular surgery consultation
   c) Hyperbaric oxygen therapy
   d) Subfascial endoscopic venous surgery

3. A 50-year-old female with an apparent venous stasis ulcer has failed to heal for three months with standard wound care treatments that included moist dressing and compression dressing. What is the next step in management of this patient?
   a) Venous surgery
   b) Venous Doppler
   c) Wound biopsy
   d) Venous reflux studies

4. Which of the following statements about surgery in venous stasis ulcer patients is true?
   a) Procedures that reduce the AVP to less than 30 mmHg may be beneficial.
   b) Procedures that increase the AVP to more than 30 mmHg may be beneficial.
   c) Ablative superficial venous surgery in venous stasis ulcers will decrease healing time.
   d) Ablative superficial venous surgery in venous stasis ulcers will not affect recurrence.

5. The water hammer effect is:
   a) Dilated veins and incompetent valves causing blood vessel congestion
   b) Water flowing through the venous valve
   c) Venous flow causing a hammerlike sound when it flows through a tight venous valve
   d) Showering of emboli through the incompetent valves

6. The most important component of venous ulcer management is:
   a) Venous valve surgery
   b) Ablative superficial venous surgery
   c) Compression
   d) Revascularization

7. The next step in the treatment of a venous ulcer patient whose ulcer worsens and increases in size after debridement is:
   a) Vascular surgery
   b) Venous surgery
   c) Hyperbaric oxygen therapy
   d) Considering a diagnosis of pyoderma gangrenosum

8. The next step in the treatment of a venous stasis ulcer patient who has not healed in more than three months, despite standard wound management, is:
   a) Hyperbaric oxygen therapy
   b) Wound biopsy
   c) Increase compression to apply lymphedema pump
   d) Negative pressure wound therapy

9. Which of the following statements about short-stretch bandages is true?
   a) They have high resting and low working pressure.
   b) They lower the risk of developing toe ischemia.
   c) They are more useful in non-ambulatory patients.
   d) They compress the lower extremity by resisting changes in force during resting.

10. All of the following statements about long-stretch bandages are true except:
    a) They are extensible.
    b) They return to original length when force is removed.
    c) They lose elasticity over time.
    d) They are more useful in ambulatory patients.

See answers on page 122.

NOTES

ANSWER KEY

1. b) A typical venous stasis ulcer usually has an irregular wound edge, shallow depth, moderate exudates, and good peripheral pulse.

2. b) In patients with mixed arteriovenous disease, treatment of only the elevated venous pressure will not succeed when significant arterial disease is present. The next step for this 67-year-old female is a vascular surgery consultation.

3. c) The next step for a patient with a venous stasis ulcer failing standard wound management for more than three months is a wound biopsy. It is important to do venous reflux studies and look for perforators or incompetent valves; however, a biopsy should be done first to rule out malignancy, pyoderma gangrenosum, or vasculitis. Venous Doppler is an important test used to check for deep venous thrombosis, but this test is usually administered before starting compression therapy when DVT is suspected. Venous surgery is a good intervention to prevent recurrence for a refractory venous stasis ulcer or a patient with reflux or incompetent perforators, but it is not the next step in this scenario.

4. a) Venous leg ulcers are also correlated with increased ambulatory venous pressures (AVP). Patients with venous leg ulcers and increased AVP may benefit from a procedure like a venous valve transplant, which reduces the AVP to less than 30 mmHg. The addition of ablative superficial venous surgery to this strategy has not been shown to affect ulcer healing, but it does reduce ulcer recurrence.

5. a) The water hammer effect is secondary to calf muscle pump dysfunction secondary to incompetent valves causing dilated veins and blood vessel congestion.

6. c) The most important component of venous ulcer management is compression. All other components are important, but compression is the most important for venous stasis ulcer management.

7. d) Pyoderma gangrenosum should be considered when ulcer size increases and when an ulcer worsens after debridement. Patients with pyoderma gangrenosum have pathergy, where any trauma will make the ulcer worse. Vascular assessment should be done on initial evaluation, and the patient should be referred to vascular surgery if the patient has mixed arteriovenous disease, which is also another differential diagnosis to consider. Hyperbaric oxygen therapy is not indicated in venous stasis ulcers. Venous surgery is indicated if the patient has reflux and perforator or valve incompetence, but a possible diagnosis of pyoderma gangrenosum is the most appropriate choice.

8. b) The next step in the treatment of a patient with a venous stasis ulcer that has not healed in more than three months despite standard wound management is a wound biopsy.

9. b) Short-stretch bandages have low resting and high working pressure, lessen the possibility of developing toe ischemia, are less useful in non-ambulatory patients, and compress the lower extremity by resisting changes in force during walking.

10. d) Long-stretch bandages are extensible bandages. They return to original length when force is removed and lose elasticity over time. Short-stretch bandages are more useful in ambulatory patients.

LYMPHEDEMA 15

Neha J. Shah, MPT, CLT
Jayesh B. Shah, MD, CWSP, FAPWCA, FACCWS

INTRODUCTION

This chapter describes lymphedema, a disease that afflicts the lymphatic system and can complicate wound healing. It most commonly affects the extremities but occasionally involves the trunk, head, or genital area. It is caused by the accumulation of protein rich lymphatic fluid in the interstitial tissue, which can lead to fibrosis and lipodermatosclerosis.

OBJECTIVES

Participants should be able to describe the function of the lymphatic system and the causes and characteristics of lymphedema, discuss the management options for lymphedema, and describe the acceptable standard of care for lymphedema.

I. Lymphedema definition

A. Lymphedema is persistent edema lasting longer than three months, with little or no response to overnight elevation or diuretics, and the associated presence of skin changes, primarily thickened skin, hyperkeratosis, and papillomatosis.

II. Epidemiology of lymphedema

A. Lymphedema resulting from filariasis, an infection by the nematode *Wuchereria bancrofti* carried by mosquitoes, affects 2% of the world's population in areas such as India, Africa, Haiti, and Malaysia.

B. In Western countries, upper-extremity lymphedema due to complications resulting from breast cancer treatment is the most common presentation associated with surgery and radiation therapy.

C. Lower-extremity lymphedema can be secondary to cancer, lymph node dissection, chronic venous disease, recurrent infection, obesity, and arthritis.

D. Cancer-related lymphedema in the lower extremities is less prevalent.

III. Function of the lymphatic system

A. Filters noxious matter, such as bacteria

B. Production of lymphocytes (WBCs), which are important for fighting infections and enhancing the body's immune capabilities

C. Regulates the concentration of protein in lymph

IV. Significance of the lymphatic system

A. Lymph time volume is the amount of lymph fluid the lymphatic system can transport in a unit of time.

B. An increase of lymph fluid due to physical activity, heat, or inflammation results in an increase in lymph time volume.

C. Lymph transport is supported by the contraction of the skeletal muscle, arterial pulsation, respiratory pressure changes, negative pressure in central veins, and external pressure, e.g., manual lymph drainage.

V. Pathophysiology of lymphedema

A. A chronic inflammatory lymphostatic disease caused by mechanical failure of the lymphatic system

B. Accumulation of protein rich fluid

C. Fluid in interstitium causes chronic inflammation and reactive fibrosis of the affected tissues

VI. Primary lymphedema

A. Congenital lymphedema (present at birth): Milroy's disease, or type IA (Figure 15.1), begins in infancy and causes lymph nodes to form abnormally. It occurs because of mutation in the FLT4 gene, which encodes the vascular endothelial growth factor receptor 3. Also included in type I lymphedema are the more rare syndromic forms, including lymphedema-distichiasis syndrome (double row of eyelashes), yellow nail syndrome, and lymphedema with ptosis—all three of which are due to mutations of the FOXC2 gene. (A table of syndromic lymphedema can be found at: https://rarediseases.org/rare-diseases/hereditary-lymphedema/.)

B. Lymphedema praecox: Meige's syndrome, or type II (Figure 15.2), often causes lymphedema around puberty, though it can occur later in life, until age 35. It is non-syndromic even though it is due to a mutation of FOXC2.

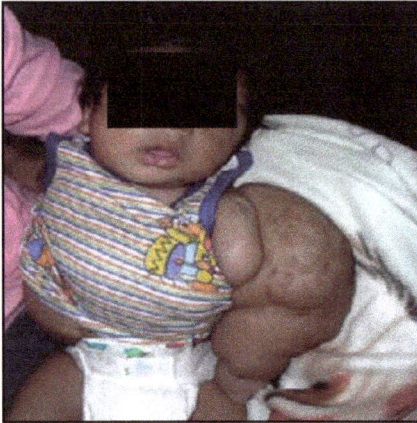

Figure 15.1: Milroy's disease, primary lymphedema.

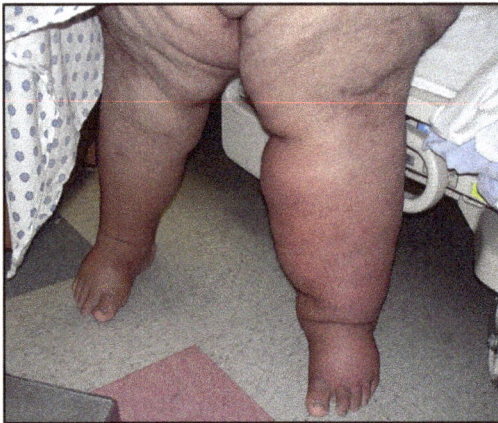

Figure 15.2: Meige's syndrome, lymphedema praecox.

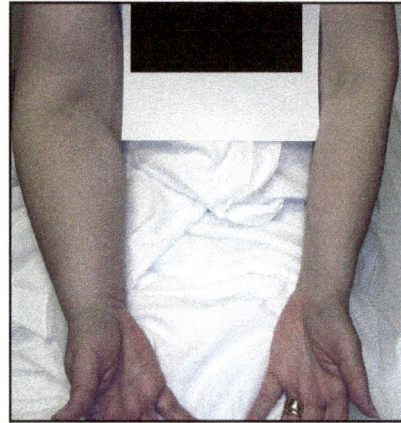

Figure 15.3a: A 55-year-old female with stage 3 breast cancer after mastectomy.

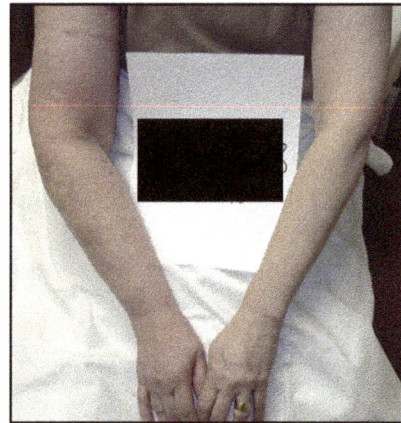

Figure 15.3b: Same patient after manual lymphatic drainage.

Most cases of hereditary lymphedema, type IA and type II, are inherited as autosomal dominant traits.

C. Late-onset lymphedema (lymphedema tarda)—this occurs rarely and usually begins after age 35.

VII. Secondary lymphedema
(Figures 15.3a and 15.3b)
A. Surgery
B. Radiation therapy
C. Trauma
D. Filariasis
E. Cancer/malignant tumors
F. Chronic venous insufficiency
G. Infection
H. Iatrogenic
I. Obesity
J. Self-induced

VIII. Stages of lymphedema
A. Latency—transport capacity reduced, no edema
B. Stage I—pitting edema, reduce with elevation, reversible
C. Stage II—pitting becomes difficult, fibrosis starts, spontaneously irreversible lymphedema
D. Stage III—no pitting, fibrosis and sclerosis, skin changes (e.g., papillomas, hyperkeratosis)

IX. Characteristics of lymphedema
A. Asymmetric
B. No pain
C. No bruising
D. Frequent cellulitis/erysipelas
E. Foot edematous
F. Positive Stemmer's sign (Figure 15.4): when a thickened cutaneous fold at the dorsum of toes or fingers cannot be lifted or is difficult to lift
G. Pitting edema

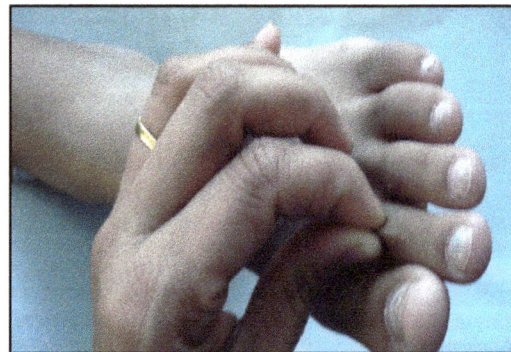

Figure 15.4: Negative Stemmer's sign.

X. Diagnosis

A. Physical exam
B. Direct lymphograph
C. Indirect lymphograph
D. Lymphoscintigraphy
E. Duplex Doppler ultrasound
F. CT scan
G. MRI

XI. Differential diagnosis

A. Lipedema—flabby swelling of legs arising from deposition of adipose tissue
   1. Characteristics
      a) Bilateral symmetrical swelling from iliac crest to ankles
      b) Dorsum of feet never involved
      c) Negative Stemmer's sign
      d) Little or no pitting
      e) No cellulitis/erysipelas
      f) Painful on palpation
      g) Bruises easily
   2. Treatment: calorie conscious low-fat, low-carb diet; exercises; complete decongestive treatment if no contraindications
B. Other differential diagnoses
   1. Chronic venous insufficiency
   2. Acute deep vein thrombosis
   3. Congestive heart failure
   4. Cardiac Edema
   5. Malignancy
   6. Myxedema
   7. Chronic regional pain syndrome (reflex sympathetic dystrophy)

XII. Treatment of Lymphedema

A. Conservative treatment—complete decongestive therapy is the most acceptable standard of care
   1. Phase I—decongestive phase, consists of manual lymph drainage (Figure 15.5), compression bandaging, exercises, skin care, nail care, and self care
   2. Phase II—maintenance phase, consists of continued use of compression garment and night bandaging

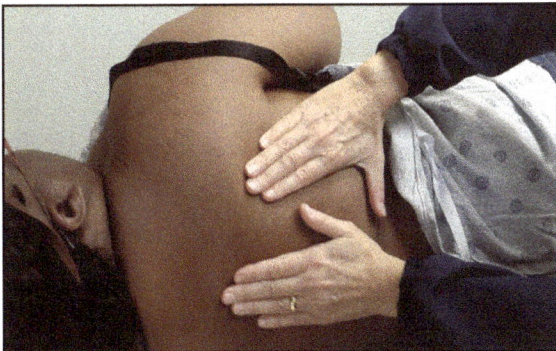

Figure 15.6: Sequential pneumatic compression pumps. Start with a pressure of 50 mmHg and increase as tolerated. Pumping should be done twice a day for 30-60 minutes.

B. Surgery—with poor results
   1. Reduction (debulking)
   2. Surgery to improve drainage
   3. Microsurgical techniques
   4. Liposuction
C. Dietary recommendations when necessary
D. Sequential pneumatic compression pumps
   1. Usually used when outpatient complete decongestive therapy is not possible due to:
      a) Patient confined to home
      b) Patient undergoing treatment for open wounds
   2. Used to maintain the reduction of lymphedema following phase I and phase II of complete decongestive therapy to maintain the reduction of lymphedema
E. Other elastic support garments—CircAid®, Juzo®
F. Newer sequential pneumatic compression pumps; thought to simulate manual lymph drainage (Figure 15.6)

XIII. Case history

A. A 35-year-old male with a history of diabetes and long-standing cellulitis of five years developed a gradual swelling and worsening of edema in his left foot. The patient was admitted again with cellulitis and a wound secondary to trauma on the medial aspect of his left leg (Figure 15.7).

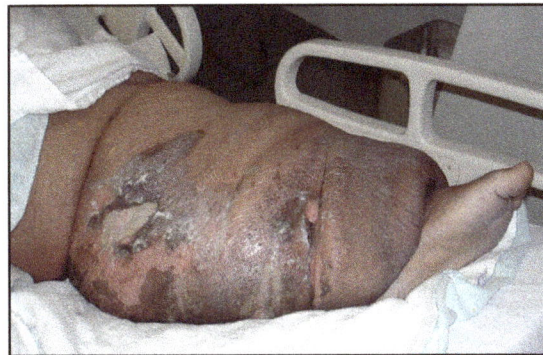

Figure 15.5: Manual lymphatic drainage.

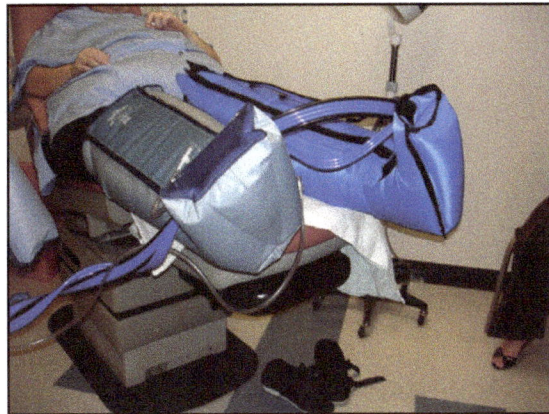

Figure 15.7: A 35-year-old male with secondary lymphedema.

B. A 72-year-old female with lymphedema due to chronic
    venous insufficiency (phlebolymphedema), before (Figure
    15.8a) and after (Figure 15.8b) manual lymphatic drain-
    age therapy.

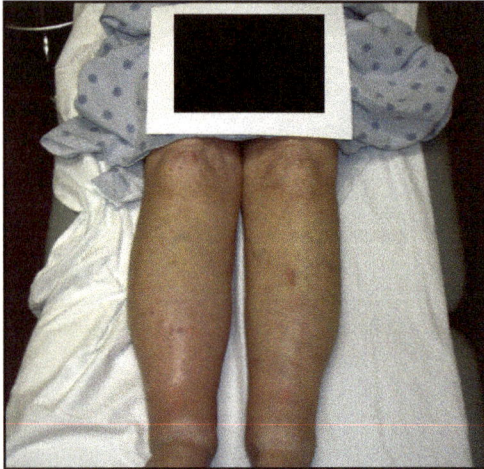

**Figure 15.8a: A 72-year-old female before manual
lymphatic drainage.**

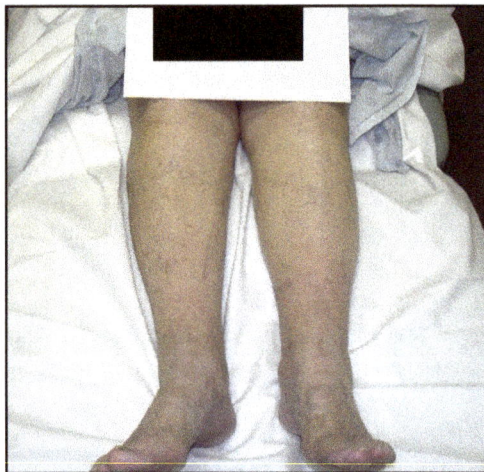

**Figure 15.8b: Same 72-year-old female after manual
lymphatic drainage.**

RESOURCES

1. Földi M, Földi E. *Földi's Textbook of Lymphology*.
    München: Elsevier; 2006.
2. McCulloch JM, Kloth LC, Feedar JA. *Wound Healing Al-
    ternatives in Management*. 2nd ed. Philadelphia: F.A. Davis
    Company; 1995.
3. Sheffield PJ, Fife CE, editors. *Wound Care Practice*. 2nd ed.
    North Palm Beach: Best Publishing Company; 2007.
4. Moore KL, Dalley AF. *Clinically Oriented Anatomy*. Phila-
    delphia: Lippincott Williams & Wilkins; 1999.
5. Krasner DL, Rodeheaver GT, Sibbold RG. *Chronic Wound
    Care*. Malvern: HMP Communications; 2001.
6. Bowker JH, Pfeifer MA. *Levin and O'Neal's The Diabetic
    Foot*. St. Louis: Mosby; 2001.

SAMPLE QUESTIONS

1. Lymphedema is a curable condition.
   a) True
   b) False

2. The most acceptable standard of care for lymphedema is:
   a) Surgery
   b) Compression pumps
   c) Complete decongestive therapy
   d) Medications

3. All of the following are acceptable treatment for lymphedema except:
   a) Manual lymphatic drainage
   b) Compression pumps
   c) Surgery
   d) Aggressive diuresis

4. All of the following statements about lymphedema are true except:
   a) Globally, the most common cause of lymphedema is filariasis.
   b) In the Western world, lymphedema is most commonly the result of cancer treatment.
   c) Lymphedema is curable with surgery.
   d) Lymphedema may be confused with lipedema.

5. All of the following statements about Meige's syndrome are true except:
   a) It occurs at puberty.
   b) It occurs shortly after birth.
   c) It usually involves the lower extremities.
   d) While there is no cure for lymphedema praecox, the condition can be managed by early diagnosis and treatment.

6. Milroy's disease is:
   a) A congenital hereditary lymphedema occurring at or shortly after birth
   b) A secondary lymphedema, secondary to *Wuchereria bancrofti*
   c) The same as lymphedema tarda
   d) A secondary lymphedema, secondary to breast cancer treatment

7. All of the following are causes of secondary lymphedema except:
   a) Filariasis
   b) Cancer
   c) Obesity
   d) Miege's syndrome

8. All of the following are characteristics of lipedema except:
   a) Bilateral symmetrical swelling from the iliac crest to the ankles
   b) Positive Stemmer's sign
   c) Little or no pitting edema
   d) Painful on palpation

9. Positive Stemmer's sign is when:
   a) A thickened cutaneous fold at the dorsum of toes or fingers cannot be lifted or is difficult to lift
   b) A cutaneous fold at the dorsum of toes or fingers that can be lifted and pinched
   c) A thickened cutaneous fold becomes sclerosed and nodular
   d) A thickened cutaneous fold has +3 pitting edema

10. All of the following are functions of the lymphatic system except:
    a) It filters noxious matter such as bacteria.
    b) It produces lymphocytes (WBCs), which are important for fighting infections and enhancing the body's immune capabilities.
    c) It regulates the concentration of protein in lymph.
    d) It helps to kill bacteria by phagocytosis.

See answers on page 129.

NOTES

ANSWER KEY

1. b) Lymphedema is not a curable condition.

2. c) The most acceptable standard of care for lymphedema is complete decongestive therapy.

3. d) Acceptable treatment for lymphedema includes manual lymphatic drainage, compression pumps, and surgery. Aggressive diuresis is not a treatment for lymphedema and is usually not effective.

4. c) Globally, the most common cause of lymphedema is filariasis. In the Western world, lymphedema is most commonly a result of cancer treatment. Lymphedema is still not curable with surgery. Lymph node transplantation microsurgery is experimental at the present time. Lymphedema may be confused with lipedema.

5. b) Meige's disease, or lymphedema praecox, often causes lymphedema around puberty, though it can occur later in life, until age 35.

6. a) Milroy's disease is a congenital hereditary lymphedema that occurs at or shortly after birth.

7. d) Filariasis, obesity, and cancer are causes of secondary lymphedema, while Meige's syndrome is congenital (primary) lymphedema.

8. b) Lipedema is usually bilateral symmetrical swelling from the iliac crest to the ankles with negative Stemmer's sign. Patients with lipedema have little or no pitting edema and experience pain on palpation.

9. a) Positive Stemmer's sign is when a thickened cutaneous fold at the dorsum of toes or fingers cannot be lifted or is difficult to lift.

10. d) Functions of the lymphatic system include filtering noxious matter, such as bacteria, the production of lymphocytes (WBCs), and the regulation of the concentration of protein in lymph. Phagocytosis is not a function of the lymphatic system.

ARTERIAL INSUFFICIENCY ULCERS 16

Jayesh B. Shah, MD, CWSP, FAPWCA, FACCWS

INTRODUCTION

This chapter describes the risk factors for peripheral arterial disease (PAD) and how to conduct a history and physical assessment of PAD. Included are the noninvasive tests for assessing atherosclerotic vascular disease (AVD), medical and surgical interventions for PAD, and an algorithm for limb salvage.

OBJECTIVES

Participants should be able to explain the risk factors for PAD, discuss the role of $TcPO_2$ in assessing PAD, and describe the ankle-brachial index (ABI) as an assessment tool for PAD.

I. Peripheral arterial disease
A. Prevalence
  1. 12 million patients in the United States go undiagnosed
  2. Of the 2.5 million patients diagnosed, only 4% are treated
B. Risk factors
  1. Smoking
  2. Diabetes and impaired glucose tolerance (IGT)
  3. Advanced age
  4. Male
  5. Hypertension
  6. Hyperlipidemia
  7. Fibrinogen
  8. Homocysteine
  9. Polycythemia
  10. Thrombocytosis
C. Protective factors
  1. Mild to moderate ethanol intake and regular exercise are considered to be protective factors
D. History
  1. Fontaine stages of peripheral artery occlusive disease (PAOD)
    a) Fontaine stage 1—asymptomatic
      i) 50% of patients
      ii) Gradual narrowing of the major limb vessel accompanied by a variable degree of collateralization
    b) Fontaine stage 2—intermittent claudication
      i) Exercise-induced cramping or tiredness of the calf, thigh, or buttock
      ii) Symptoms are highly reproducible and relieved with rest
      iii) Measured by
        (1) Distance at which there is onset of pain
        (2) Maximal walking distance
    c) Fontaine stage 3—rest pain
      i) Usually nocturnal
      ii) Mainly in the metatarsal and instep area
      iii) Grave's sign: insufficient blood/nutrition for skin
    d) Fontaine stage 4—necrosis and/or gangrene due to total occlusion of below knee vessels (Figure 16.1)

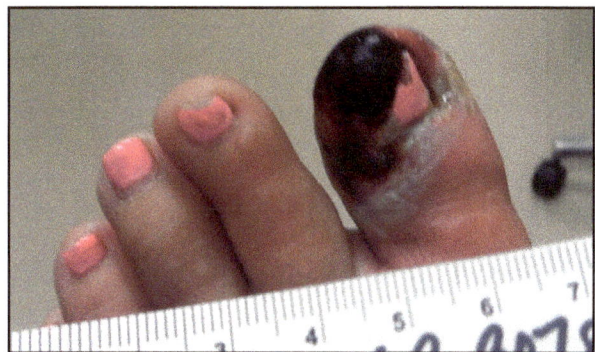

Figure 16.1: Fontaine stage 4—ulceration and gangrene.

Table 16.1: Fontaine stages of peripheral artery occlusive disease.

	FONTAINE		RUTHERFORD		
STAGE	DESCRIPTION	GRADE	CLINICAL FEATURES	OBJECTIVE/CRITERIA	CATEGORY
1	Asymptomatic	0	Asymptomatic No hemodynamically significant diagnosis	Normal treadmill or reactive to hyperemia test	0
2	Intermittent claudication	1	Mild claudication	Completes treadmill exercise, AP after ex >50 mmHg but at least 20 mmHg lower than resting value	1
2	Intermittent claudication	1	Moderate claudication		2
2	Intermittent claudication	1	Severe claudication	Cannot complete treadmill exercise and AP after exercise <50 mmHg	3
3	Ischemic rest pain	2	Ischemic rest pain	Resting AP <40 mmHg, flat or barely pulsatile ankle or metatarsal PVR: TP <40 mmHg	4
4	Ulceration/gangrene	3	Minor tissue loss, non-healing ulcer Focal gangrene with diffuse pedal ischemia	Resting AP <60 mmHg, flat or barely pulsatile ankle or metatarsal PVR: TP <40 mmHg	5
4	Ulceration/gangrene	3	Major tissue loss extending above TM level Functional foot no longer salvageable	Resting AP <60 mmHg, flat or barely pulsatile ankle or metatarsal PVR: TP <40 mmHg	6

E. Physical
1. 5 P's
   a) Pulseless
   b) Pain/numbness
   c) Poikilothermia (coolness)
   d) Pallor
   e) Paresthesia
2. Skin temperature
   a) Cool to touch
      i) Distal cooler than proximal
      ii) Affected side cooler than unaffected side
   b) Warm to touch (normal color)
      i) Good collateral flow
3. Pulses
   a) Simple scale
      i) 0 = absent
      ii) 1+ = palpable, but diminished
      iii) 2+ = normal
   b) Diminished or absent femoral pulses signify aortoiliac occlusive disease
   c) Exaggerated popliteal pulse suggests aneurysm
   d) Dorsalis pedis pulse may be congenitally absent—10%
   e) Posterior tibialis pulse may be congenitally absent—2%
4. Trophic changes (Figure 16.2)
   a) Dry skin
   b) Atrophy of skin and muscles
   c) Loss of distal pulp turgor

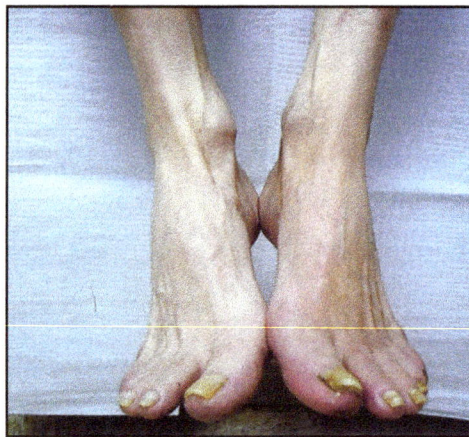

Figure 16.2: Trophic changes.

   d) Absence of hair
   e) Shiny
   f) Dependent rubor and elevation pallor
   g) Cyanosis—more severe, decreased flow
5. Ulcerations in arterial insufficiency patients (Figure 16.3)
   a) Location
      i) Toes, interdigital, heel, lateral malleolus
   b) Appearance
      i) Pale, irregular, dry, poor granulation, necrosis
6. Toenails in arterial insufficiency patients (Figure 16.3)
   a) Hard
   b) Brittle

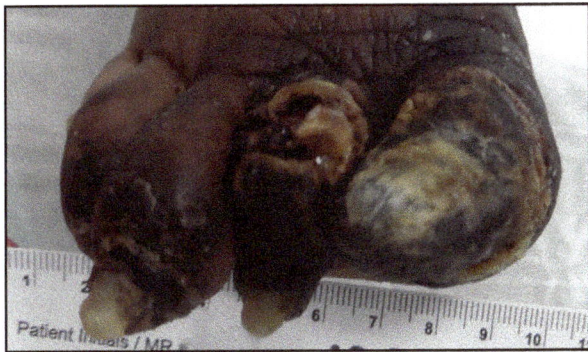

Figure 16.3: Arterial insufficiency.

c) Thickened
d) Ridged
e) Deformed
F. Examine for poor circulation
1. Rubor of dependency
a) Note color of the foot at rest
b) Elevate extremity and hold for 60 seconds. Foot elevation produces skin pallor in patients with ischemic skin (Buerger's sign)
c) Place extremity back on the surface and note time for color to reappear
d) When dependent, the ischemic limb will have a red or ruddy color, which is called dependent rubor or reactive hyperemia (Goldflam's sign)
2. Capillary refill time—rate at which blood refills empty capillaries
a) Press soft pad of finger or toe until it turns white
b) Release pressure and note time for color to return
c) Normal capillary refill time is <3 seconds
3. Claudication—exercise-induced cramping or tiredness of calf, thigh, or buttock
a) Measured by distance
i) Onset of pain
ii) Maximal walking distance
4. Venous filling time
a) Patient should sit up quickly and dangle leg
b) Time the flushing and venous filling of the lower extremities
i) Normal (flush immediate and filling 10 seconds)
ii) Severe ischemia (flush greater than 20 seconds; filling greater than 30 seconds)
5. The paradox of functional microvascular disease
a) A failing pedal wound in a patient with diabetes who has palpable pulses inches away
G. Examine for microvascular disease
1. It is not uncommon for small vessels in the toe to show evidence of ischemia, even though DP/PT pulses are present and adequate.
2. Large and small vessel disease does not progress at the same rate.

II. Noninvasive tests for peripheral artery occlusive disease (PAOD)
A. Common tests
1. Ankle-brachial index (ABI)
2. Doppler studies
3. Magnetic resonance angiography
4. TcPO$_2$
5. Skin perfusion studies
6. Segmental pressures
B. Ankle-brachial index
1. Value interpretation
a) >1.2 = Non-compressible vessels
b) 0.9–1.2 = Normal range
c) 0.75–0.90 = Moderate disease
d) 0.50–0.75 = Severe disease
e) <0.5 = Ischemic gangrene necrosis likely
2. Symptoms associated with ABI
a) 0.6-0.9 = Mild claudication
b) 0.3-0.6 = Severe claudication
c) <0.3 = Rest pain/ischemic ulcer
3. ABI may become abnormal with exercise
C. Toe-brachial index
1. Ratio of toe perfusion pressure (mmHg) to brachial perfusion pressure (mmHg)
a) Normal = >0.7
b) Abnormal = <0.5
2. More accurate than ABI in diabetics with calcified (non-compressible) blood vessels
3. A photoplethysmographic transducer taped to a toe emits infrared light that indicates returning blood flow when an occlusive cuff is released
4. Toe-brachial index interpretation (Table 16.2)

Table 16.2: Toe-brachial index interpretation.

RANGE	INTERPRETATION
>0.7	Normal
0.5–0.7	Mild
0.35–0.5	Moderate
<0.35 and toe pressure 40 mmHg	Moderate–severe
<0.35 and toe pressure <30 mmHg	Severe

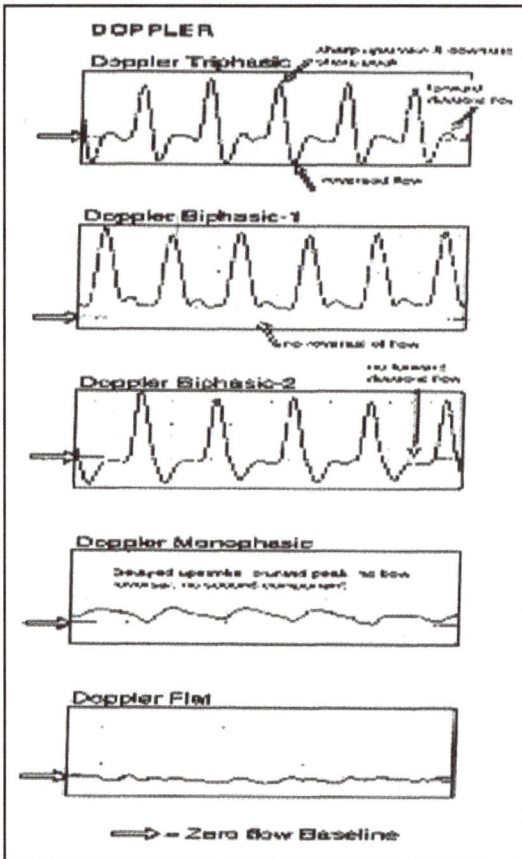

Figure 16.4: Doppler.

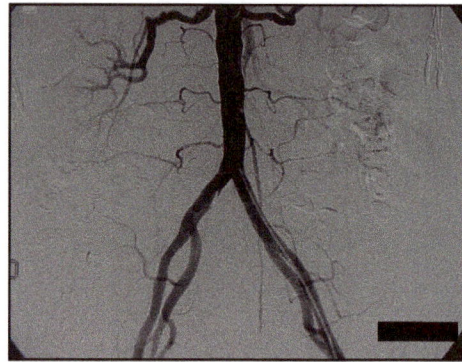

Figure 16.5a: Arteriogram with typical PAD in diabetics showing aortoiliac vessels.

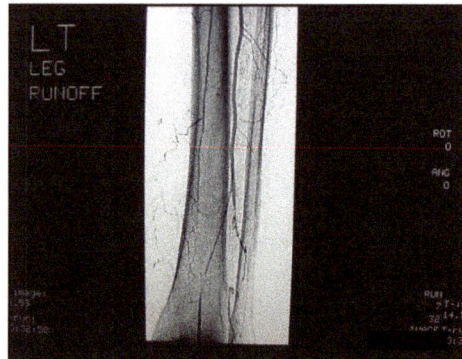

Figure 16.5b: Femoropopliteal artery.

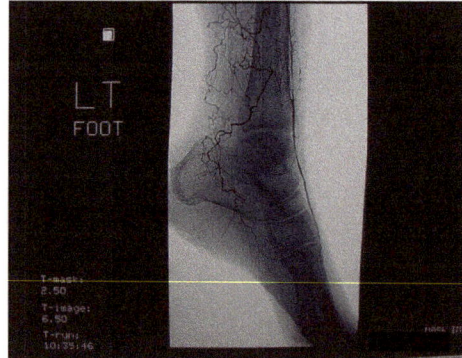

Figure 16.5c: Anterior tibial, posterior tibial, and dorsalis pedis vessels.

D. Doppler (Figure 16.4)
   1. Triphasic (normal)
   2. Biphasic
   3. Monophasic
   4. Blunted
   5. No flow
E. Magnetic resonance arteriography (MRA)
   1. Pros
     a) Less expensive
     b) Noninvasive
     c) No ionizing radiation or dye
   2. Cons
     a) Artifacts
     b) Pacemaker, orbital metallic foreign body (FB) contraindicated
F. Arteriogram (Figures 16.5a–16.5c)
   1. Gold standard
   2. Ordered prior to all vascular surgery
   3. Potential complications
     a) Dye allergies
     b) Renal disease
   4. Difference between diabetic and non-diabetic vascular disease (Table 16.3)

Table 16.3: Diabetic vs. non-diabetic vascular disease.

	DIABETIC	NON-DIABETIC
Clinical	More common, affects younger patients	Less common, affects older patients
Male/female	M = F	M > F
Occlusion	Multisegmental	Single segment
Lower extremities	Both	Unilateral
Vessels involved	Tibial/peroneal	Aortic, iliac, femoral

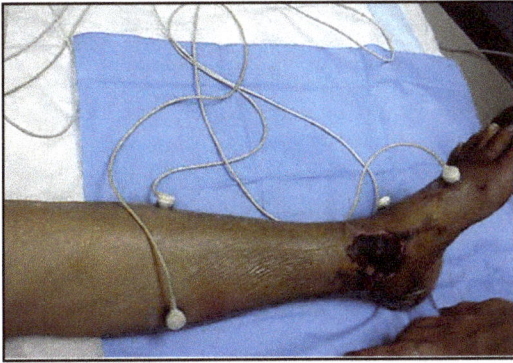

Figure 16.6: Transcutaneous tissue oxygen studies.

G. Transcutaneous oximetry ($TcPO_2$) (Figure 16.6)
1. Advantages
   a) Physiologic measurement
   b) Painless
   c) Better predictor of healing than Doppler
   d) Cheap, fast
   e) Can calculate an index using peripheral/chest value
2. Disadvantages
   a) Not anatomic
   b) Not commonly available
   c) Gross measurement (influenced by infection, edema, volume, etc.)
   d) Cannot be used on toes or plantar feet
3. Reasons for $TcPO_2$ studies
   a) Evaluate arterial status
   b) Evaluate for wound healing potential
   c) Predict amputation level healing
   d) Predict efficacy of HBOT
4. $TcPO_2$ criteria for diagnosis of critical limb ischemia
   a) Ankle systolic pressure less than 60 mmHg
   b) Supine $TcPO_2$ less than 10-15 mmHg
   c) Dependent $TcPO_2$ less than 40-45 mmHg
5. How to use oximetry as an aid to assess wound healing potential and select HBOT candidates (9)
   a) Questions
      i) Is wound healing complicated by severe hypoxia?
         (1) Hypoxia exists if there is a baseline air value of <40 mmHg.
         (2) Thirty-eight studies since 1982 suggest that hypoxia sufficient to impair or prevent wound healing is defined as $TcPO_2$ <40 mmHg.
         (3) Find the degree of hypoxia (Table 16.4).

Table 16.4: Degrees of hypoxia.

$TcPO_2$	ASSESSMENT
>40 mmHg	Adequate for healing
21-40 mmHg	Moderate hypoxia
0-20 mmHg	Severe hypoxia

   b) Does the patient's wound respond to respired oxygen?
      i) 100% oxygen challenge.
      ii) For hypoxia to be considered reversible and the patient considered a possible candidate for HBOT treatments, oxygen tensions should reach at least 40 mmHg and the percent change from baseline should be at least 50%.
      iii) If either of these conditions is not met, then the probability of success is low.
   c) Does the patient's wound site respond to hyperbaric oxygen?
      i) HBO values should rise above normobaric oxygen values and should achieve >200 mmHg (some hyperbaricists use >100 mmHg).
      ii) In-chamber TCOM is the best single predictor of healing.
         (1) In-chamber <100 mmHg: only 18% benefitted
         (2) In-chamber 490-700 mmHg: 78.3% benefitted
         (3) Despite an air TCOM of <20 mmHg, 64% (164/256) of patients were helped (this may demonstrate the efficacy of HBOT)
   e) Is the patient's wound at the point where it will heal without further HBOT?
      i) Repeat $TcPO_2$ evaluation on air at 1 atm abs at 3-4 week intervals.
      ii) Baseline values should be normal (>40 mmHg) when healing process is in place.

III. Medical intervention for PAD
A. Lifestyle modification
   1. Smoking cessation
   2. Exercise
   3. Lipoprotein and cholesterol modification
B. Medications
   1. Aspirin (antiplatelet effect)
   2. Pletal (cilostazol)
      a) Decreases platelet aggregation
      b) Acts as a vasodilator
      c) May facilitate an increase in exercise capacity
      d) Cannot be used in patients with heart failure
   3. Plavix (clopidogrel)
      a) Inhibits the binding of adenosine triphosphate (ATP)
      b) Antiplatelet effect
      c) Slightly better than aspirin in comparative study

IV. Surgical intervention for PAD

A. Endarterectomy and bypass.

B. Aortobifemoral bypass has long term records for occlusive disease of aorta and iliac arteries.

C. Bypass utilizing autogenous vein is preferred reconstruction for femoral, popliteal, and tibial occlusive disease (prosthetic materials are used when vein is not available).

D. Endovascular procedures including balloon angioplasty, stenting, atherectomy, and thrombolysis.
   1. More successful for focal stenoses in larger vessels with good runoff

V. Hyperbaric oxygen therapy (HBOT)

A. UHMS Definition: use of 100% oxygen at pressures greater than 1.0 atm abs. Current information indicates that pressurization should be at least 1.4 atm abs.

B. HBOT is adjunctive therapy to
   1. Surgical debridement
   2. Local wound care
   3. Antibiotic therapy
   4. Establishment of adequate blood flow
   5. Off-loading

VI. Pathway for Arterial Ulcer Management
(Refer to Chapter 32, Pathway 9, page 298)

RESOURCES

1. McCulloch JM, Kloth LC, Feedar JA. *Wound Healing Alternatives in Management*. 2nd ed. Philadelphia: F.A. Davis Company; 1995.

2. Sheffield PJ, Fife CE (editors). *Wound Care Practice*. 2nd ed. North Palm Beach: Best Publishing Company; 2007.

3. Chaurasia BD. *B.D. Chaurasia's Handbook of General Anatomy*. New Delhi: CBS Publishers & Distributors; 1985.

4. Moore KL, Dalley AF. *Clinically Oriented Anatomy*. Philadelphia: Lippincott Williams & Wilkins; 1999.

5. Krasner DL, Rodeheaver GT, Sibbold RG. *Chronic Wound Care*. Malvern: HMP Communications; 2001.

6. Bowker JH, Pfeifer MA. *Levin and O'Neal's The Diabetic Foot*. St. Louis: Mosby; 2001.

7. Scheffler A et al. Influence of clinical findings, positional maneuvers, and systolic ankle arterial pressure on $TcPO_2$ in PAOD. *Eur J F Clin Invest*. 1992; 22:420-6.

8. Sheffield PJ. Measuring tissue oxygen tension: a review. *Undersea Hyperb Med*. 1998; 25(3):179-88.

9. Dietz D, Sheffield PJ. Non-invasive wound assessment tools. In: Sheffield PJ, Fife CE, editors. *Wound Care Practice*. 2nd ed. North Palm Beach: Best Publishing Company; 2007: 129-74.

10. Fife CE, Buyukcakir C, Otto, GH, et al. The predictive value of transcutaneous oxygen tension measurement in diabetic lower extremity ulcers treated with hyperbaric oxygen therapy: a retrospective analysis of 1,144 patients. *Wound Repair Regen*. 2002; 10:198-207.

11. Fife CE, Smart DR, Sheffield PJ, et al. Transcutaneous oximetry in clinical practice: consensus statements from an expert panel based on evidence. *Undersea Hyperb Med*. 2009; 36(1):43-53.

SAMPLE QUESTIONS

1. A 48-year-old male with a history of third toe gangrene subsequent to a vascular bypass and third toe amputation is not healing at the amputation site. The patient's $TcPO_2$, taken post-amputation, shows an average oxygen value of 20 mmHg at the transmetatarsal level with a good response to 100% oxygen. This indicates the patient has:
   a) Small vessel disease
   b) Macrovascular disease
   c) Normal circulation
   d) Either a or b

2. A 48-year-old male with type 2 DM comes in for evaluation of a non-healing wound. The patient's ABI shows a value >1.2 on both legs. This is because the patient has:
   a) Normal circulation
   b) Small vessel disease
   c) Calcified vessels
   d) Large vessel disease

3. All of the following are risk factors for PAD except:
   a) Smoking
   b) Diabetes
   c) Thrombocytopenia
   d) Hyperlipidemia

4. An 87-year-old diabetic male with non-healable gangrenous ulcers in multiple toes in both extremities due to inadequate blood flow should have local wound care that includes:
   a) Negative pressure wound therapy
   b) Compression therapy
   c) Aggressive local debridement to bleeding tissue
   d) Local antiseptics such as a povidone iodine and chlorhexidine

5. Surgical interventions for arterial ulcers include all of the following except:
   a) Endarterectomy
   b) Valvuloplasty
   c) Femoropopliteal bypass and distal bypass
   d) Aortobifemoral bypass

6. Which of the following signs is associated with arterial ulcers?
   a) Goldflam's sign
   b) Homan's sign
   c) Stemmer's sign
   d) Buerger's sign
   e) Both a and d

7. Arterial ulcers are most likely associated with:
   a) Spider veins
   b) Lipodermatosclerosis
   c) Dependent rubor
   d) Edema

8. All of the following drugs have been shown to be effective in the medical treatment of patients with arterial disease except:
   a) Pentoxifylline
   b) Aspirin
   c) Cilostazol
   d) Clopidogrel

9. All of the following statements about cilostazol are accurate except:
   a) It decreases platelet aggregation.
   b) It acts as a vasodilator.
   c) It may facilitate an increase in exercise capacity.
   d) It can be safely used in patients with heart failure.

10. Clopidogrel was found to be better than which of these drugs in the treatment of arterial disease?
    a) Aspirin
    b) Pentoxifylline
    c) Cilostazol
    d) None of the above

See answers on page 139.

NOTES

ANSWER KEY

1. d) According to the UHMS consensus statement, a TcPO$_2$ of less than 40 mmHg is considered hypoxic, which may indicate arterial disease. A patient with hypoxia may have small vessel disease or large vessel disease but will usually not have normal circulation.

2. c) ABIs are not reliable in patients with diabetes because of calcified vessels. ABI of >1.2 indicates noncompressible vessels secondary to calcified vessels in a diabetic patient.

3. c) Risk factors for PAD include smoking, diabetes, thrombocytosis (not thrombocytopenia), and hyperlipidemia.

4. d) In patients with non-healable gangrenous ulcers where arterial flow cannot be improved, it is appropriate to use local antiseptics such as a povidone iodine and chlorhexidine. Negative pressure wound therapy is contraindicated in nondebrided wounds with 100% gangrenous tissue. Compression therapy is not indicated in patients with arterial disease where arterial flow cannot be improved. Aggressive local debridement in patients with no arterial flow could possibly make the wound worse.

5. b) Surgical interventions of arterial ulcers include endarterectomy, aortobifemoral bypass, distal bypass, and femoropopliteal bypass. Valvuloplasty is not a surgical procedure for patients with arterial ulcers.

6. e) Buerger's sign is when foot elevation produces skin pallor in patients with ischemic skin. Goldflam's sign is when the ischemic limb in dependent position has a red or ruddy color, which is also called dependent rubor or reactive hyperemia. Both Beurger's sign and Goldflam's sign are used to diagnose arterial disease. Stemmer's sign is used to diagnose lymphedema, and Homan's sign is used to diagnose deep venous thrombosis.

7. c) Arterial ulcers are most likely associated with dependent rubor. Lipodermatosclerosis, spider veins, and edema are associated with venous stasis ulcers.

8. a) Pentoxifylline was found to be as good as a placebo in treating arterial disease. Aspirin, clopidogrel, and cilostazol all have been shown to be effective in the medical treatment of patients with arterial disease.

9. d) Cilostazol should not be used in patients with congestive heart failure as it decreases platelet aggregation, acts as a vasodilator, and may facilitate an increase in exercise capacity.

10. a) In a comparative study, clopidogrel was found to be slightly better than aspirin in the treatment of arterial disease.

BURNS 17

Rasa Silenas, MD

INTRODUCTION

The burn wound is a complex injury that results in over 40,000 hospitalizations and 3,400 deaths in the United States annually. This chapter will address burn mechanisms and incidence rates, victim demographics, the rule of nines, phases of burn management, surgical burn management, IV resuscitation, wound management by degree of burn, and high-risk anatomical areas for burns.

OBJECTIVES

Participants should be able to define first-, second-, third-, and fourth-degree burns; list conditions for which patients require admission to a burn center; list three high risk burn areas on the body; and discuss when cellular and/or tissue based products (CTPs) are appropriate to use in burn management.

I. Mechanisms and incidence rate (2)

A. Thermal burns
1. Flame—most common type, 44%
2. Scald—33%
3. Contact—e.g., irons, radiators, melted plastics, 9%
B. Electrical burns—4%
C. Chemical burns—3% (be alert for eye burns) (Figures 17.1a–17.1c)

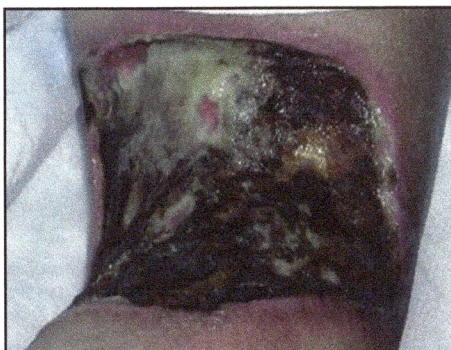

Figure 17.1a: Initial presentation of a patient with an IV infiltration of dopamine, causing chemical burns.

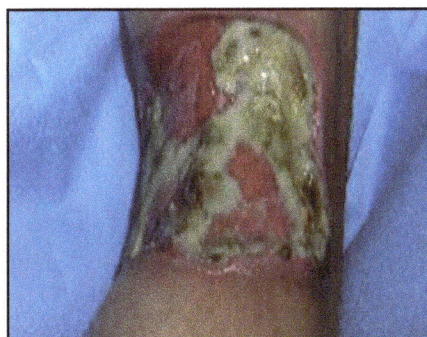

Figure 17.1b: Two weeks after enzymatic debridement and HBOT.

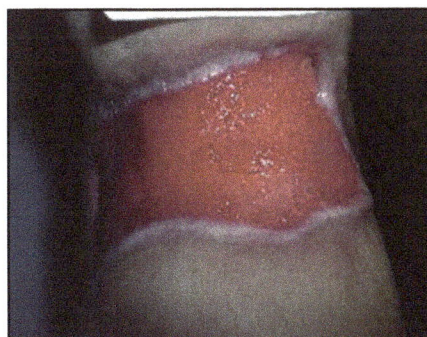

Figure 17.1c: Six weeks after enzymatic debridement and HBOT.

D. Radiation burns (solar—sunburn; ionizing) (Figure 17.2)

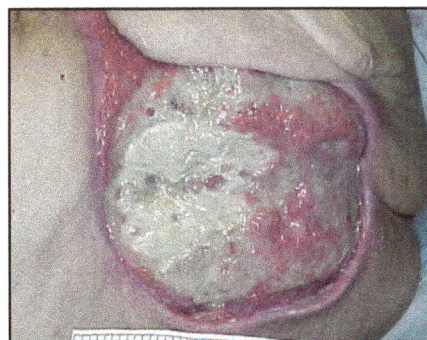

Figure 17.2: Radiation injury on the sacral region after radiation therapy for uterine cancer.

E. Depths
  1. First-degree burn: epidermal (painful, red, unblistered; not associated with major metabolic insult; not counted in burn surface area assessment) (Figure 17.3).

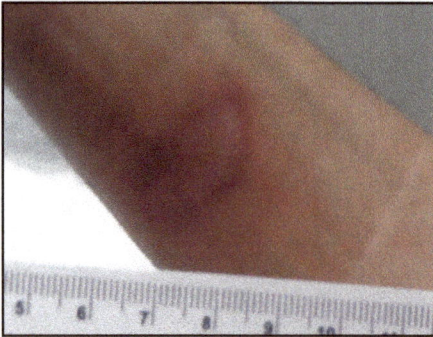

Figure 17.3: First-degree burn on right arm with redness and blistering.

  2. Second-degree burn: dermal (painful, red, blistered; healing potential depends on depth of dermal injury and presence of dermal appendages, e.g., hair follicles, sweat glands) (Figure 17.4). Superficial second-degree burns heal in two to three weeks with relatively little scarring. Deep partial-thickness burns take >3 weeks to heal and may scar heavily. These may be hard to differentiate from third-degree burns.

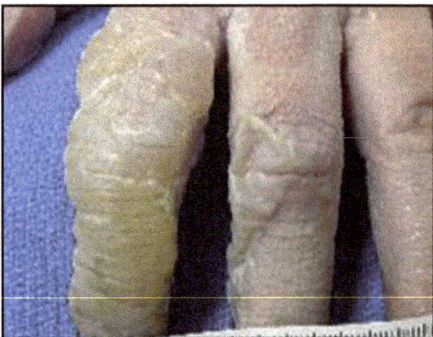

Figure 17.4: Second-degree burn.

  3. Third-degree burn: full skin thickness (often not painful due to destruction of nerve receptors); skin is dry, leathery, possibly charred (inelastic—may cause compartment syndrome or restrict respirations; surgical resurfacing required) (Figures 17.5a and 17.5b).
  4. Fourth-degree burn: extension into muscle and bone (surgical reconstruction required) (Figure 17.6).
F. Zones (4)
  1. Zone of coagulation—irreversibly nonviable tissue.
  2. Zone of ischemia—periwound tissue at risk for progression to irreversible damage due to circulatory impairment by edema or release of inflammatory factors from zone of coagulation.
  3. Zone of hyperemia—surrounding tissues without injury, which become hyperemic but will survive.

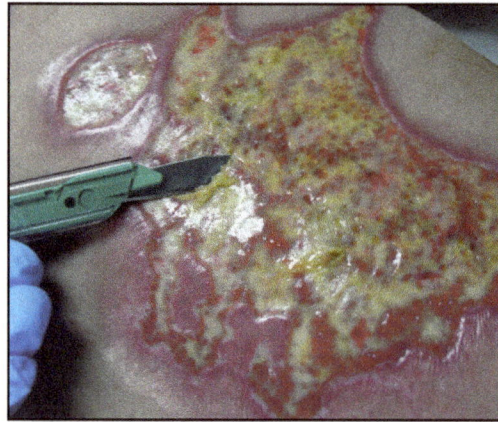

Figure 17.5a: Third-degree burns.

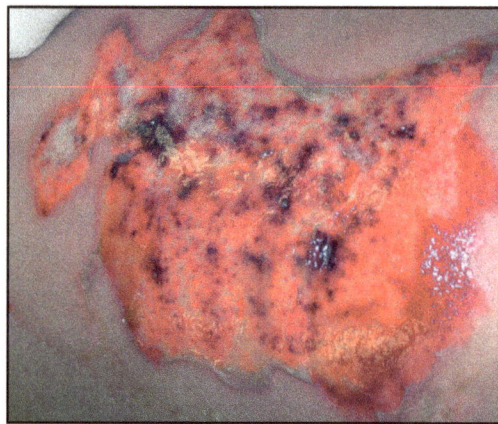

Figure 17.5b: Third-degree burns post-debridement.

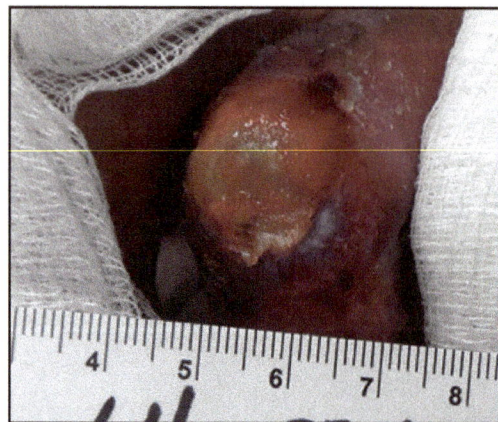

Figure 17.6: A fourth-degree burn of the fourth finger, involving the proximal interphalangeal joint, in a diabetic patient. This wound will require amputation of the finger.

G. Classification by total body surface area (TBSA)
  1. Of all reported admissions, 4% are for burns >40% TBSA (2)
  2. Rule of nines (6) (Figure 17.7)

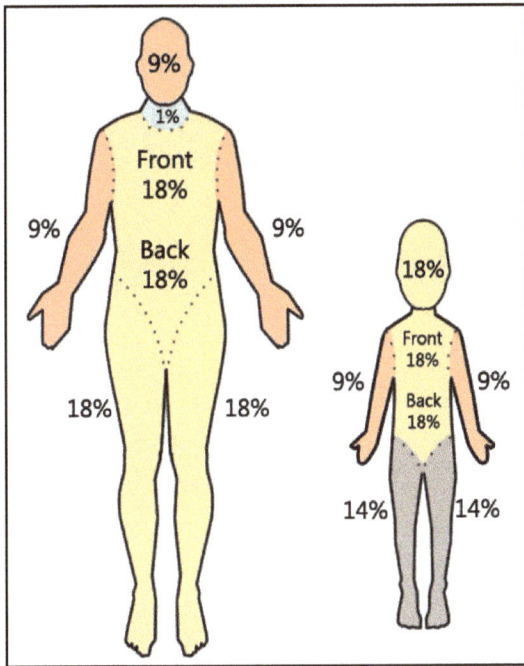

Figure 17.7: Rule of nines; adult body (left) and child's body (right).

II. Demographics

A. 450,000 burns receive medical treatment each year in the United States (1)
B. Annual burn deaths: 3,400 (2)
C. Hospitalizations: 40,000/year (30,000/year to burn centers)
   1. Survival of admitted burns overall >95%
D. Gender: 69% male
E. Ethnicity: 59% Caucasian, 20% African American, 14% Hispanic
F. Causes (all age groups): flame 43%, scald 34%, electrical 4%, other 19%
   1. Scalds predominate in children <5 years old (1)
G. Place of injury: home 72%, job 9%, other 19% (2)
H. Age distribution and risks (1)
   1. Highest incidence: working-age males (20-60 years old)
   2. Highest mortality: risk of death from major burns increases sharply in patients over 50 years old and inpatients with inhalation injury
I. Factors affecting severity
   1. Skin thickness—same burn thickness (in mm) in children and elderly results in deeper layers than in younger adults
   2. Strength/agility—ability to escape
   3. Fluid volume—smaller bodies with lower blood volume are more vulnerable to fluid loss
   4. Underlying medical conditions may complicate burn management
J. Patients requiring burn center admission (3)
   1. Need for IV resuscitation
      a) Burns >10% TBSA

2. Special nursing needs
   a) Face/neck
   b) Hands/feet
   c) Perineum
   d) Children requiring qualified personnel or equipment not available in referring facility
3. Need for surgery or specialized hospital care
   a) Full-thickness burns requiring grafting
   b) Associated injuries requiring hospital care
4. Concurrent medical conditions as cause of burn injury, e.g., stroke while smoking
5. Concurrent medical conditions complicating burn care, e.g., diabetes, asthma, immune compromise
6. Inhalation injury or other respiratory compromise
7. Electrical burns, including lightning
   a) Possible cardiac and/or neurological injury
   b) Possible extensive muscle/visceral injury without visible skin injury
   c) Possible compartment syndrome
8. Chemical burns
   a) May involve systemic toxicity
   b) Severity may not be initially visible
9. Possible child or elder abuse

III. Phases
A. Emergent
   1. Stop burning process
   2. Ensure airway—breathing—circulation (ABC)
   3. Establish IV access
   4. Estimate burn surface area
   5. Baseline weight and vital signs
   6. Escharotomy as needed
B. Acute
   1. Transfer to burn center as needed
   2. Respiratory and circulatory support; consider CO poisoning and inhalation injury
   3. Surgical debridement and reconstruction
   4. Nutritional support
C. Rehabilitation
   1. Range of motion exercise and preservation of muscle tone
   2. Scar management
      a) Compression garments, splints, silicone sheets
   3. Psychological and social support

IV. Surgical management in burns
A. Escharotomy
   1. For constriction of circulation or respiratory excursion by circumferential full-thickness burns; may be performed at bedside without need of anesthetic
B. Fasciotomy
   1. Indicated for compartment syndrome from deep tissue burns, associated trauma, or electrical injury
   2. Split-thickness skin grafts and flaps (refer to Chapter 22, pages 195-196)

V. IV resuscitation

A. Considerations
1. Initiate fluid resuscitation promptly to avoid shock. (4)
   a) Third space losses are greatest in the first 12 hours.
   b) Need at least one large bore IV—beware of dislodgement by edema.
   c) Use warmed fluids to prevent hypothermia.
   d) Weigh the patient on admission, if possible.
   e) Monitor the patient's vital signs, urine, and nasogastric output closely.
2. Parkland formula (4)
   a) Ringer's lactate 4 ml/kg/% TBSA, administer half in first eight hours after injury, half in the next 16 hours
   b) Monitor and modify according to urine output and vital signs
3. Other formulae used at some centers to reduce edema in high-volume resuscitations
   a) PlasmaLyte®
   b) Hypertonic saline
   c) Albumin
   d) Dextran

VI. Top five acute complications of major burns (2)

A. Pneumonia
B. Cellulitis
C. Urinary tract infection
D. Respiratory failure
E. Wound infection

VII. Wound management

A. Second degree: superficial dermal injury
1. Leave intact blisters alone unless they interfere with movement.
2. Cleanse and debride broken blisters.
3. Apply nonadherent dressing or cellular and/or tissue based products (CTPs).
4. On hands, face, and perineum, apply a water-soluble topical antibiotic.
B. Second degree: deep dermal injury
1. May not blister; hard to distinguish from full thickness burn.
2. Cleanse and apply silver product with bulky nonadherent dressing.
3. Candidate for CTPs.
4. Candidate for surgical grafting.
C. Third degree
1. Cleanse, apply silver product and bulky dressing
2. Early surgical debridement and grafting
3. CTPs if grafting must be delayed

VIII. Topical agents

A. Silver preparations are the most commonly used topical burn care agents (8)
1. Silver sulfadiazine cream
   a) Broad spectrum bactericidal activity against burn pathogens
   b) Soothing vehicle
   c) Not for use in pregnant women, newborns, or sulfa-allergic patients
2. Mafenide
   a) Better penetration of eschar
   b) Carbonic anhydrase inhibitor: monitor acid-base balance
B. Antibiotic ointments: suitable for minor burns
1. Bacitracin
2. Triple antibiotic ointment
3. Gentamycin
4. Mupirocin—reserve for confirmed methicillin resistant staphylococcal infection
C. Home remedies (5)
1. Aloe vera
2. Honey
3. Butter (oils should not be used)

IX. Cellular and/or tissue based products (CTPs) (4,7)

A. Temporary wound covers
1. Types
   a) Human donor skin
   b) Animal skin (typically frozen pig skin)
   c) Combination biological/bioengineered products
2. Advantages over dressings
   a) Reduce fluid and thermal loss
   b) Reduce bacterial contamination
   c) May provide healing properties
   d) May deliver wound healing factors
3. Indications
   a) Indeterminate depth burns, especially in specialized tissues
   b) Wounds too extensive to be covered in one stage by available autogenous skin grafts
   c) Uncertain viability of debrided burn bed
   d) Suspected infection of burn bed

X. High-risk areas

A. Face/neck
1. Be especially alert for eye injury and airway compromise.
2. Use a conservative approach to debridement to preserve specialized tissues.
3. Manage with a topical antibiotic or silver agent with or without dressing.
4. Avoid pressure on the cartilage of ears and nose.
5. CTPs are valuable resources.
6. Pay attention to splinting and compression to minimize contractures.

B. Hands/feet
   1. Palms and soles are less likely to need surgical resurfacing due to thickness.
   2. Wrap digits separately to prevent adhesions.
   3. Consider CTPs for pain control.
   4. Elevate for edema control.
   5. Use aggressive splinting and range of motion exercises to prevent contractures.
   6. May need escharotomy or fasciotomy for circumferential injury.
C. Perineum
   1. Edema may interfere with urethral function.
   2. High infection risk
   3. Manage with topical agents with or without loose diaper-type dressing.
   4. Be alert for social factors contributing to injury, e.g., abuse, debility, and dementia.

RESOURCES

1. American Burn Association. National Burn Repository 2012. Report of Data from 2002-2011. Chicago: American Burn Association; 2012. Accessed at: http://www.ameriburn.org/2012NBRAnnualReport.pdf.
2. American Burn Association. Burn Incidence and Treatment in the US: 2013. Fact Sheet. Chicago: American Burn Association; 2013. Accessed at: http://www.ameriburn.org/resources_factsheet.php.
3. American Burn Association. Burn Unit Referral Criteria. Chicago: American Burn Association; 1999. Accessed at: http://www.ameriburn.org/BurnUnitReferral.pdf.
4. Chester NP. Skin substitutes in burn care. *Wounds*. 2003; 20(7):203-5.
5. Cochrane Library. Cochrane & Evidence Aid: resources for burns [Internet]. 2014. Accessed at: http://www.cochranelibrary.com/app/content/special-collections/article/?doi=10.1002/%28ISSN%2914651858%28CAT%29EvidenceAidFreeaccesstoreviews%28VI%29SC000018.
6. Hettiaratchy S, Papini R. Initial management of a major burn: II—assessment and resuscitation. *BMJ*. 2004 Jul 10; 329(7457):101-3.
7. Kagan RJ, Peck MD, et al. Surgical management of the burn wound and use of skin substitutes: an expert panel white paper. *J Burn Care Res.* 2013; 34(2):60-79. Accessed at: http://www.ucdenver.edu/academics/colleges/medicalschool/departments/surgery/divisions/GITES/burn/Documents/American%20Burn%20Association%20White%20Paper.pdf.
8. Silver Sulfadiazine [Internet]. 2014. Accessed at: http://www.drugs.com/monograph/silver-sulfadiazine.html.

SAMPLE QUESTIONS

1. All of the following insults need admission to a burn center except:
   a) A 33-year-old male construction worker with 1% TBSA roofing tar burns to the dorsum of his right foot.
   b) A 2-year-old male with 3% TBSA scald burns in a glove pattern on his right hand and forearm.
   c) A 55-year-old female in good previous health with 20% TBSA burns from a house fire.
   d) A 12-year-old male with a 7% TBSA burn on his chest and upper abdomen from a clothing fire after playing with firecrackers on his driveway.
   e) A 45-year-old male with a <1% TBSA burn on his right index finger tip and a 1% TBSA burn on his left buttock after touching an exposed electrical wire.
   f) An 84-year-old widower living alone with mild dementia with a 4% TBSA grease burn of his left forearm.

2. Cellular and/or tissue based products (CTPs) are appropriate for use in which of the following scenarios?
   a) Managing pain from sunburn in a 16-year-old female
   b) Deep second-degree burns on the face of a 5-year-old female
   c) A lye burn to the perineal area in a 20-year-old schizophrenic male
   d) A third-degree scald burn of the lower abdomen and mons pubis in a 70-year-old female

3. Which of the following topical agents is appropriate for superficial second-degree burns?
   a) Silver sulfadiazine cream
   b) Aloe vera
   c) Honey
   d) Mupirocin ointment

4. Which of the following statements about superficial partial-thickness burns is true?
   a) They appear waxy white.
   b) They are typically painful.
   c) They involve only the epidermis.
   d) They never convert to full-thickness injury.

5. A 60-year-old male with a history of type 2 diabetes mellitus, hypertension, peripheral vascular disease, and end stage renal disease developed hot water burns. The patient underwent complete sloughing of the epidermis and dermis. What degree of burn does this patient have?
   a) First-degree burn
   b) Second-degree burn
   c) Third-degree burn
   d) Fourth-degree burn

6. A healthy 55-year-old female is brought to the emergency room one hour after falling in the shower. She has painful, blanching, unblistered redness (30%) and painful blistering (5%) of her hip and anterior thighs. Appropriate management would be:
   a) Outpatient care with silvadene and nonadherent bulky dressings
   b) Community hospital admission with early excision and CTPs
   c) Burn center referral and resuscitation with Parkland formula
   d) Burn center referral with early excision and skin grafting

7. Which of the following locations is the most likely place for a burn injury to occur?
   a) High school chemistry laboratory
   b) Construction site
   c) Interstate highway
   d) A home kitchen

8. A 48-year-old male who had received a kidney transplant for polycystic kidney disease has a 7% TBSA burn on his chest and arms after his clothing caught fire in a barbecue accident. Where should he be treated?
   a) Home
   b) Community hospital
   c) Burn center
   d) Hospice

9. A 36-year-old male is rescued, unconscious, from his bed by firefighters during a house fire. He is intubated in the field, an intravenous line is inserted, and fluids are started. At the burn center, he is evaluated as having 40% TBSA burns on his torso and legs. The complication for which he is at highest risk is:
   a) Hypovolemic shock
   b) Pneumonia
   c) Wound sepsis
   d) Unrecognized femoral fracture

10. A 25-year-old female spilled a can of paint stripper and cleaned it up without using gloves, washing her hands shortly after. Half an hour later she is experiencing painful, blanching red patches on her palms, dorsal hands, and right cheek, and her right eye is painful and hypersensitive to light. The label on the can shows lye as the principal ingredient. Concerns include all of the following except:
    a) Conjunctival burns
    b) Evolution to a greater depth injury over time
    c) Loss of range of motion in the hand
    d) Compartment syndrome

See answers on page 148.

NOTES

ANSWER KEY

1. d) Burn center referral is indicated for burns >10% TBSA, burns of high risk areas, situations of suspected abuse, or when social factors limit a patient's ability to administer self care. Otherwise, thermal burns of <10% TBSA in noncritical areas can usually be managed in community hospitals or on an outpatient basis.

2. b) Facial burns are often not excised to avoid sacrificing specialized skin. Deep partial-thickness burns may be managed with cellular and/or tissue based products to reduce pain and accelerate healing.

3. a) Silver sulfadiazine cream is one of the most commonly used topical agents for burn care. The use of aloe vera or honey is not supported by evidence. Additionally, mupirocin ointment should be reserved for methicillin-resistant staphylococcal infections.

4. b) Preservation of the dermis in a partial-thickness burn means that sensory innervation is not destroyed.

5. c) Loss of epidermis and dermis is characteristic of a third-degree burn.

6. a) Blanching redness without blisters indicates a first-degree burn, which is not included in calculating TBSA. This patient has a 5% partial-thickness burn, which appears superficial and can be expected to heal in three weeks with topical care.

7. d) More burn injuries occur at home than in any other location.

8. c) The patient taking immunosuppression medications should be managed in a burn center due to his increased risk of infection.

9. b) The complication with the highest incidence in major burn patients is pneumonia.

10. d) Chemical injuries may develop a greater depth of injury than what appears on initial presentation. Splash events may cause burns of the eyes. Hand burns carry a risk of stiffness unless they are properly splinted and managed with range of motion exercises. Compartment syndrome is more characteristic of electrical burns.

PRESSURE ULCER PREVENTION AND SKIN CARE ISSUES 18

Dianne Rudolph, RN, GNP-BC, DNP, CWOCN
Jesse Cantu, RN, BSN, CWS, FACCWS

INTRODUCTION

In order to prevent pressure ulcers it is important to identify patients at risk and select the proper protocol for wound prevention and treatment. Risk of pressure ulcer development can be assessed by the Braden scale, Norton scale, and Waterlow scale. The National Pressure Ulcer Advisory Panel (NPUAP) serves as the authoritative voice for improved patient outcomes in pressure ulcer prevention and treatment. The NPUAP pressure ulcer staging system will be discussed.

OBJECTIVES

Participants should be able to describe three tools for assessing pressure ulcer risk, list six common pressure ulcer sites, and discuss the NPUAP Pressure Ulcer Staging system.

I. Incidence and prevalence of pressure ulcers
A. Scope of the problem varies widely per NPUAP
B. Acute care hospitals
   1. 4.7–32% of hospitalized patients may develop a pressure ulcer. Incidence is higher in ICUs. Overall incidence of new pressure ulcers in acute care is approximately 7%.
   2. Two thirds of hospital-acquired pressure ulcers (HAPUs) occur during the first week of hospitalization in the ICU.
C. Long-term care facilities: 2.3–28% (average 10%) of patients develop pressure ulceration
D. Home care: up to 29% of patients may develop a pressure ulcer
E. 257,412 cases of stage III and IV ulcers per year
F. Pain: pressure ulcers are often associated with severe pain
G. Death: about 60,000 patients die as a direct result of pressure ulcers each year
H. Costs
   1. Monetary cost
      a) Pressure ulcers cost $9.1–11.6 billion per year in the United States.
      b) Cost in individual patient care can range from $20,900 to 151,700 per ulcer.
      c) Medicare estimated that in 2007, each pressure ulcer added $43,180 in costs to a hospital stay.
   2. Non-monetary costs
      a) Emotional and psychological stress
      b) Loss of independence and control
      c) Physical and social stress
      d) Support systems/caregiver fatigue
   3. Cost because of lawsuits
      a) 17,000 lawsuits are related to pressure ulcers yearly.
      b) It is the second most common claim after wrongful death, more prevalent than falls or emotional distress.

II. Pathophysiology
A. Definition of pressure ulcer (NPUAP) (Figure 18.1)

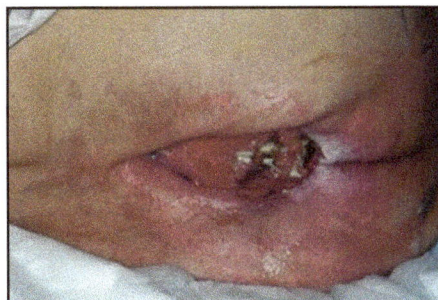

Figure 18.1: Pressure ulcer on buttocks.

   1. Localized injury to the skin and/or underlying tissue is usually over a bony prominence as a result of pressure, or pressure in combination with shear and/or friction. A number of contributing or confounding factors are also associated with pressure ulcers; the significance of these factors is yet to be elucidated (Figure 18.2).
   2. Factors that contribute to pressure ulcer development:
      a) Pressure
      b) Shear
      c) Friction
      d) Moisture

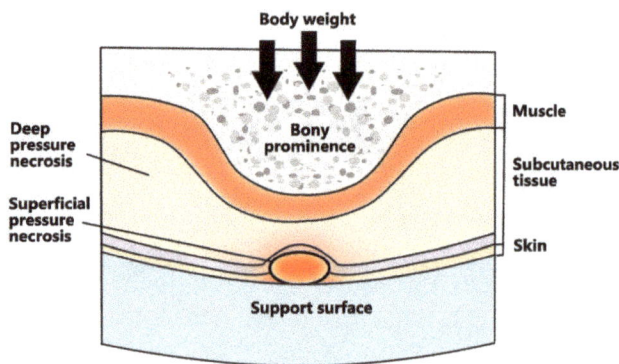

Figure 18.2: Pathophysiology of a pressure ulcer.

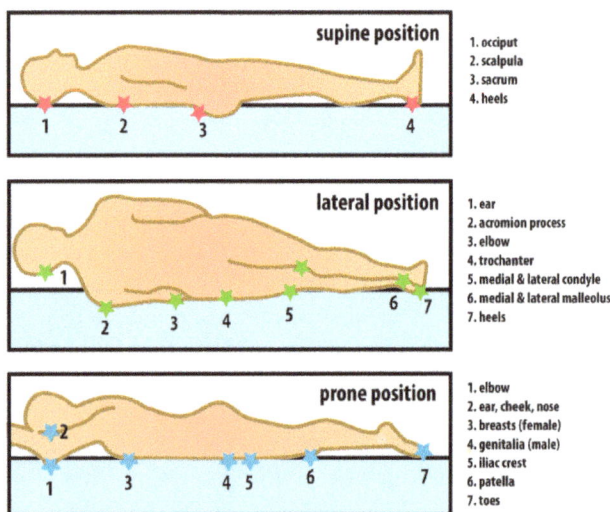

Figure 18.3: Common sites of pressure ulcers.
Adapted from the Tissue Viability Society.

B. Common sites
1. 70% of ulcers in bedbound patients occur in the sacral or heel areas (Figure 18.3).
2. Ischial tuberosities are common ulcer sites in wheelchair-bound patients.

III. Pressure ulcer stages (NPUAP staging definitions)
A. Suspected deep tissue injury (Figures 18.4a and 18.4b)
1. Purple or maroon localized area of discolored intact skin or blood-filled blister due to damage of underlying soft tissue from pressure and/or shear. The area may be preceded by tissue that is painful, firm, mushy, boggy, or warmer or cooler compared to adjacent tissue.
2. Further description: deep tissue injury may be difficult to detect in individuals with dark skin tones. Evolution may include a thin blister over a dark wound bed. The wound may further evolve and become covered by thin eschar. Evolution may be rapid, exposing additional layers of tissue even with optimal treatment.

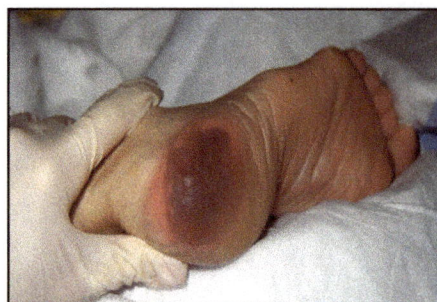

Figure 18.4a: Deep tissue injury on heel.

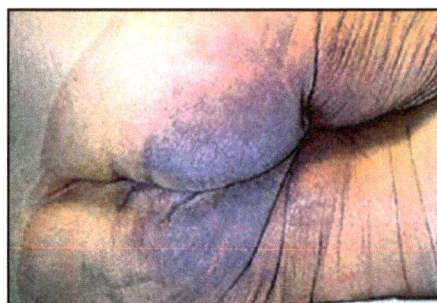

Figure 18.4b: Deep tissue injury on buttocks.

B. Stage I pressure ulcer (Figures 18.5a and 18.5b)
1. Intact skin with non-blanchable redness of a localized area, usually over a bony prominence. Darkly pigmented skin may not have visible blanching; its color may differ from the surrounding area.
2. Further description: the area may be painful, firm, soft, or warmer or cooler as compared to adjacent tissue. Stage I may be difficult to detect in individuals with dark skin tones. May indicate at-risk individuals (a heralding sign of risk).

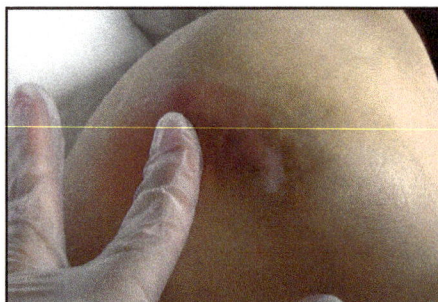

Figure 18.5a: Stage I pressure ulcer; checking for blanching redness on right buttock.

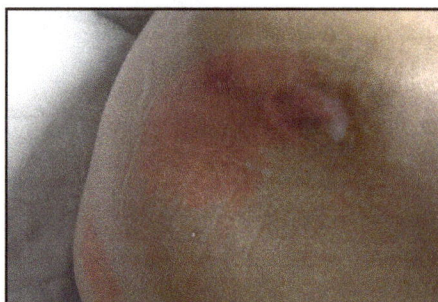

Figure 18.5b: Stage I pressure ulcer above exhibits non-blanchable redness.

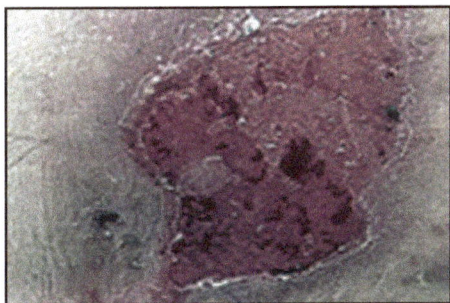
Figure 18.6a: Stage II pressure ulcer on sacrum.

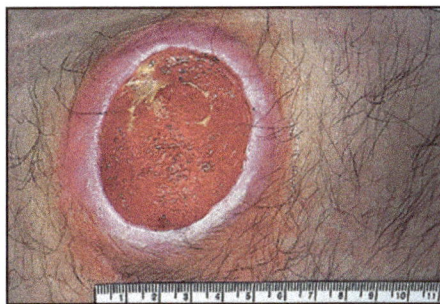
Figure 18.7a: Stage III pressure ulcer on sacrum.

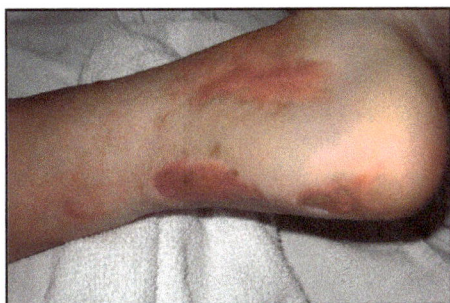
Figure 18.6b: Stage II pressure ulcer on heel.

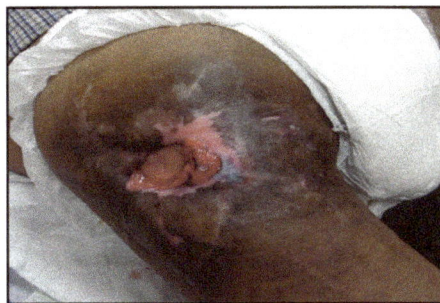
Figure 18.7b: Stage III pressure ulcer on ischium.

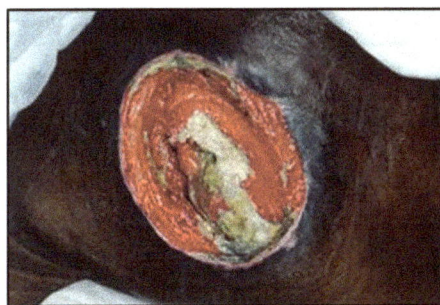
Figure 18.8a: Stage IV pressure ulcer on ischium.

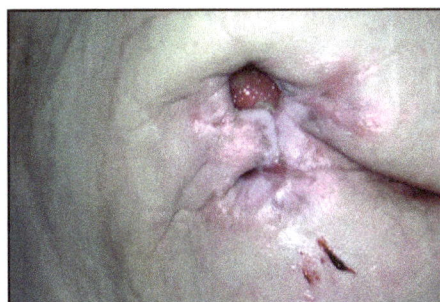
Figure 18.8b: Stage IV pressure ulcer on sacrum and coccyx.

C. Stage II pressure ulcer (Figures 18.6a and 18.6b)
   1. Partial thickness loss of dermis presenting as a shallow open ulcer with a red pink wound bed without slough. May also present as an intact or open/ruptured serum-filled blister.
   2. Further description: presents as a shiny or dry shallow ulcer without slough or bruising. (Bruising indicates suspected deep tissue injury.) This stage should not be used to describe skin tears, tape burns, perineal dermatitis, maceration, or excoriation.

D. Stage III pressure ulcer (Figures 18.7a and 18.7b)
   1. Full-thickness tissue loss. Subcutaneous fat may be visible, but bone, tendon, or muscle is not exposed. Slough may be present but does not obscure the depth of tissue loss. May include undermining and tunneling.
   2. Further description: the depth of a stage III pressure ulcer varies by anatomical location. The bridge of the nose, ear, occiput, and malleolus do not have subcutaneous tissue, and stage III ulcers can be shallow. In contrast, areas of significant adiposity can develop extremely deep stage III pressure ulcers. Bone/tendon is not visible or directly palpable.

E. Stage IV pressure ulcer (Figures 18.8a and 18.8b)
   1. Full-thickness tissue loss with exposed bone, tendon, or muscle. Slough or eschar may be present on some parts of the wound bed; often includes undermining and tunneling.
   2. Further description: the depth of a stage IV pressure ulcer varies by anatomical location. The bridge of the nose, ear, occiput and malleolus do not have subcutaneous tissue, and these ulcers can be shallow. Stage IV ulcers can extend into muscle and/or supporting structures (e.g., fascia, tendon, or joint capsule), making osteomyelitis possible. Exposed bone/tendon is visible or directly palpable.

F. Unstageable pressure ulcer (Figures 18.9a and 18.9b)
   1. Full-thickness tissue loss in which the base of the ulcer is covered by slough (yellow, tan, gray, green, or brown) and/or eschar (tan, brown, or black) in the wound bed.

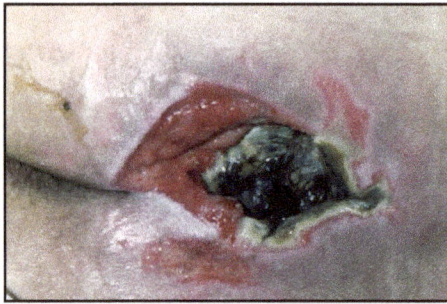

Figure 18.9a: Unstageable ulcer on sacrum.

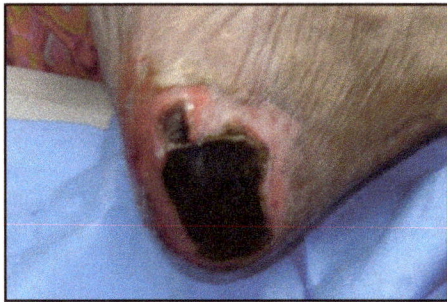

Figure 18.9b: Unstageable ulcer on left heel.

    2. Further description: until enough slough and/or eschar is removed to expose the base of the wound, the true depth (and therefore stage) cannot be determined. Stable (dry, adherent, intact without erythema or fluctuance) eschar on the heels serves as the body's natural biological cover and should not be removed.

G. Limitations of staging
    1. A stage I wound may be superficial or deep.
    2. If the wound base is not visible, it cannot be staged.
    3. Staging is only applicable to pressure ulcers.
    4. Reverse staging should not be used to describe the healing of pressure ulcers.
    5. The body is unable to regenerate certain tissues (fat, fascia, muscle); therefore, reverse staging is inaccurate when used as a parameter for wound healing.

IV. Best practices for pressure ulcer prevention

A. Assessment
    1. There is no universally agreed upon best approach for conducting a risk assessment; however, expert consensus suggests that the approach be structured to facilitate consideration of all relevant risk factors.
B. Identify patients at risk
C. Manage tissue loads/off-loading
D. Friction and shear forces
E. Manage moisture/incontinence
F. Skin care and early treatment
G. Nutrition
H. Host factors/comorbidities
I. Education
J. Team/interdisciplinary approach

V. Risk assessment scales

A. Braden scale
    1. Sensory perception
    2. Activity
    3. Mobility
    4. Skin moisture
    5. Friction and shear
    6. Nutrition
    7. The lower the score, the higher the risk
    8. 18 or less: high risk older adult
    9. Note: if a patient presents with a pressure ulcer, he/she is automatically considered high risk
B. Norton scale
    1. Physical condition
    2. Mental condition
    3. Activity
    4. Mobility
    5. Incontinence
    6. Greater than 18: low risk
    7. Less than 10: very high risk
C. Waterlow scale
    1. Build
    2. Skin type
    3. Sex
    4. Malnutrition screening
    5. Continence
    6. Mobility
    7. Tissue malnutrition/neurological deficit/trauma/surgery
    8. Score of 10: at risk
    9. Score of 20: high risk
D. Conclusion
    1. According to Pancorbo-Hidalgo et al.(1), of these scales, the Braden scale has the best validity and reliability indicators across numerous studies and settings. Both the Braden and Norton scales predict pressure ulcer development better than nurses' clinical judgment. The Waterlow scale is highly sensitive but does not predict pressure ulcer development. The use of such a scale may improve preventative intervention but may not decrease pressure ulcer incidence.

VI. Manage tissue loads

A. Positioning and turning: 30/30 rule; avoid head of bed (HOB) elevation >30 degrees, and do not turn more than 30 degrees side to side.
    1. To decrease friction and shear, the head of the bed should normally be maintained at 30 degrees, except when the patient eating, at which time it is raised to approximately 90 degrees to prevent aspiration. Keeping the patient in an upright position puts pressure on the coccyx, diminishing blood flow—a key ingredient in skin breakdown. When turning side to side, the angle should also be only 30 degrees. Propping patients too far on their sides creates pressure points on the hip and trochanter.

B. Pillows/bolsters as needed: separate bone from bone and skin from skin
C. Use of draw sheets
D. Trapezes if indicated
E. Support surfaces
   1. Group 1, if at risk: multilayer foam
   2. Group 2 for multiple stage II ulcers
   3. Low air loss mattress (Figure 18.10), alternating pressure pads, ROHO cushions for stage III or IV pressure ulcers
   4. Air fluidized therapy: works through immersion (Figure 18.11)
   5. Continue to turn and reposition the individual regardless of the support surface in use
   6. Establish turning frequency based on the characteristics of the support surface and the individual's response
F. Wheelchair cushions
   1. Select a cushion that effectively redistributes the pressure away from the pressure ulcer.

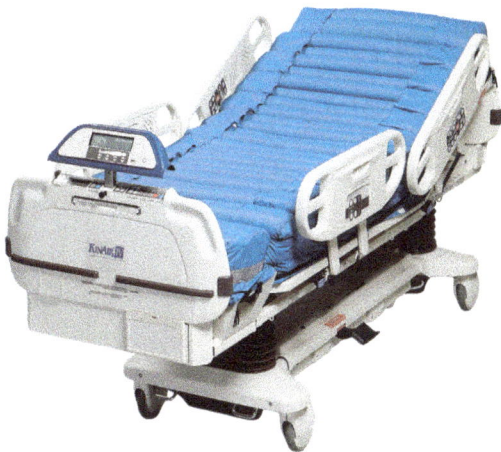

Figure 18.10: KinAir® IV low air loss mattress.
Photo courtesy of ArjoHuntleigh.

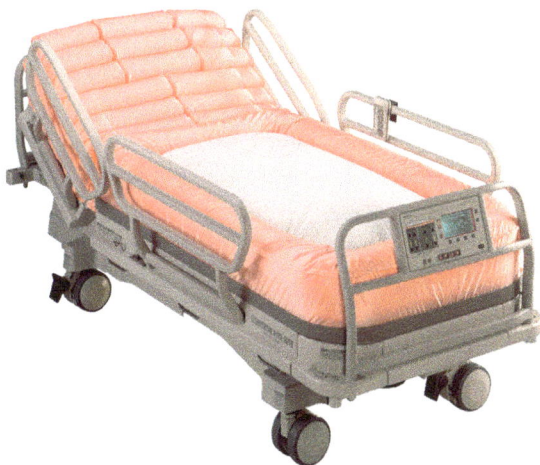

Figure 18.11: Clinitron® Rite Hite® Air Fluidized Therapy Unit. Photo courtesy of Hill-Rom Services, Inc.

   2. Cushion construction achieves pressure redistribution in one of two basic methods: immersion/envelopment or redirection/off-loading.
   3. Some options include foams, gels, low air loss, and pillows.
   4. Do not use donuts.
G. Heels
   1. Heels are subject to pressure ulcer development even with a support surface.
   2. Heel protectors may offer a false sense of security.
   3. Heel flotation is the goal.
   4. Use heel suspension devices that elevate and off-load the heel completely in such a way as to distribute the weight of the leg along the calf without placing pressure on the Achilles tendon.
H. Managing tissue load in patients with medical devices
   1. Consider adults with medical devices to be at risk for pressure ulcers.
   2. Oxygen tubing/masks, splints, casts, antithrombic devices, and compression hose can contribute to the formation of pressure ulcers.
   3. Ensure proper fit of device and monitor for excessive moisture, edema, or early signs of tissue injury.
I. Medically unpreventable pressure ulcers
   1. Kennedy ulcer—a pressure ulcer that some people get as they are dying, usually within the last 8-12 hours of life (Figure 18.12).

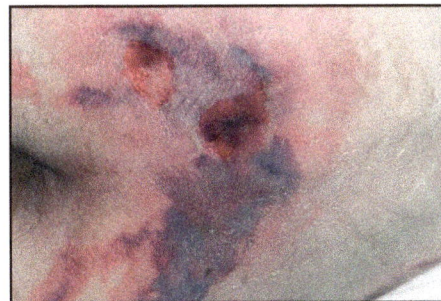

Figure 18.12: Kennedy ulcer.

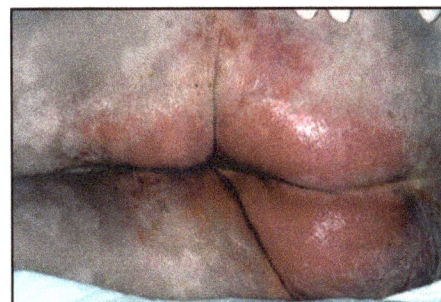

Figure 18.13: Skin irritation from moisture/incontinence.

J. Moisture/incontinence (Figure 18.13)
   1. Toileting programs as indicated
   2. Foley: document rationale
   3. Frequent perineal care and use of moisture barriers: zinc oxide, dimethicone, petrolatum, or combination of trypsin/balsam peru (Xenaderm™)

4. Breathable pads, minimize diapers in bed
5. Treat intertriginous areas: topical antifungals
6. Evaluate need for colostomy or urostomy
K. Nutrition
   1. Protein-energy malnutrition: increased protein turn-over, protein deficiency, decreased caloric intake, and increased caloric needs due to stress or illness can lead to unintentional weight loss and skin break-down.
   2. Elderly patients are at greatest risk for nutritional issues and pressure ulcer because of:
     a) Decreased lean body mass
     b) Decreased skin elasticity
     c) Loss of subcutaneous fat cushion
     d) Dental issues
     e) Dysphagia
     f) Anorexia of aging
     g) Cognitive decline
     h) Polypharmacy
     i) Social factors
   3. Physical assessment (refer to Chapter 12)
   4. Nutritional assessment (refer to Chapter 12)
     a) Check anthropometrics, BMI
     b) Calorie count, dietary recall, food preferences
     c) Prealbumin and albumin, BMP
   5. Nutritional therapy and supplementation (refer to Chapter 12)
     a) Provide 30 to 35 kcalories/kg body weight for adults at risk of a pressure ulcer who are assessed as being at risk of malnutrition.
     b) 1.5 g/kg body weight of protein
     c) Vitamin C, zinc, etc.
L. Manage host factors
   1. Comorbid conditions
   2. Diabetes
   3. Anemia
   4. Peripheral vascular disease
   5. Venous disease
   6. Insensate/limited mobility
   7. Medications: anticoagulants, steroids, NSAIDs
   8. Obesity/malnutrition
   9. Psychosocial
   10. Infection/sepsis
   11. Immunosuppression
   12. Pain
   13. Microclimate
M. Education
   1. Team approach: physician, NP, PA, WOCN, RN, LVN, CNA, RD, PT/OT, case management, administration
   2. Ongoing assessment of learning needs
   3. Ongoing education (NPUAP curriculum for pressure ulcer prevention and treatment)
   4. Present on admission: critical for both physicians and nursing
   5. Staff education on staging
   6. Common vocabulary and language
   7. Use standardized forms for documentation
   8. Establish consistent methods of communication
   9. Information sharing/networking: what works in other facilities/settings?
   10. Risk assessment tools (i.e., Braden scale) upon admission and at routine intervals
   11. Comprehensive assessment tools, flow charts or algorithms, bundles, or mnemonics
   12. Measurement/quantification of wound healing progress (PUSH tool—Pressure Ulcer Scale for Healing)
   13. Approach should be systematic
N. Patient education
   1. Easily available generic reading materials
   2. Modify as needed for specific population needs
   3. Multilingual and at appropriate reading level
   4. Involve patient and family in care, including decision making where appropriate
   5. Incorporate culturally sensitive care

RESOURCES

1. Pancorbo-Hidalgo PL, Garcia-Fernandez FP, Lopez-Medina IM, Alvarez-Nieto C. Risk assessment scales for pressure ulcer prevention: a systematic review. *J Adv Nurs*. 2006; 54(1):94-110.

2. Reddy M, et al. Preventing pressure ulcers: a systematic review. *JAMA*. 2006; 296(8):974-84.

3. Fife CE. Pressure ulcers: towards a new understanding of an old problem. In: Sheffield PJ, Fife CE, editors. *Wound Care Practice*. 2nd ed. North Palm Beach: Best Publishing Company; 2007: 431-66.

4. Broussard CL. Interventions in managing pressure ulcers. In: Sheffield PJ, Fife CE, editors. *Wound Care Practice*. 2nd ed. North Palm Beach: Best Publishing Company; 2007: 467-84.

5. Stansby G, Avital L, Jones K, Marsden G. Prevention and management of pressure ulcers in primary and secondary care: a summary of NICE guidance. *BMJ*. 2014 Apr 23; 348:g2592 doi: 10.1136/bmj.g2592.

6. AWMA. *Pan Pacific Clinical Practice Guideline for the Prevention and Management of Pressure Injury*. Osborne Park: Cambridge Media; 2012.

7. Are we ready for this? Preventing Pressure ulcers in hospitals: a toolkit for improving quality of care [Internet]. 2014 [cited 2014 Nov 11]. Accessed at: http://www.ahrq.gov/professionals/systems/long-term-care/resources/pressure-ulcers/pressureulcertoolkit/putool1.html.

8. Flike K. Pressure ulcer prevention in the ICU: a case study. *Crit Care Nurs Q*. 2013; 36(4):415-20. DOI: 10.1097/CNQ.0b013e3182a1eae2.

9. National Pressure Ulcer Advisory Panel. NPUAP Prevention and Treatment of Pressure Ulcers: 2014 Clinical Practice Guidelines [Internet]. 2014 [cited 2014 Nov 11]. Accessed at: http://www.npuap.org/resources/educational-and-clinical-resources/prevention-and-treatment-of-pressure-ulcers-clinical-practice-guideline/.

SAMPLE QUESTIONS

1. Pressure reduction can occur by all of the following except:
   a) Turning a patient at least every two hours
   b) Lifting the heels to avoid contact with the surface
   c) Raising the head of the bed to 45 degrees
   d) Placing pillows or wedges between the legs
   e) Positioning the patient

2. The most common pressure ulcer site is the:
   a) Ankle
   b) Elbow
   c) Sacrum
   d) Shoulder

3. The best validity and reliability pressure ulcer risk assessment tool is the:
   a) Braden scale
   b) Norton scale
   c) Waterlow scale

4. Pressure ulcers can occur as a result of which of the following medical devices?
   a) Casts
   b) Oxygen tubing
   c) Compression stockings
   d) Both a and b
   e) All of the above

5. For adequate healing to occur, the recommended daily protein intake for a 55 kg woman would be:
   a) 55 grams
   b) 83 grams
   c) 162 grams
   d) None of the above

6. For patients with urinary or fecal incontinence, which of the following products would be recommended for preventing further skin breakdown?
   a) A urea-based skin product
   b) A topical antifungal agent
   c) Dimethicone
   d) Hydrogel-based products

7. Which of the following patients is at the greatest risk for skin breakdown?
   a) A 75-year-old undergoing hip surgery for a fracture
   b) A 55-year-old with a prealbumin of 24 and a lower-extremity cast
   c) A 45-year-old paraplegic with existing pressure ulcers
   d) All of the above

8. Which of the following statements is true regarding pressure ulcer prevention strategies?
   a) Pressure ulcer prevention strategies should be aimed at the specific needs of the patient.
   b) Frequent smaller position changes are preferable to major repositioning every two to three hours.
   c) Friction, shear, and moisture are as important as pressure redistribution in preventing pressure ulcers.
   d) All of the above statements are true.

9. Elderly patients are at the greatest risk for nutritional issues and pressure ulcer because of:
   a) Presence of subcutaneous fat cushion
   b) Well-fitted dentures
   c) Bulimia of aging
   d) Polypharmacy

10. All of the following are limitations of pressure ulcer staging except:
   a) The descriptions of stage I pressure ulcers and deep tissue injury are the same.
   b) If the wound base is not visible, it cannot be staged.
   c) Staging is only applicable to pressure ulcers.
   d) Reverse staging should not be used to describe the healing of pressure ulcers.

See answers on page 158.

NOTES

ANSWER KEY

1. c) Pressure reduction can occur by turning a patient at least every two hours, lifting the heels to avoid contact with the surface, raising the head of the bed to 30 degrees (not 45 degrees), placing pillows or wedges between the legs, and positioning the patient.

2. c) The most common pressure ulcer site is the sacrum.

3. a) The best validity and reliability pressure ulcer risk assessment tool is the Braden scale.

4. e) Oxygen tubing/masks, splints, casts, antithrombic devices, and compression hose can all contribute to the formation of pressure ulcers.

5. b) For adequate healing to occur, the recommended daily protein intake is 1.5 gm/kg of body weight; therefore, a 55 kg woman would require around 83 grams of protein.

6. c) Frequent perineal care and use of moisture barriers is recommended in patients with urinary and stool incontinence, and the use of moisture barriers like zinc oxide, dimethicone, petrolatum, or a combination of trypsin/balsam peru (Xenaderm™) may help prevent skin breakdown.

7. c) All of the patients in question are at risk for developing pressure ulcers, but the 45-year-old paraplegic has the highest risk. This patient will have problems with all the factors listed in the Braden scale risk assessment for pressure ulcers, including sensory perception, moisture, activity, mobility, nutrition, and friction and sheer.

8. d) Pressure ulcer prevention strategies include all of the choices listed: strategies are specific and customized to the needs of the patient; frequent smaller position changes are preferable to major repositioning every two to three hours; and friction, shear, and moisture are as important as pressure redistribution in preventing pressure ulcers.

9. d) Elderly patients are at the greatest risk for nutritional issues and pressure ulcer because of the loss of subcutaneous fat. Dental issues are also a major reason for nutritional issues in elderly patients, but well-fitted dentures usually help patients to eat. Anorexia of aging, not bulimia, is a problem that causes nutritional issues in elderly patients.

10. a) The descriptions of stage I wounds and deep tissue injury are not the same—a stage I ulcer is described as intact skin with non-blanchable redness of a localized area over a bony prominence, while deep tissue injury is a purple or maroon localized area of discolored intact skin or blood-filled blister due to damage of underlying soft tissue from pressure and/or sheer. The other limitations listed are accurate.

DIABETIC ULCER: DIAGNOSIS AND MANAGEMENT 19

Javier La Fontaine, DPM, MS
Kathren McCarty, DPM, MS, FACFAS

INTRODUCTION

This chapter addresses the pathophysiology of diabetic ulcerations, the types of diabetic ulcers (neuropathic, neuroischemic, and ischemic), how to evaluate diabetic wound patients, and the management options for diabetic foot ulcers. Surgical management options include elective foot surgery, prophylactic foot surgery, curative foot surgery, and emergent foot surgery.

OBJECTIVES

Participants should be able to discuss the risk factors for ulceration, contrast the types of amputations (digital, ray, transmetatarsal, Lisfranc, Chopart, Syme, and transtibial), and discuss the wound care protocol recommended after four weeks of insufficient healing.

I. Diabetic ulcer diagnosis
A. Epidemiology of diabetes
  1. 120,000 amputations a year in the United States
  2. Two-thirds of those amputations are attributed to diabetic complications
  3. 85% of all diabetic amputations are preceded by ulceration (Figure 19.1)

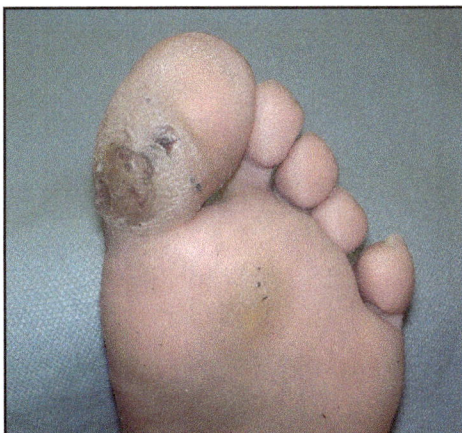

Figure 19.1: Diabetic preulcer at the hallux.

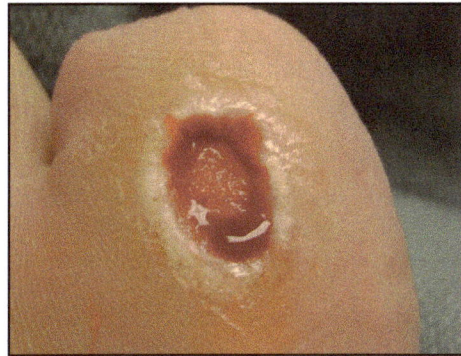

Figure 19.2: Neuropathic diabetic foot ulceration.

B. Pathophysiology of diabetic foot ulceration (Figure 19.2)
  1. Diabetes plays a significant role in the development of plantar pedal ulceration.
  2. Neuropathy, vasculopathy, and deformity are essential for the development of a neuropathic ulceration.
  3. Neuropathy is the most important single independent risk factor.
  4. Neuropathy leads to loss of protective sensation.
  5. Neuropathy leads to deformities via motor neuropathy of intrinsic muscle of the foot. Therefore, deformities, such as hammertoes, will predispose the foot to areas of increased pressure, which in this case would be the dorsum of the toe and the metatarsal head of the respective toe via retrograde force. In the presence of neuropathy the area of pressure will develop callus and subsequently become an ulcer.
  6. Neuropathy, especially autonomic, promotes anhidrosis, which causes dryness of skin and fissures. Both ulcers and fissures, along with vascular disease, place the patient at risk for infection and gangrene.
C. Evaluating a diabetic wound patient
  1. Poorly controlled diabetes is associated with the development of end organ disease such as arteriovascular disease and peripheral neuropathy. However, the data linking hemoglobin A1c to healing are not strong. Current guidelines suggest that attempting to lower A1c below 7 may be associated with death in older patients. Therefore, while glucose control is

always an important component of diabetes management, the possible benefit of very tight glucose control on healing should be weighed against the proven risk of adverse events.

2. Pertinent medical history should be gathered in relation to cardiovascular disease. Patients with a history of coronary artery disease, stroke, and smoking may have significant peripheral vascular disease, and further vascular evaluation is warranted.

3. A complete evaluation of the wound is essential to formulate a treatment plan.

4. Assessment of the contralateral limb should be done as well to screen and compare pathology with the affected limb.

5. The first assessment of vascular status should be done by palpation of the dorsalis pedis and posterior tibial pulse.

6. Non-invasive arterial evaluation should be performed in all patients with non-healing wounds or on patients over age 50 with a history of diabetes. This can be done using the ankle-brachial index or other noninvasive methods such as transcutaneous oximetry or skin perfusion pressure.

7. Palpable pulses may be unreliable in diabetic patients because of Monckeberg's sclerosis (calcification of the tunica media of vessel wall).

8. Neuropathy should be assessed as well. Monofilament, vibration, and deep tendon reflexes should be tested to assess the severity of neuropathy.
   a) Peripheral neuropathy screening for loss of protective sensation can be accomplished using the Semmes-Weinstein 5.07 monofilament and deep tendon reflex testing vibration with 128 Hz tuning fork.

9. There is evidence that neuropathy may have an effect on autoregulation of capillaries and, therefore, poor oxygenation at the wound base.

10. Infection should be ruled out in diabetic wounds (Figure 19.3). Although erythema, swelling, heat, and pain are classic signs of infection, it is not always the case in the diabetic wound.

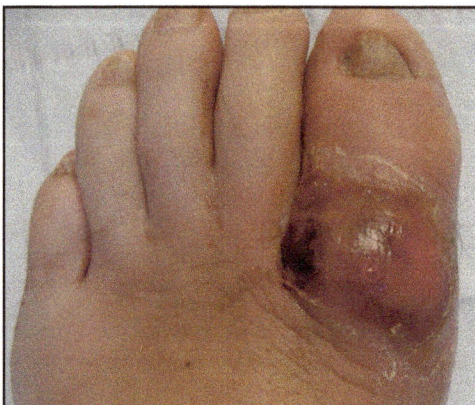

Figure 19.4: Inflammation secondary to repetitive stress.

11. Inflammation is commonly seen in neuropathic ulcers because of repetitive stress, which occurs in the development of the ulcer, as well as an excessive inflammatory response observed in neuropathic limbs (Figure 19.4).
    a) For example, Charcot neuroarthropathy may simulate an underlying bone infection when in reality there is no infection.

12. If infection is suspected, deep cultures are preferred.

13. The deformity that is causing the ulcer should be evaluated.

14. Identification of the deformity is not only important for wound healing, but also to prevent recurrence.

15. Structural deformities, such as bunions, hammertoes, and limited joint mobility, need to be recognized for the management of these wounds.

16. The increased pressure observed is directly proportional to the severity of the deformity.

D. Types of diabetic ulcers
   1. There are three types of ulceration the healthcare professional will encounter.
      a) Neuropathic ulcer (Figure 19.5)—the neuropathic ulcer is painless with a hyperkeratotic rim and red granular base. Maceration is usually present underneath the hyperkeratosis. It occurs in locations where there is increased pressure, commonly the plantar aspect of the foot.

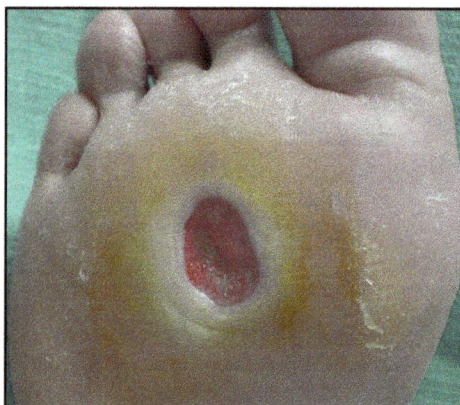

Figure 19.3: Diabetic foot infection.

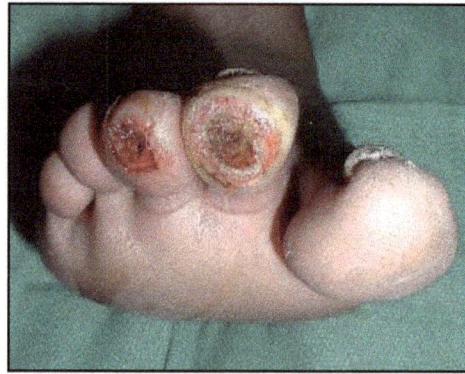

Figure 19.5: Neuropathic ulcer.

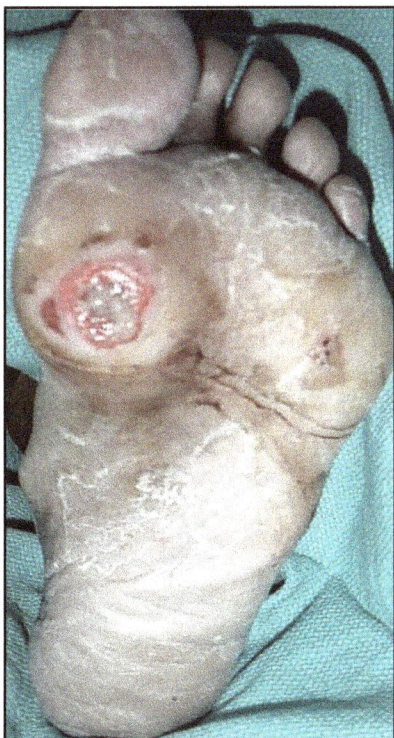

Figure 19.6: Neuroischemic ulceration.

b) Neuroischemic ulcer (Figure 19.6)—the neuroischemic ulcer is the most difficult ulcer to treat in the foot. It has characteristics of the neuropathic ulcer, but microvascular disease makes this ulcer a challenge to heal. Often noninvasive arterial studies demonstrate mild macrovascular disease. The appearance of the foot is consistent with signs of vascular disease as well as severe neuropathy. The wound base is pink in color mixed with a fibrinous type tissue that recurs even with sharp debridement.

c) Ischemic ulcer (Figure 19.7)—the ischemic ulcer has a yellowish or grayish base with a margin that bleeds for a short period of time. This sign is deceptive as the clinician may believe that the

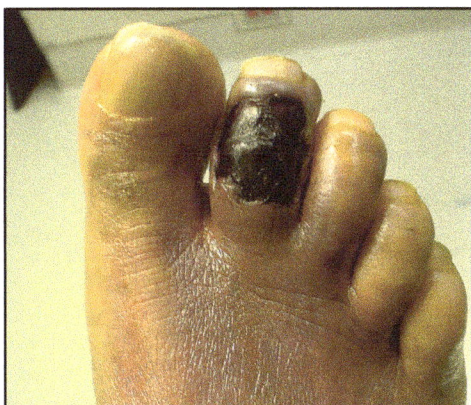

Figure 19.7: Ischemic ulcer.

wound is well perfused. It is usually painful since the patient may present with rest pain as well. Vascular consultation is imperative for the treatment of this type of wound.

E. Prevention of diabetic foot ulceration
1. Universal standards of clinical prevention and treatment of ulcerations must be established to ultimately decrease the rate of infection, amputation, and mortality of patients with diabetes. Foot biomechanics, structure, and skin integrity should be evaluated.
2. Diabetic patients are more prone to onychomycosis, cutaneous infections, and deformity.
3. It has been shown that prescriptive shoe wear, shoe inserts and cushions, and debridement of calluses are crucial for decreasing plantar pressures and redistributing pressure loads.
4. It has been shown that prophylactic foot surgeries can be effective in preventing foot ulcers in diabetic patients when indicated.

II. Management of diabetic foot ulcers

A. Treatment of diabetic foot ulceration
1. Consistent wound measurement
2. Glucose control
3. Surgical debridement
4. Antibiotics
5. Off-loading
6. Moist wound environment
7. Advanced wound care therapies
8. Vascular and surgical reconstruction
9. Bed rest or limited activity; cutout felt pads and total contact casting should be used to off-load these wounds.
10. If after approximately four weeks the wound care protocol is producing insufficient healing, the treatment must be reassessed; determine if edema, blood supply, and/or nutrition are preventing the healing process.
a) Alternative therapies such as cellular tissue products should be employed.
b) Hyperbaric oxygen therapy may help in ulcer healing and provide a significant reduction in the risk of major amputation.
11. After appropriate wound care and debridement, an off-loading modality should be chosen to transfer or decrease the plantar pressure from one specific location to the rest of the plantar aspect of the foot in balanced redistribution. Bony prominences, edema, previous amputation, wound location, and wound care all play important parts in the decision-making process for off-loading.

B. Surgical management in diabetic wound patients
1. Sometimes surgical intervention may be necessary. The role of surgical management is a viable option when it comes to successfully treating recurrent diabetic ulcerations, infections, and other related

complications that exist in the foot and ankle. In regard to surgical intervention for the diabetic foot, Armstrong and Frykberg have offered the following classifications.

    a) Class I: elective foot surgery, performed to treat a painful deformity in a patient without loss of protective sensation

    b) Class II: prophylactic foot surgery, performed to reduce the risk of ulceration or reulceration in patients with a loss of protective sensation, but without an open wound

    c) Class III: curative foot surgery, performed to assist in healing an open wound

    d) Class IV: emergent foot surgery, performed to arrest or limit the progression of acute infection

2. Whether surgical intervention is curative, prophylactic, or elective, the patient with diabetes should be fully assessed preoperatively for the degree of deformity, history of ulcerations, general physical condition, vascular status, and impairment of glucose control.

3. When surgery is emergent, the primary surgical intervention should be done immediately with staged additional procedures to follow after the above considerations have been addressed.

4. Prophylactic and elective surgery can successfully prevent future ulcerations. Withholding surgical management of deformities in the well-controlled diabetic patient may place the foot at future risk for ulceration and amputation.

5. Failure to remove the deformity can prove more dangerous than the judicious use of surgery to relieve bony pressure.

C. Elective surgery

  1. There are several goals for elective surgery candidates:

    a) Prevention of recurrent ulceration

    b) Reduction of pressure, primarily over bony prominences

    c) Establishment of a functional foot

D. Amputation is usually reserved for emergent cases to treat severe infection.

  1. Amputation and plastic surgery techniques may actually be used to cure persistent problem wounds and improve quality of life (QOL).

  2. Several recent studies have shown that patients may prefer and enjoy a better QOL with amputation and a closed surgical site versus continual, wearisome treatments for a chronic or recurrent open wound.

  3. Surgeons must weigh many considerations in order to successfully plan the appropriate level of amputation. These factors include tissue viability (e.g., presence of ulcerations, tissue deficits), micro- and macrovascular circulation, anatomy and biomechanical function, cardiac demand and energy expenditure, and rehabilitation potential.

4. Also, the reality that one amputation can lead to another in the future due to the creation of biomechanical abnormalities or a worsening of disease must be considered.

5. Maintaining toe-off and propulsion in the gait cycle to reduce transfer pressures to adjacent metatarsals and digits should be achieved, if possible.

6. The levels of amputation in the lower extremity include: digital (Figure 19.8), ray (Figure 19.9), transmetatarsal (Figures 19.10a and 19.10b), Lisfranc (Figure 19.11), Chopart (Figure 19.12), Syme (Figure 19.13), and transtibial (Figure 19.14).

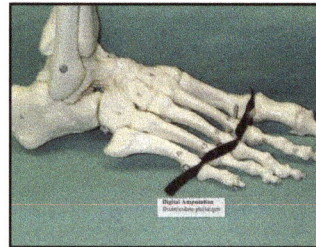

Figure 19.8: Digital amputation.

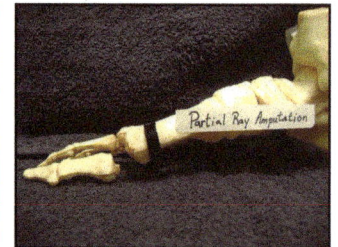

Figure 19.9: Partial ray amputation.

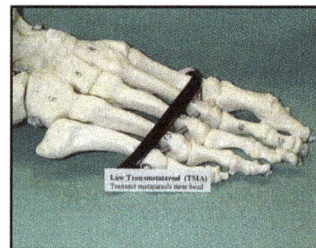

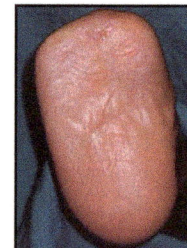

Figures 19.10a, b: Low transmetatarsal amputation.

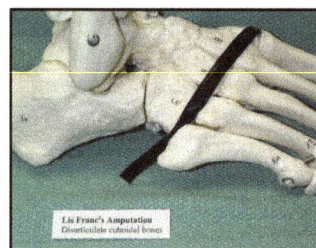

Figure 19.11: Lisfranc amputation.

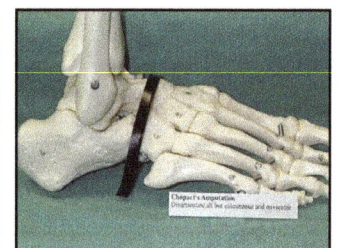

Figure 19.12: Chopart amputation.

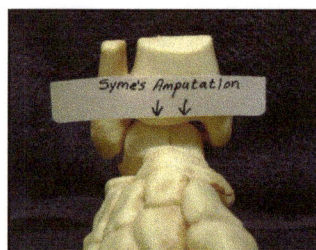

Figure 19.13: Syme amputation.

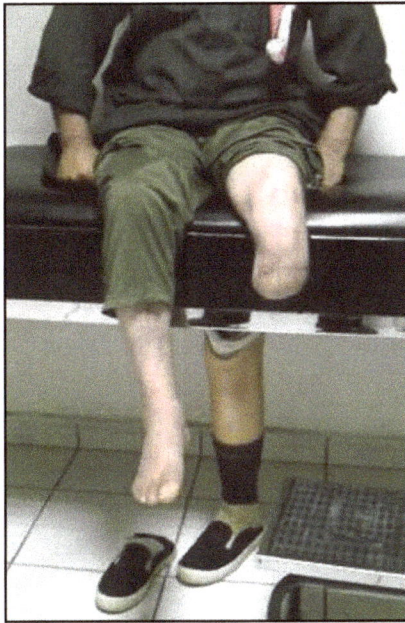

Figure 19.14: Transtibial amputation (BKA).

E. Some other possible surgeries include:
    1. First ray surgery (e.g., Keller arthroplasty, bunionectomy, sesamoidectomy, first metatarsal osteotomy)
    2. First metatarsal-medial cuneiform fusion
    3. Digital surgery (e.g., hammertoe repair, lesser metatarsal osteotomy, resection of a lesser metatarsal head, nail avulsion for ingrown nails), exostectomy
    4. Midfoot and rear foot arthrodesis
    5. Achilles tendon lengthening
F. Following surgery, appropriate accommodative or off-loading shoe gear must be fabricated and used daily to prevent future ulceration (refer to Chapter 20).

RESOURCES

1. Frykberg RG, Armstrong DG, Giurini J, et al. Diabetic foot disorders: a clinical practice guideline. American College of Foot and Ankle Surgeons. *J Foot Ankle Surg*. 2000; 39(5 Suppl):S1-60.
2. Armstrong DG, Lavery LA, Harkless LB. University of Texas classification system for diabetic foot wounds. *Diabetes Care*. 1998; 21:855-9.
3. Kahn KH, Derksen TA, Steinberg JS. Diabetic foot wounds. In: Sheffield PJ, Fife CE, editors. *Wound Care Practice*. 2nd ed. North Palm Beach: Best Publishing Company; 2007: 405-30.
4. Bosker GW, LaFontine J. Orthotics and prosthetics in wound care. In: Sheffield PJ, Fife CE, editors. *Wound Care Practice*. 2nd ed. North Palm Beach: Best Publishing Company; 2007: 901-20.
5. Malone M, Bowling FL, Gannass A, Jude EB, Boulton AJ. Deep wound cultures correlate well with bone biopsy culture in diabetic foot osteomyelitis. *Diabetes Metab Res Rev*. 2013 Oct; 29(7):546-50.
6. La Fontaine J, Harkless LB, Davis CE, Allen MA, Shireman PK. Current concepts in diabetic microvascular dysfunction. *J Am Podiatr Med Assoc*. 2006 May-Jun; 96(3):245-52.
7. Infectious Diseases Society of America. IDSA Infections by Organ System: Diabetic Foot Infections [Internet]. 2012. Accessed at: http://www.idsociety.org/Organ_System/#DiabeticFootInfections.

SAMPLE QUESTIONS

1. What percentage of diabetic foot amputations is preceded by ulcers?
   a) 35%
   b) 50%
   c) 75%
   d) 85%

2. The most important single independent risk factor for ulceration is:
   a) Peripheral vascular disease
   b) Neuropathy
   c) Foot deformity
   d) History of prior amputations

3. Advanced wound modalities might be considered if a diabetic wound is not progressing after _____ of standard wound care.
   a) Two weeks
   b) Four weeks
   c) Six weeks
   d) Eight weeks

4. The Semmes-Weinstein test is used to assess:
   a) Blood flow to the feet
   b) Protective sensation of the feet
   c) Pressure on the feet
   d) Temperature of the feet

5. All of the following are treatments are considered standards of care for foot ulcers with adequate blood flow except:
   a) Debridement
   b) Off-loading
   c) Antibiotics
   d) Glucose control

6. Which of the following can lead to an ulcer in the presence of neuropathy and vascular disease?
   a) Hammertoe
   b) Anhidrosis
   c) Callus
   d) All of the above

7. The most important method of treatment to heal a plantar foot ulcer is:
   a) Moisturizer
   b) Off-loading
   c) Collagenase
   d) A swab culture

8. When foot ulcers continue to recur and obvious deformity exists, the best option is:
   a) Casting
   b) Diabetic shoes
   c) Surgical correction
   d) Dressing changes and hope it does not get infected

9. Sometimes palpable pulses are unreliable in the diabetic patient because of:
   a) Loss of protective sensation
   b) The diabetes
   c) Monckeberg's sclerosis
   d) Lack of pedal hair

10. A patient presents to the emergency room and upon evaluation is diagnosed with gas gangrene. The podiatrist determined he has to perform surgery immediately. What is the class of surgery?
    a) Elective
    b) Emergent
    c) Curative
    d) Prophylactic

See answers on page 166.

NOTES

ANSWER KEY

1. d) 85% of diabetic foot amputations are preceded by ulcers.

2. b) The most important single independent risk factor for ulceration is neuropathy. Patients with neuropathy do not feel sensation, and ulceration occurs when patients do not wear any protective footwear.

3. b) Advanced wound modalities may be considered if a diabetic wound is not progressing after standard wound management for four weeks.

4. b) The Semmes-Weinstein test is used to assess the protective sensation of feet.

5. c) Among the treatments listed, debridement, off-loading, and glucose control are considered standards of care for foot ulcers with adequate blood flow. Antibiotics are required only when infection is present. (7)

6. d) Hammer toe, anhidrosis, and callus can lead to an ulcer in the presence of neuropathy and vascular disease. Any area at risk to develop an open wound will be complicated with vascular disease.

7. b) The most important treatment to heal a plantar foot ulcer is off-loading. Plantar foot ulcers will not heal with persistent trauma at the wound base. Moisturizer is needed for dry, cracked skin common to diabetics, but it is not a treatment to heal plantar foot ulcers. Collagenase is used for enzymatic debridement, which may be necessary in the treatment of diabetic plantar foot ulcers, but it is not the most important treatment. Swab culture is necessary if a diabetic foot ulcer is infected.

8. c) When foot ulcers continue to recur and obvious deformity exists, the best option is surgical correction. Rigid foot deformities often cannot be off-loaded properly. Casting is good for healing diabetic foot ulcers but will not prevent reoccurrence. Diabetic shoes are good for prevention; however, when foot ulcers continue to reoccur secondary to foot deformity they are not the best choice for prevention. Dressing changes are necessary for healing diabetic foot ulcers, not to prevent ulceration in the presence of foot deformities.

9. c) Palpable pulses may be unreliable in the diabetic patient because of Monckeberg's sclerosis; the calcification of the media makes the arterial wall easily palpable even with diminished blood flow.

10. b) As gas gangrene is a limb threatening infection, it is considered an emergent procedure.

OFF-LOADING DIABETIC FOOT ULCERS: ORTHOTICS 20

Elias R. Cheleuitte, DPM, FACFAS

INTRODUCTION

This chapter discusses practical criteria for selecting an appropriate off-loading modality for a diabetic foot ulcer. The focus is on the advantages and disadvantages of various off-loading modalities, including casting, walkers, shoes, splints, chairs, walking aids, and other assistive devices.

OBJECTIVES

Participants should be able to identify and describe the biomechanical etiology of tissue breakdown, describe the selection criteria for the use of various off-loading modalities, and understand the role that activity plays in ulcer recurrence.

I. Foot ulceration
A. Mechanisms of injury (Figures 20.1 and 20.2)

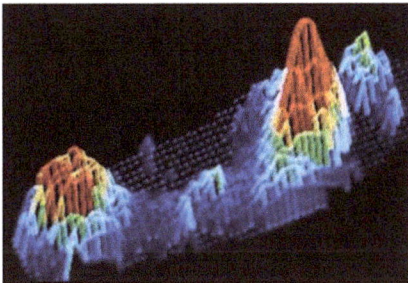

Figure 20.1: In-shoe pressure measurements showing peak plantar pressure points on the foot.

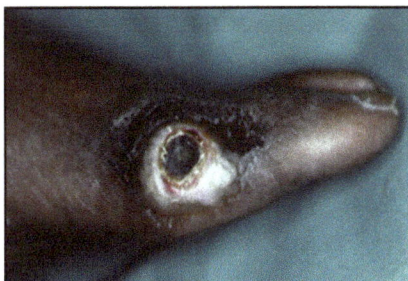

Figure 20.2: Ulceration due to repetitive pressure.

Table 20.1: Risk factors for foot ulceration.

	ODDS RATIO	p VALUE
Loss of protective sensation	15.2	<0.001
History of previous amputation	10.0	<0.02
Elevated plantar pressure (>65 N/cm^2)	5.9	<0.001
One or more subjective symptoms of neuropathy	5.1	<0.02
Hallux rigidus, hallux valgus, toe deformity	3.3	<0.03
Poor diabetes control (glycohemoglobin >9%)	3.2	<0.03
Duration of diabetes >10 years	3.0	<0.04
Male gender	2.7	<0.05

1. Low pressure—constant exposure
2. Moderate pressure—repetitive exposure
3. High pressure—single exposure
B. Etiology of diabetic foot ulcerations (Figure 20.3)
   1. Areas of moderate to high pressure
   2. Repetitive microtrauma
   3. Peripheral sensory neuropathy
   4. Thermal stress, inflammation
   5. Tissue breakdown

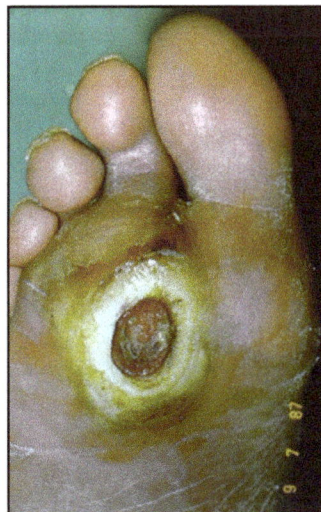

Figure 20.3: Diabetic foot ulceration due to plantar pressure.

C. In 1963, a very early off-loading article concluded that providing an equal distribution of plantar pressures in the foot was the key factor in healing neuropathic ulcerations. To this day, practical off-loading of the diabetic foot ulcer remains a challenge for all wound care specialists.

D. Up to 50% of people with diabetes will eventually lose sensation in their feet. It is vital to off-load these patients, but the fact that the patients can't judge if they have obtained adequate plantar pressure relief proves to be a challenge.

II. Off-loading
A. Methods to off-load the foot (Figure 20.4)

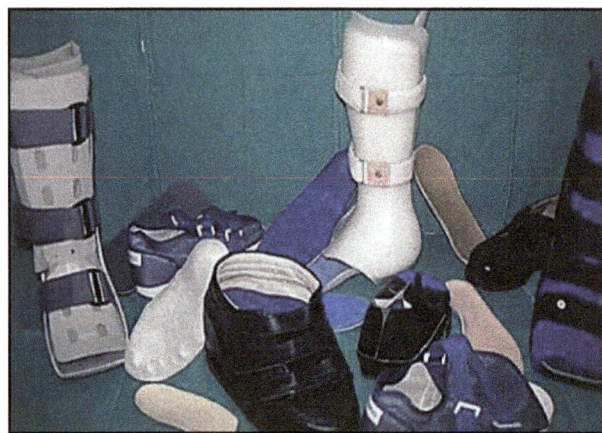

Figure 20.4: Common methods to off-load the foot.

1. Bed rest
2. Wheelchair
3. Crutches
4. Total contact cast (TCC)
5. Charcot restraint orthotic walker (CROW)
6. Integrated prosthetic and orthotic system (IPOS)
7. Surgical/post-op shoe
8. Healing sandal
9. Removable cam walkers

B. Consideration and patient selection for off-loading modalities should include:
1. Location of ulceration
2. Home environment
3. Functional capabilities of patient
4. Patient compliance plays a major role in our success of modality.
5. Presence of infection
6. Vascular status

C. Total contact cast: long considered the gold standard of off-loading modalities (Figure 20.5)
1. Advantages
   a) Forced compliance
   b) Shortens stride length
   c) Decreases cadence
   d) Reduces activity
   e) Reduces peak plantar pressures
   f) Reimbursable by Medicare and others

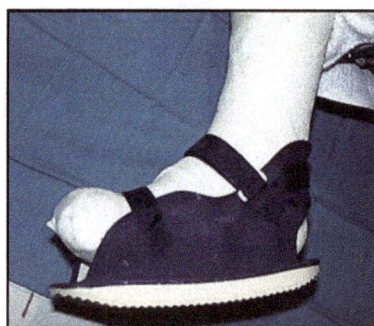

Figure 20.5: Total contact cast.

2. Why are total contact casts not widely used?
   a) Patient concerns
      i) Claustrophobia
      ii) Hot
      iii) Heavy
      iv) Disrupts sleep
      v) Difficult to bathe
   b) Physician concerns
      i) Wound surveillance
      ii) Requires specialized training
      iii) Time commitment
      iv) Cost of materials
      v) Reimbursement
      vi) Topicals
3. Contraindications
   a) Infection
   b) Severe peripheral vascular disease (PVD)
   c) Instability and/or difficulty ambulating
D. Charcot restraint orthotic walker (CROW) (Figure 20.6)
1. Advantages
   a) User-friendly
   b) Reusable device
   c) Permits wound surveillance
   d) Permits local wound care
   e) Patient acceptance
   f) Durable
   g) Can be fitted to very deformed feet

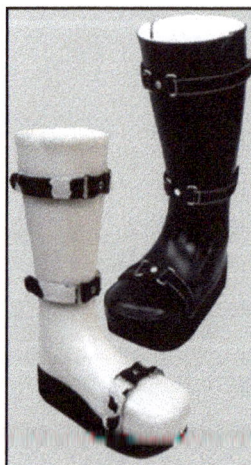

Figure 20.6: Charcot restraint orthotic walker (CROW).

2. Disadvantages
   a) Expensive
   b) Requires specialized equipment and prosthetist/ pedorthist to fabricate
   c) Typically two to four weeks fabrication time
   d) Often requires adjustments due to patient edema
   e) Can cause ulceration if poorly fabricated
   f) Not as effective off-loading as other modalities
E. Integrated prosthetic and orthotic system (IPOS)
   1. Advantages
      a) Designed for forefoot ulcerations
      b) 10 degrees of dorsiflexion and heel elevated 4 cm for forefoot off-loading
   2. Disadvantages
      a) Balance with the shoe can be an issue
F. Healing sandal
   1. Advantages
      a) Total contact orthotic made of plastozote
      b) Ulcerated area cut out to off-load
   2. Disadvantages
      a) Poor control of foot motion increases stress at ulceration site
G. Removable cam walkers (Figure 20.7)
   1. Advantages
      a) User-friendly
      b) Reusable device
      c) Permits wound surveillance
      d) Permits local wound care
      e) Patient acceptance
   2. Disadvantages
      a) Sometimes less effective off-loading than TCCs
      b) Patient compliance
      c) Durability of device
      d) Not currently reimbursable under Medicare for diabetic foot ulcers

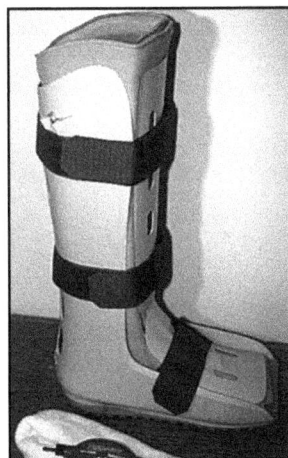

Figure 20.7. Removable cam walker.

III. Summary

A. Off-loading is a very important aspect of wound healing that is sometimes undervalued and overlooked.
B. Diabetic foot ulcers are often caused by a combination of pressure and strain to the plantar aspect of the foot. Good off-loading requires reduction of both of these forces.
C. There is not one perfect device for off-loading; however, there are many options available to find an appropriate fit for each patient.
D The likelihood of DFU healing is increased with off-loading adherence. Current evidence favors the use of nonremovable casts or fixed ankle walking braces as optimum off-loading modalities. There currently exists a gap between what the evidence supports regarding the efficacy of DFU off-loading and what is performed in clinical practice despite expert consensus on the standard of care. (24)

RESOURCES

1. Bosker GW, La Fontaine J. Orthotics and prosthetics in wound care. In: Sheffield PJ, Fife CE, editors. *Wound Care Practice.* 2nd ed. North Palm Beach: Best Publishing Company; 2007: 901-20.

2. Armstrong DG, Lavery LA. Elevated peak plantar pressures in patients who have Charcot arthropathy. *J Bone Joint Surg Am.* 1998 Mar; 80(3):365-9.

3. Lavery LA, Vela SA, Lavery DC, Quebedeaux TL. Reducing dynamic foot pressures in high-risk diabetic subjects with foot ulcerations. A comparison of treatments. *Diabetes Care.* 1996; 19(8):818-21.

4. Pecoraro RE, Reiber GE, Burgess EM. Pathways to diabetic limb amputation: basis for prevention. *Diabetes Care.* 1990; 13(5):513-21.

5. Reiber GE, Vileikyte L, Boyko EJ, et al. Causal pathways for incident lower-extremity ulcers in patients with diabetes from two settings. *Diabetes Care.* 1999; 22(1)157-62.

6. Bauman JH, Girling JP, Brand PW. Plantar pressures and trophic ulceration: an evaluation of footwear. *J Bone Joint Surg.* 1963; 45B(4):652-73.

7. Cavanagh PR, Bus SA. Offloading the diabetic foot for ulcer prevention and healing. *J Am Podiatr Med Assoc.* 2010; 52(3Suppl):37S-43S.

8. Landsman AS, Meaney DF, Cargill RS, et al. High strain rate tissue deformation: a theory on the mechanical etiology of diabetic foot ulcerations. *J Am Podiatr Med Assoc.* 1995; 85(10):519-27.

9. Zou D, Mueller MJ, Lott DJ. Effect of peak pressure and pressure gradient on subsurface shear stresses in the neuropathic foot. *J Biomech.* 2007; 40(4):883-90.

10. Pound N, Chipchase S, Treece K, et al. Ulcer-free survival following management of foot ulcers in diabetes. *Diabet Med.* 2005; 22(10):1306-9.

11. Snyder RJ, Kirsner RS, Warriner RA, et al. Consensus recommendations of advancing the standard of care for treating neuropathic foot ulcers in patients with diabetes. *Ostomy Wound Manage.* 2010; 56(4Suppl):S1-24.

12. Lavery LA, Armstrong DG, Wunderlich RP, et al. Risk factors for foot infections in individuals with diabetes. *Diabetes Care.* 2006; 29(6):1288-93.

13. Hanft J, et al. The use of the custom molded healing sandal for the treatment of plantar diabetic foot ulcerations. Abstract presented at: Joint Annual Meeting and Scientific Seminar, American College of Foot and Ankle Surgeons; 2000 February 8-12, Miami, FL.

14. Van Deursen R. Footwear for the neuropathic patient: offloading and stability. *Diabetes Metab Res Rev.* 2008; 24(Suppl1):S96-100.

15. Snyder RJ, Lanier KK. Diabetes: offloading difficult wounds. *Lower Ext Rev.* 2009. Accessed at: http://lermagazine.com/article/diabetes-offloading-difficult-wounds.

16. Hanft J, et al. The use of the fixed ankle walker for the treatment of plantar diabetic foot ulcerations. Abstract presented at: Joint Annual Meeting and Scientific Semi-

nar, American College of Foot and Ankle Surgeons; 2000 February 8-12, Miami, FL.

17. Armstrong DG, Lavery LA, Kimbriel HR, Nixon BP, Boulton AJ. Activity patterns of patients with diabetic foot ulceration. Patients with active ulcerations may not adhere to a standard pressure offloading regiment. *Diabetes Care.* 2003; 26(9):2595-97.

18. Searle A, Campbell R, Tallon D, Fitzgerald A, Vedhara K. A qualitative approach to understanding the experience of ulceration and healing in the diabetic foot: patient and podiatrist perspective. *Wounds.* 2005; 17(1):16-26.

19. Crews RT, Armstrong DG, Boulton AJ. A method for assessing offloading compliance. *JAPMA.* 2009; 99(1):100-3.

20. Aperqvist J, Larsson J, Agardh CD. Long-term prognosis for diabetic patients with foot ulcers. *J Int Med.* 1993; 233(6)485-91.

21. McGuire J. Diabetes: options for offloading. *Lower Ext Rev.* 2011. Accessed at: http://lermagazine.com/article/diabetes-options-for-offloading.

22. Zgonis T, editor. *Surgical Reconstruction of the Diabetic Foot and Ankle.* Philadelphia: Lippincott Williams & Wilkins; 2009.

23. Wunderlich RP. Off-loading diabetic foot wounds/ orthotics. In: Shah JB, Sheffield PJ, Fife CE, editors. *Wound Care Certification Study Guide.* North Palm Beach: Best Publishing Company; 2007: 163-7.

24. Snyder RJ, Frykberg RG, Rogers LC, Applewhite AJ, Bell D, Bohn G, Fife CE, Jensen J, Wilcox, J. The management of diabetic foot ulcers through optimal off-loading; building consensus guidelines and practical recommendations to improve outcomes. *J Am Podiatr Med Assoc.* 2014; 104(6):555-67.

SAMPLE QUESTIONS

1. Which is a common etiology of diabetic foot ulcerations?
   a) Repetitive microtrauma
   b) Peripheral neuropathy
   c) Areas of high pressure
   d) All of the above

2. Which modality is best suited for forefoot plantar diabetic ulceration?
   a) Healing sandal
   b) Cam walker
   c) IPOS
   d) PO shoe

3. Which is the highest risk factor for diabetic foot ulceration?
   a) Poor glycemic control
   b) Increased plantar pressure
   c) Loss of plantar sensation
   d) PVD

4. Which modality is considered the gold standard in off-loading diabetic foot ulcerations?
   a) Total contact cast
   b) Healing sandal
   c) CROW device
   d) PO shoe

5. All of the following factors require consideration before choosing an off-loading modality except:
   a) Location of ulceration
   b) Patient functional capabilities
   c) Patient insulin dependency
   d) Vascular studies

6. All of the following statements about TCCs are true except:
   a) It decreases cadence.
   b) It reduces activity level.
   c) It reduces peak plantar pressures.
   d) It is not reimbursed by Medicare/insurances.

7. Contraindications of TCC use include all of the following except:
   a) Infection
   b) Severe PVD
   c) Instability or difficulty ambulating
   d) Heel ulcerations

8. The disadvantage of using a CROW device includes:
   a) It requires adjustments.
   b) It doesn't permit for local wound care.
   c) It is expensive.
   d) Both a and c

9. Diabetic ulcerations can commonly be found:
   a) Around the ankle
   b) On the plantar surface of the foot
   c) On the dorsum of the foot
   d) Over the sacrum

10. Which of the following statements about TCCs is true?
    a) It is a method of relieving pressure on the foot.
    b) It is a special cast for fractures due to Charcot neuro-osteoarthropathy.
    c) It is recommended for use over infected diabetic foot ulcers.
    d) It is removable.

See answers on page 173.

NOTES

ANSWER KEY

1. d) A common etiology of diabetic foot ulcerations is usually repetitive microtrauma at areas of high pressure in patients with peripheral neuropathy.

2. c) IPOS (integrated prosthetic and orthotic system) is best suited to off-load diabetic forefoot ulceration. The healing sandal and cam walker are also used to off-load diabetic ulcers; however, IPOS is best suited for off-loading diabetic forefoot ulcers. The PO shoe is not able to off-load forefoot ulcers.

3. c) Loss of protective sensation in the plantar foot (neuropathy) is the highest risk factor for the diabetic foot ulcer.

4. a) TCC (total contact casting) is considered the gold standard for off-loading diabetic foot ulcers.

5. c) Before choosing an off-loading device it is important to look at the location of the ulcer, the functional capabilities of patient, and the patient's vascular status. Insulin dependency is not a factor in the choice of an off-loading device.

6. d) The TCC decreases cadence, reduces activity level, reduces peak plantar pressures, and is reimbursed by Medicare/insurances.

7. d) Contraindications for TCC use include infection, severe PVD, and instability or difficulty ambulating. Heel ulcerations are not a contraindication for the use of TCCs.

8. d) The disadvantages of a CROW device include required adjustments and high cost. The device does allow for local wound care.

9. b) Diabetic ulcerations can commonly be found on the plantar surface of the foot.

10. a) TCC is a method of relieving pressure on the foot. It is contraindicated in infected diabetic foot ulcers, is not removable by the patient, and is not a special cast for fractures due to Charcot neuroosteoarthropathy.

DERMATOLOGY REVIEW AND UNUSUAL WOUNDS

21

Rajendra S. Singh, MD
Jayesh B. Shah, MD, CWSP, FAPWCA, FACCWS

INTRODUCTION

This chapter reviews the basic morphology of skin disease and dermatological considerations for the healing of skin lesions. Included are examples of unusual wounds, such as malignant wounds, vasculitic wounds, and infectious wounds. Key diagnostic features are included for the history and physical examination.

OBJECTIVES

Participants should be able to identify the clues that point to possible malignancy, describe a vasculitic wound, and discuss how to evaluate an unusual wound.

I. Basic morphology of skin disease

A. Macule—a circumscribed, flat non-palpable lesion that is flush with the level of surrounding normal skin, usually smaller than 10 mm in diameter (Figure 21.1a)

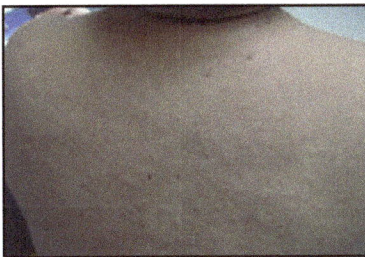

Figure 21.1a: Macule.

B. Patch—a flat, non-palpable lesion that is flush with the level of surrounding normal skin and greater than 10 mm in diameter (Figure 21.1b)

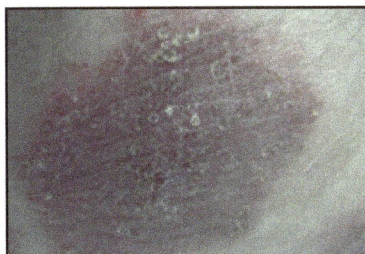

Figure 21.1b: Patch.

C. Papule—a superficial, circumscribed dome-shaped or flat-topped palpable lesion elevated above the skin surface and less than 10 mm in diameter (Figure 21.1c)

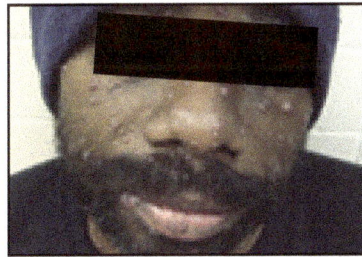

Figure 21.1c: Papule.

D. Plaque—a lesion that rises slightly above the surface of the skin, usually greater than 10 mm in diameter (Figure 21.1d)

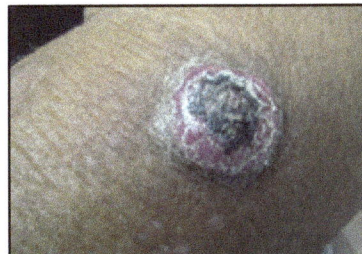

Figure 21.1d: Plaque.

E. Nodule—a firm lesion that is thicker or deeper than the average plaque or papule (Figure 21.1e)

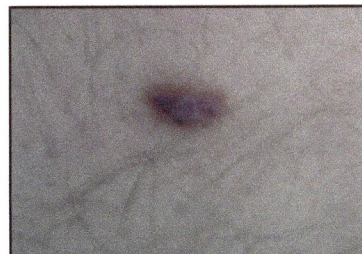

Figure 21.1e: Nodule.

F. Vesicle—an elevated lesion that contains clear fluid and less than 10 mm in diameter (Figure 21.1f)

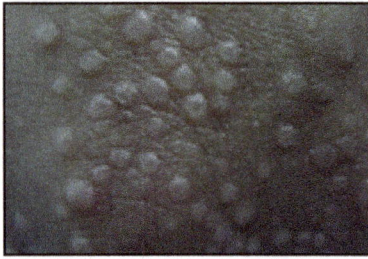

Figure 21.1f: Vesicles.

G. Bulla—an elevated lesion that contains clear fluid, usually larger than 10 mm in diameter (Figure 21.1g)

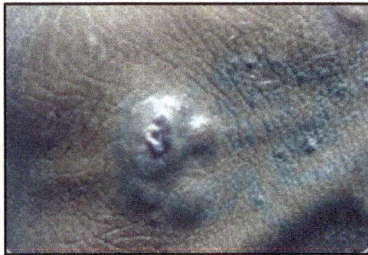

Figure 21.1g: Bulla.

H. Pustule—an elevated lesion that contains pus (Figure 21.1h)

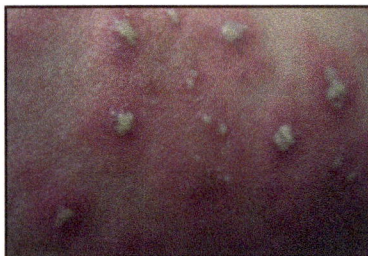

Figure 21.1h: Pustules.

II. Skin lesions
A. Overview
1. Benign lesions
2. Premalignant and malignant epidermal tumors
3. Tumors of the dermis
4. Melanocytic lesions
5. Inflammatory dermatoses
6. Blistering dermatoses
7. Infections
8. Arthropod bites, stings, and infestations
9. Miscellaneous conditions
B. Benign skin lesions
1. Seborrheic keratosis (Figure 21.2)

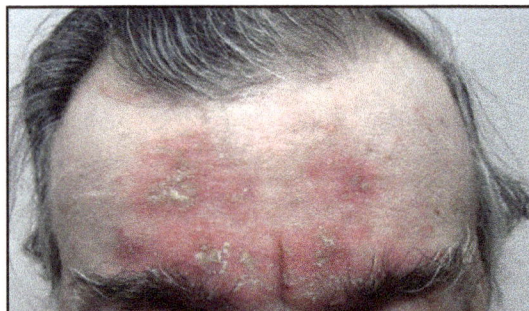

Figure 21.2: Seborrheic keratosis.

a) Benign hyperplastic tumor of the epidermis, which is more common in older individuals
b) Usually affects the trunk, head and neck, extremities; only hair-bearing skin
c) Clinically presents as exophytic, sharply demarcated, pigmented lesions that protrude above the skin's surface; appear to be stuck to the skin. They can be single or multiple, soft, and tan-black.
d) Treatment options include freezing and surgical curettage.
2. Seborrheic dermatitis (Figure 21.3)

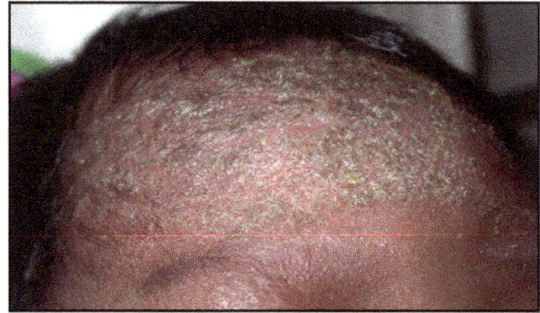

Figure 21.3: Seborrheic dermatitis.

a) Characteristic sites of involvement include scalp, ears, face, central chest, and intertriginous areas.
b) Can be a cutaneous sign of HIV infection
c) Clinical features include macules and papules on an erythematous, often greasy base, typically with extensive scaling and crusting.
d) Treatment options include use of topical azoles, either as shampoo or cream, along with low-potency corticosteroids and emollients.
3. Actinic keratosis (Figure 21.4)

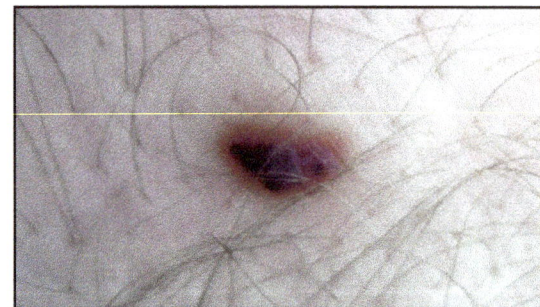

Figure 21.4: Actinic keratosis.

a) A common precancerous intraepidermal neoplasm of actinically damaged skin characterized by variable atypia of keratinocytes.
b) Clinically presents as ill-defined, white-red scaly macules or slightly elevated papules or plaques, found mostly in older patients.
c) Cryosurgery is the mainstay of treatment; new modalities under investigation include photodynamic therapy, immunomodulation, and drugs that target genetic defects.

C. Pre-malignant and malignant epidermal tumors
1. Clues of malignancy
   a) Unusual locations
   b) Asymmetric lesion
   c) Granulation extending over the border
   d) Exuberant granulation tissue or callus
   e) Purple-red color around ulcer
   f) Ulcer in center of pigmented lesion
   g) History of repeated trauma
   h) Wound with no obvious etiology
   i) Rolled-out edges
   j) Fungating growth
   k) Wound secondary to burns, trauma, radiotherapy, and diabetes
2. Basal cell carcinoma
   a) The most common type of skin cancer, affecting one in every six Americans
   b) Malignancy arising from epidermal basal cells
   c) Clinically presents as pearly red macule, papule, nodule, or plaque, most commonly on sun exposed skin
   d) Presents as a wound, outgrows its blood supply, erodes, and subsequently ulcerates
   e) Multiple variants including nodular basal cell carcinoma with papules present
   f) Treatment is usually biopsy and excision
   g) Close follow-up for additional lesions
   h) Case studies
      i) A 72-year-old female with a 10-year-old non-healing wound on her right leg was diagnosed with basal cell cancer on biopsy (Figure 21.5a).

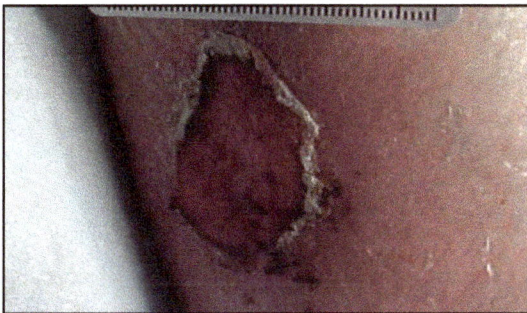
Figure 21.5b: Basal cell cancer on back.

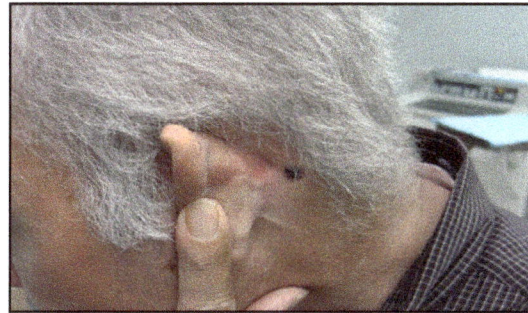
Figure 21.5c: Basal cell carcinoma on back of ear.

   e) Usually present as a red papule, nodule or plaque, commonly hyperkeratotic or ulcerated
   f) Composes 20% of all primary malignancies
   g) Can metastasize
   h) May be caused by ultraviolet light exposure
   i) Mohs surgery (microscopically controlled surgery); need to assess regional lymph nodes and excise any lymph nodes or obtain fine needle aspiration (FNA) of any potential problematic areas.
   j) Case studies
      i) An 80-year-old female, with a small wound on her left hand that continued to grow, was diagnosed with squamous cell cancer on biopsy (Figure 21.6a).

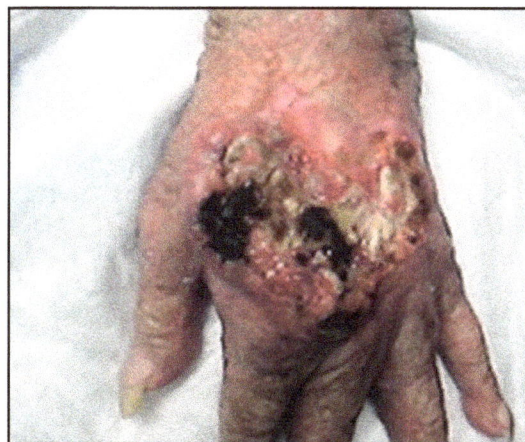
Figure 21.5a: Basal cell cancer on a right leg.

      ii) A 62-year-old male with a non-healing wound on his back was diagnosed with basal cell cancer on biopsy (Figure 21.5b).
      iii) A 65-year-old male with a plaque-like lesion behind his ear (Figure 21.5c).
3. Squamous cell cancer
   a) Malignant neoplasm of keratinizing epidermal cells
   b) Grows rapidly
   c) Marjolin reported that chronic wound underwent malignant changes
   d) Second most common form of skin cancer

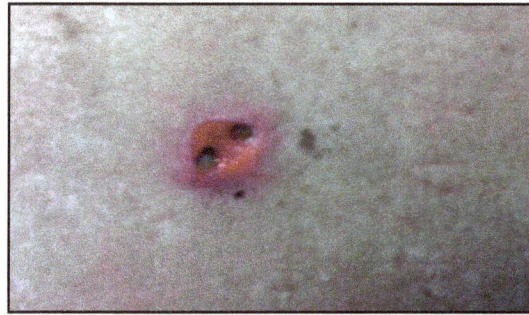
Figure 21.6a: Squamous cell cancer on left dorsal hand.

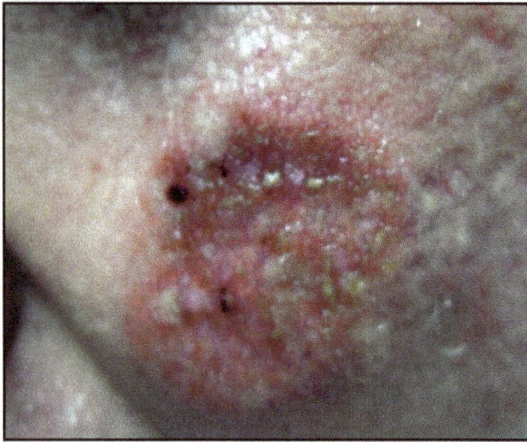

Figure 21.6b: Bowen's disease; precancerous squamous cell carcinoma.

ii) A 50-year-old female with Bowen's disease and squamous cell cancer *in situ* (Figure 21.6b).

4. Kaposi's sarcoma
   a) Malignant tumor of the lymphocytic and epithelial cells linked to herpetic viruses as well as HIV.
   b) Lesions are slightly raised, over-elongated, and poorly demarcated with rust or purple red maculae or patches.
   c) Treatments include highly active antiretroviral therapy (HAART), local radiation therapy, cryotherapy, chemotherapy, and alitretinoin gel.
   d) Case study
      i) A 32-year-old diabetic Hispanic male, HIV negative, presents with multiple wounds on foot (Figures 21.7a and 21.7b).

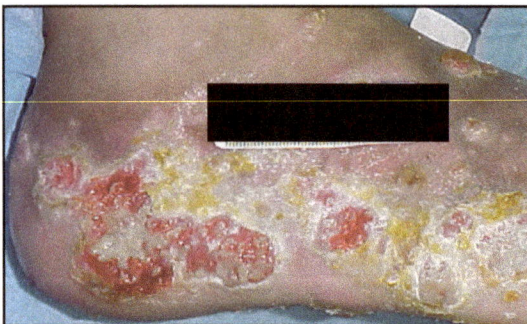

Figure 21.7a: Kaposi's sarcoma of right foot on initial presentation.

5. T-cell lymphoma (Figure 21.8)
   a) Patients with T-cell lymphoma rarely present with ulceration.
   b) Treatment remains chemotherapy and local wound care.
6. Non-Hodgkins lymphoma
   a) Ulcerative lymphoma is associated with poor prognosis.
   b) Mainly seen in immunocompromised patients.

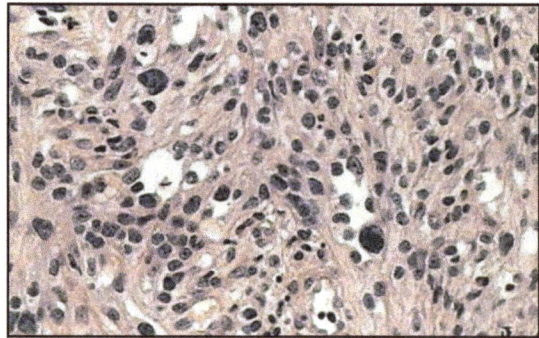

Figure 21.7b: Microscopic exam of Kaposi's sarcoma patient showing abnormal nuclei.

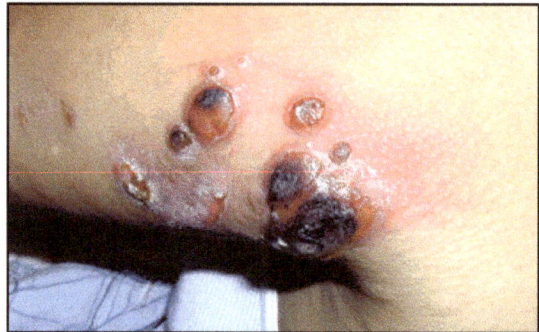

Figure 21.8: T-cell lymphoma.

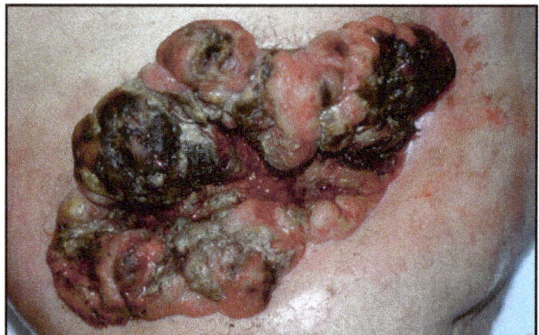

Figure 21.9: A 53-year-old with fungating growth on the left thigh draining purulent material with no improvement on antibiotics. Biopsy suggests soft tissue sarcoma.

7. Soft tissue sarcoma (Figure 21.9)
   a) High grade cancer arising from leg muscle
   b) Necrotic core can be "gas-like"
   c) Requires tissue biopsy
D. Tumors of the dermis
   1. Dermatofibroma (Figure 21.10)
      a) Fibrohistiocytic tumor of the dermis
      b) Most commonly seen on the lower extremities
      c) Clinically presents as firm, mildly elevated to dome-shaped brownish nodules
      d) Surgical excision is often employed to rule out melanocytic lesions
   2. Dermatofibrosarcoma protuberans
      a) Mesenchymal neoplasm of dermis and subcutis
      b) Generally regarded as a superficial low grade sarcoma

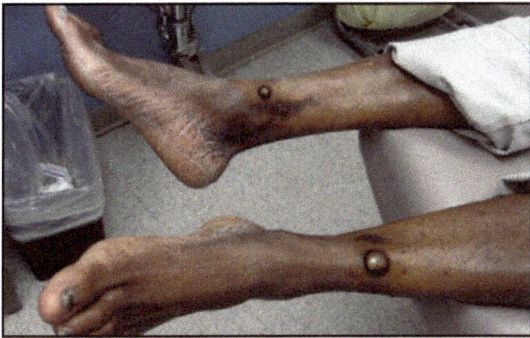

Figure 21.10: Dermatofibroma.

    c) Clinically presents on the trunk of young to middle age adults as a large nodule or plaque, often with multiple protuberances.

    d) Treatment options include wide local excision and Mohs surgery.

E. Melanocytic lesions

  1. Melanocytic nevus (Figure 21.11)

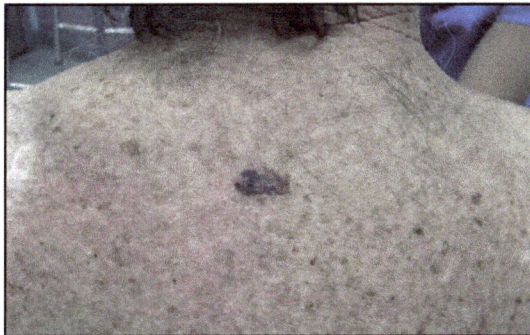

Figure 21.11: Melanocytic nevus.

    a) Extremely common lesion found almost anywhere and at any age

    b) Can be junctional, intradermal, or compound nevus (pigmented lesion of the skin)

    c) Indications for removal include a changing nevus, atypical clinical appearance suspicious for melanoma, cosmetic reasons, and features of irritation

  2. Dysplastic nevi (Figure 21.12)

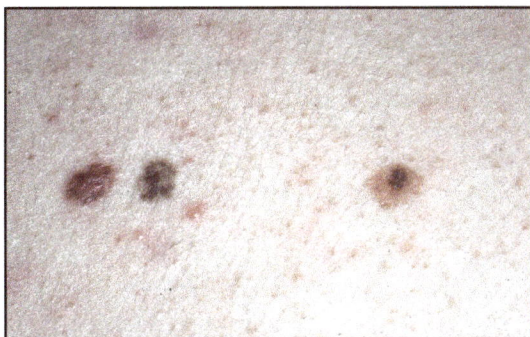

Figure 21.12: Dysplastic nevi.

    a) A common, controversial clinical designation for nevi that have morphological changes such as asymmetry, color variations, indistinct or notched borders

    b) Usually presents as pigmented macules, papules, or plaques

    c) Most common on the scalp and trunk, mostly in older children and young adults

    d) Surgical excision for ruling out melanoma is the preferred treatment option

  3. Malignant melanoma (Figure 21.13)

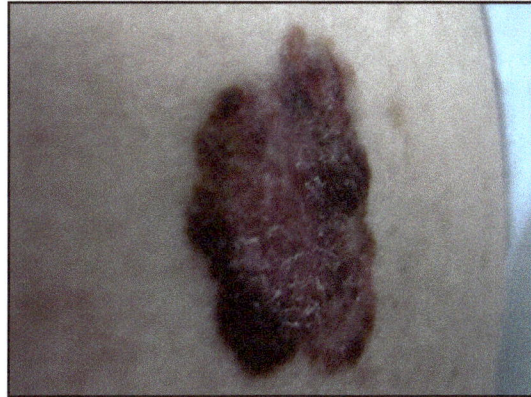

Figure 21.13: Malignant melanoma.

    a) Tumor of melanocytes is the most lethal form of cancer; multiple types

    b) Prognostic indicators

      i) Breslow's depth—describes how deeply tumor cells have invaded (depth measured by micrometer)

      ii) Presence of ulceration

      iii) Staging—Clark's level marks the invasion of malignant melanoma through the skin layers to the subcutaneous fat layer. Each successive level indicates a worsening prognosis

        (1) Level 1: confined to epidermis (*in situ*)

        (2) Level 2: invasion into papillary dermis

        (3) Level 3: tumor filling papillary dermis and compressing the reticular dermis

        (4) Level 4: invasion of reticular dermis (localized)

        (5) Level 5: invasion of subcutaneous tissue (regionalized by direct extension)

    c) Types of malignant melanoma

      i) Superficial spreading malignant melanoma

      ii) Nodular melanoma

      iii) Acral lentiginous melanoma

      iv) Amelanotic melanoma

      v) Minimal deviation melanoma

      vi) Desmoplatic melanoma

F. Inflammatory dermatoses

  1. Acute eczematous dermatitis

    a) Different clinical forms include:

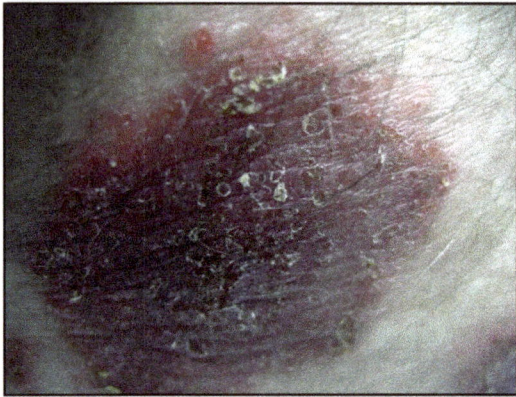

Figure 21.14a: Contact dermatitis on back after application of medication patch.

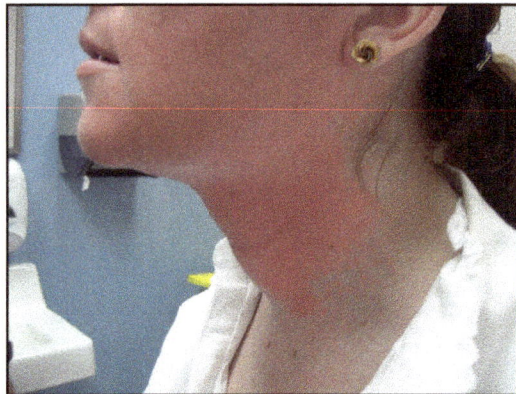

Figure 21.14b: Contact dermatitis on face after wearing jewelry.

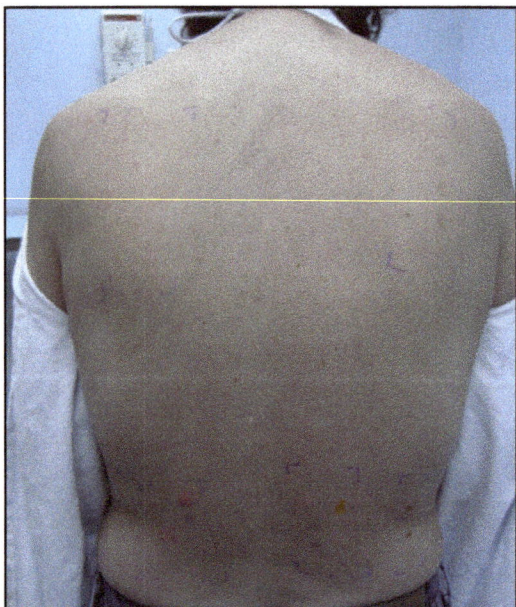

Figure 21.14c: Patch testing.

       i)   Allergic contact dermatitis (Figures 21.14a -21.14c)
       ii)   Atopic dermatitis
       iii)   Primary irritant dermatitis
       iv)   Photo eczematous dermatitis
       v)   Drug-related eczematous dermatitis

    b)   Clinically characterized by red papulovesicular oozing and crusted lesions early on that, with persistence, develop into raised scaling plaques with poorly defined scaling.

    c)   Patch testing remains the gold standard for diagnosis in allergic contact dermatitis.

    d)   Avoidance of irritants and topical corticosteroids are often the first line of treatment for most of these disorders.

2.   Erythema multiforme (Figure 21.15)

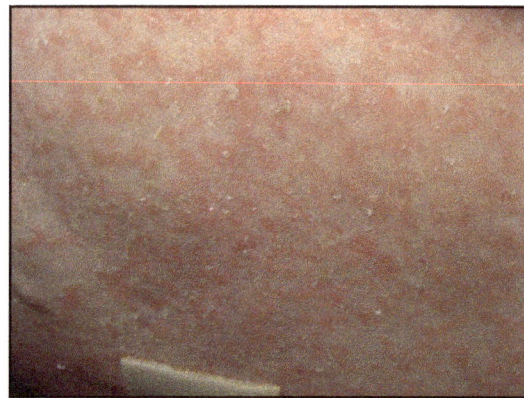

Figure 21.15: Erythema multiforme.

    a)   Most common sites of involvement include extremities and face.

    b)   Clinically characterized by abrupt onset of popular target lesions.

    c)   Vast majority of lesions appear within 24 hours.

    d)   A preceding herpes simplex virus (HSV) infection is the most common precipitating factor, rarely drugs.

    e)   Treatment options include topical and systemic treatment of acute eruption with antiseptic/antiviral agents, as well as prophylactic treatment of recurrent disease.

3.   Psoriasis

    a)   Most common sites of involvement are the scalp, elbows, and knees, followed by the nails, hands, feet, and trunk.

    b)   Clinically characterized by sharply demarcated, scaly erythematous plaques and occasionally sterile pustules.

    c)   Treatment options include phototherapy, vitamin D3 analogues, corticosteroids, topical retinoids, methotrexate, and recently introduced biologic agents such as etanercept and infliximab.

4. Lichen planus
   a) Most common sites of involvement include wrists, forearm, lower extremities, presacral areas, hair, nails, and mucous membranes.
   b) Clinically characterized by flat topped violaceous papules and plaques; variants include annular, bullous, hypertrophic, inverse, linear, ulcerative, drug-induced, and lichen planopilaris
   c) Treatment options include topical, intralesional, and systemic corticosteroids; retinoids; narrow-band ultraviolet B (UVB); psoralen and ultraviolet A (PUVA) light therapy; topical calcineurin inhibitors; and for severe cases, oral cyclosporine.
5. Lupus erythematous (Figures 21.16a and 21.16b)

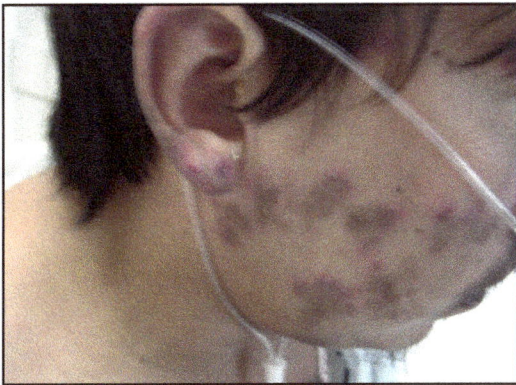

Figure 21.16a: Lupus erythematous with rash on face.

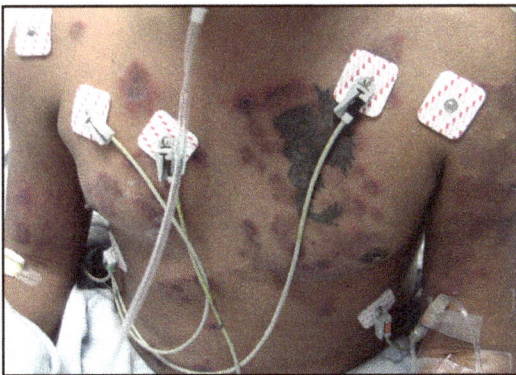

Figure 21.16b: Rash on chest and both arms in patient with lupus.

   a) Cutaneous lupus is a common autoimmune disorder.
   b) Cutaneous lesions usually consist of:
      i) Poorly defined malar erythema
      ii) Large, sharply demarcated erythematous scaling plaques
      iii) Usually on sun-exposed skin
      iv) Eight times more common in females
   c) Topical, intralesional, and systemic corticosteroids are the mainstays of treatment.
      i) Antimalarial therapies, gold, dapsone, and newer biological agents have been used with variable success.

G. Blistering dermatosis
   1. Blistering dermatosis pemphigus
      a) Autoimmune blistering diseases resulting from loss of integrity of normal intercellular attachments within the epidermis and mucous epithelium.
      b) Divided into three major forms:
         i) Pemphigus vulgaris
            (1) The most common form, which involves the mucosa and skin, especially of the scalp, face, axilla, groins, trunk, and points of pressure.
         ii) Pemphigus foliaceus
         iii) Paraneoplastic pemphigus
      c) Patients usually present with painful oral mucosal erosions and flaccid blisters, erosions, crusts, and macular erythema in areas of skin involvement.
      d) Diagnosis confirmed by demonstration of IgG autoantibodies against the cell surface of intraepidermal keratinocytes by immunofluorescence.
      e) Treatment consists of systemic corticosteroids and immunosuppressive therapy.
   2. Bullous pemphigoid
      a) Most common of the autoimmune blistering diseases.
      b) Predominantly affects the elderly.
      c) Common sites of involvement include inner aspects of thighs, flexor aspects of forearms, axilla, groin, and oral involvement.
      d) Clinically, patients can present with urticarial plaques with intense pruritis to widespread tense bulla filled with clear fluid.
      e) Diagnosis confirmed by presence of linear deposits of IgG and/or C3 along the dermal-epidermal junction on direct immunofluorescence.
      f) Treatment options include systemic corticosteroids and immunosuppressive therapy.
   3. Dermatitis herpetiformis (DH) (Figure 21.17)

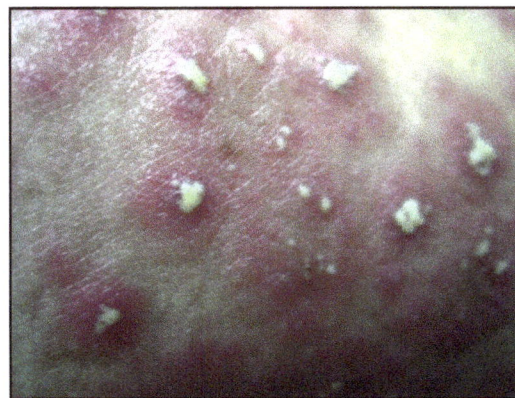

Figure 21.17: Dermatitis herpetiformis.

      a) DH is a cutaneous manifestation of celiac disease and is associated with gluten sensitivity in virtually all cases.

b) Lesions characteristically occur bilaterally and involve, preferentially, the extensor surfaces, elbows, knees, upper back, and buttocks.

c) Treatment includes dapsone and a gluten-free diet.

H. Infections
  1. Verruca (Figure 21.18)

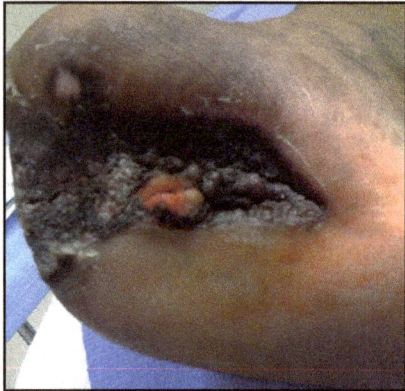

Figure 21.18: Verruca vulgaris.

a) Common lesion of childhood and adolescents.

b) Verrucous papules caused by infection with HPV.

c) Most common subtype is verruca vulgaris; other types include plantar warts, verruca plana, and condyloma acuminatum.

d) Treatment options include cryotherapy, trichloracetic acid application, electrosurgery, curettage, surgical excision, and topical cytotoxic therapy.

  2. Superficial fungal infections (Figure 21.19)

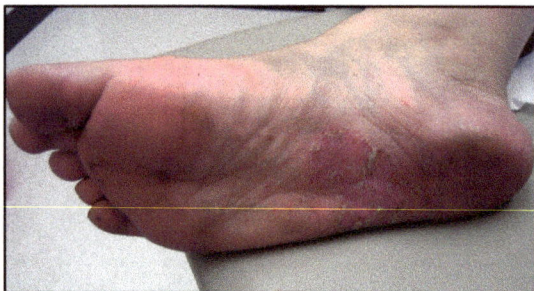

Figure 21.19: Tinea infections of the foot.

a) Superficial fungal infections are confined to the stratum corneum.

b) Causative organisms include one of three genera of dermatophytes (*Microsporum, Epidermophyton,* and *Trichophyton*).

c) Characteristic clinical presentations include:
  i) Tinea capitis (scalp)
  ii) Tinea barbae (beard)
  iii) Tinea corporis (body)
  iv) Tinea cruris (genital area)
  v) Tinea pedis (feet)
  vi) Onychomycosis (nail)

d) Clinical presentation includes scaly, erythematous plaques, often annular, rarely vesicular or pustular.

e) Potassium hydroxide (KOH) prep shows branching septate hyphae.

f) Topical antifungals are the mainstay of treatment.

I. Arthropod bites, stings, and infestations
  1. Arachnida (spiders, scorpions, ticks, and mites), insects (lice, bedbugs, fleas, wasps, bees, and mosquitoes), and chilopoda (centipedes) are the main groups affecting humans.
    a) Usually present as red papules, nodules, or pustules at the site of bite or sting.
  2. Arachnida and insect bites (ants, spiders, chiggers, fleas, bed bugs)
    a) Bites—typical appearance.
    b) Most insect bites are not serious.
    c) Necrotic skin lesions can be caused by any insect.
    d) Brown recluse spider (*Loxosceles reclusa*) bites:
      i) Difficult to diagnose
      ii) Spider usually not seen (80%)
        (1) 20% have seen spider
        (2) 12% bring spider into hospital
      iii) Bite is a minor sting or burn, typically occurring while cleaning closets, attics, or wood piles.
      iv) Bite severity is based on venom load and host immune response.
      v) 10% progress to necrosis
      vi) Venom—complex
        (1) Water soluble; spreads rapidly, has eight enzymes
        (2) Main enzyme: sphingomyelinase D
      vii) Treatment
        (1) Antibiotics
        (2) Dapsone (within 24 hours of bite)
          (a) Inhibits neutrophil migration
          (b) Not in G6PD deficiency
        (3) Debridement
        (4) Possible HBOT
      viii) Spider bite case history
        (1) An 80-year-old diabetic male with a spider bite on presentation, after debridement, and after HBOT (Figures 21.20a–21.20c).

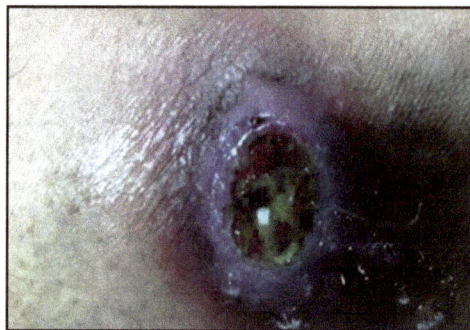

Figure 21.20a: A 50-year-old diabetic male with spider bite. Note the necrotizing wound with surrounding induration and erythema.

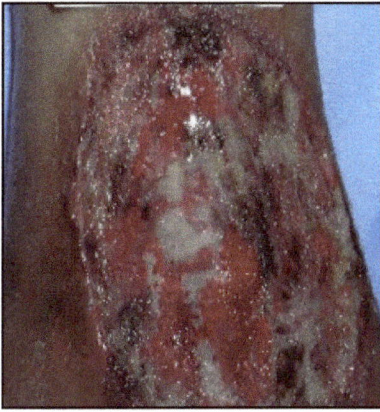

Figure 21.20b: Spider bite after debridement.

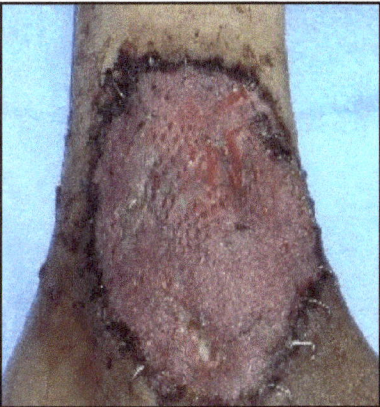

Figure 21.20c: Wound after HBOT and split thickness skin graft.

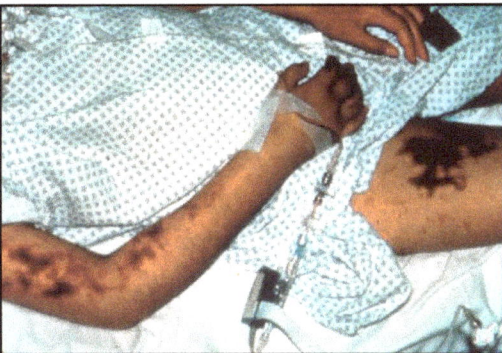

Figure 21.21: Antiphospholipid syndrome.

J. Miscellaneous conditions
1. Antiphospholipid syndrome (Figure 21.21)
    a) Associated with multiple systemic diseases
    b) Involves both lupus anticoagulant and or anticardiolipin antibodies
2. Vasculitis
    a) Key features
        i) Purpura
        ii) Livedo reticularis
        iii) Arthritis
        iv) Painful lesions
        v) Systemic symptoms
        vi) Skin lesions

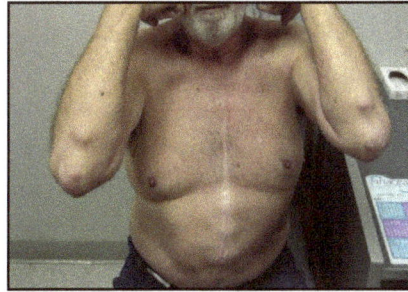

Figure 21.22a: Nodules.

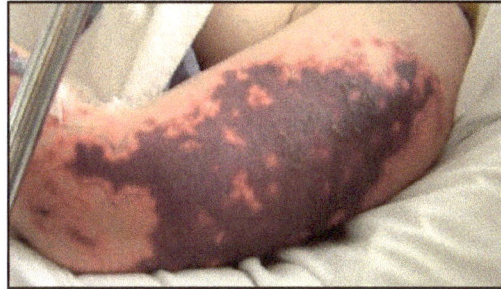

Figure 21.22b: Vasculitis.

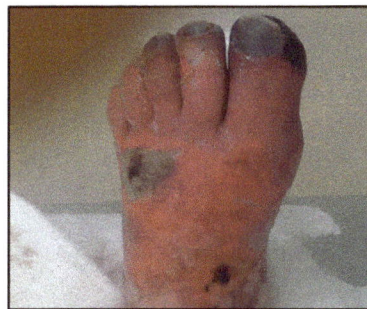

Figure 21.23: Microthrombotic disease.

        vii) Nodules (Figure 21.22a)
        viii) Tissue necrosis (Figure 21.22b)
3. Microthrombotic disease (Figure 21.23)
    a) Key features
        i) Livedo reticularis
        ii) Intense pain, clearly out proportion to the size of the wound
        iii) Eschar often present
        iv) Purple color of the surrounding skin
        v) Cyanosis
4. Coumadin necrosis (Figure 21.24)
    a) Usually appears within first week of starting warfarin (Coumadin) therapy.
    b) Protein C deficiency
    c) Usually appears on trunk
5. Hydroxyurea-related ulcers
    a) Hydroxyurea is an antineoplastic agent commonly used to treat myeloproliferative disorders and other nonneoplastic conditions.
    b) Dermatologic side effects of hydroxyurea are fairly common and include:
        i) Hyperpigmentation
        ii) Scaling

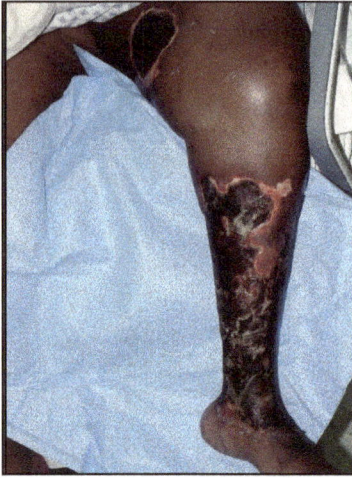

Figure 21.24: Leg and thigh ulcers diagnosed with coumadin necrosis. Photo courtesy of Mary Hirsch.

    iii) Erythema
    iv   Desquamation of the face and hands and partial alopecia
    v) A less well-described and less well-characterized complication is leg ulcers
    vi) Case study: hydroxyurea-induced ulcerations
        (1) A 70-year-old female with polycythemia vera on hydroxyurea with painful wounds for the last three months that have not improved with compression therapy. Biopsy shows stasis ulceration (Figure 21.25).

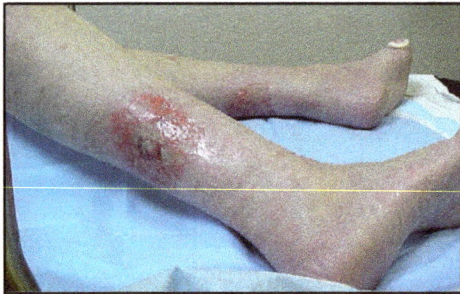

Figure 21.25: Hydroxyurea-induced ulceration.

  6. Cutaneous calcinosis
    a) Nonbypassable
    b) Low tissue oxygenation (TcPO$_2$)
    c) Abnormal calcium/phosphorus product
    d) May benefit from low calcium hemodialysis
    e) May need parathyroidectomy
    f) IV sodium thiosulfate may be helpful
    g) Usually gets worse with aggressive debridement
    h) Electrical stimulation and HBOT may help
    i) Case study: cutaneous calcinosis
        i) A 65-year-old female with type 2 DM and ESRD on dialysis for >10 years suddenly presents with painful superficial skin necrosis (Figures 21.26a and 21.26b).

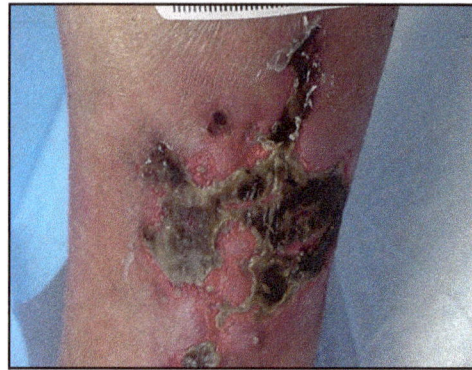

Figure 21.26a: Initial presentation of Calciphylaxis.

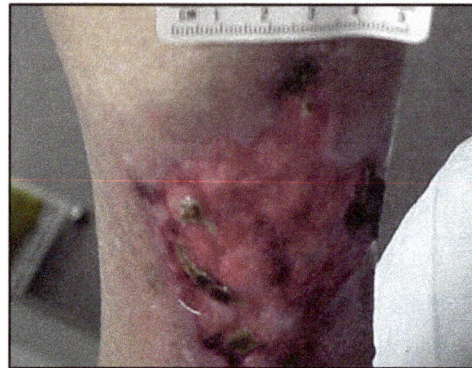

Figure 21.26b: Wound two weeks after electrical stimulation and enzymatic debridement.

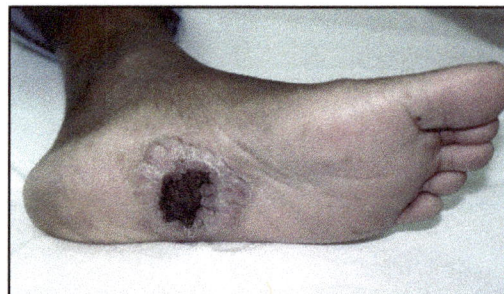

Figure 21.27: Keloid and pigmented plantar STSG. Photo courtesy of Mary Hirsch.

  7. Scars and keloids (Figure 21.27)
    a) Scars can present initially as red papules and plaques, which later become lighter tan and sometimes indurated.
    b) Some anatomic locations are more prone to develop hypertrophic scars and keloids.
    c) Some individuals have a genetic predisposition for developing keloids.
    d) Keloids differ from hypertrophic scars by growing beyond the margins of the original wound.
    e) Histological features include dermal fibrosis in scars and hypertrophic scars while keloids show the presence of keloidal collagen.
    f) Treatment options include surgical excision and high potency topical and intralesional corticosteroids.

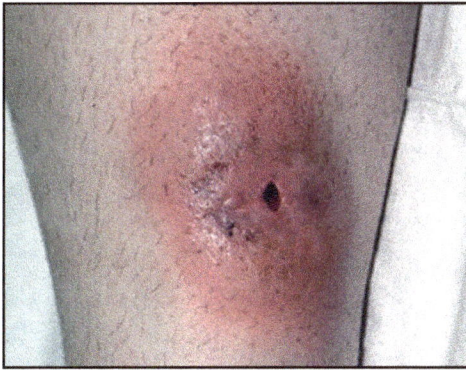

Figure 21.28a: Initial presentation in a patient with pyoderma gangrenosum. Photo courtesy of Mary Hirsch.

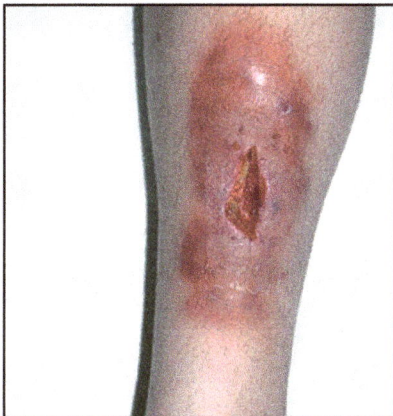

Figure 21.28b: Worsening after debridement.
Photo courtesy of Mary Hirsch.

8. Pyoderma gangrenosum (Figures 21.28a and 21.28b)
   a) Very painful
   b) Blister starts small
   c) Mainly skin involved
   d) Necrotic
   e) Crops of lesions at different stage of healing or development
   f) Autoimmune disorder
   g) Associated with ulcerative colitis (UC) and Crohn's disease
   h) Worse with debridement (pathergy)
   i) Treatment is steroid therapy
   j) Protect wound
9. Factitious disorder (Figure 21.29)

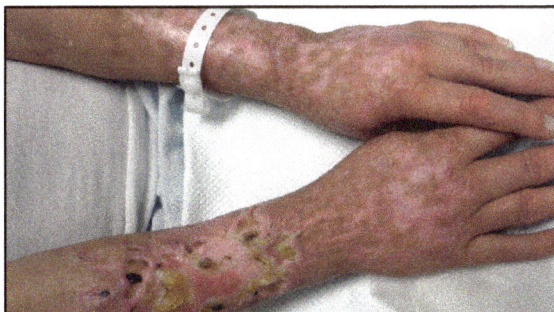

Figure 21.29: Patient with multiple self-inflicted wounds.

a) Associated with psychiatric disorders.
b) Ulcers have geometric edges and good granulation tissue.
c) Patients have an unexplained urge to harm themselves.
d) Psychiatry consult and putting on a dressing that cannot be easily removed by the patient is the recommended treatment.
10. Scleroderma (Figure 21.30)

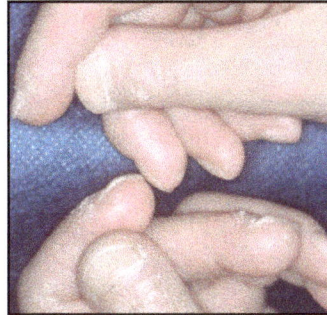

Figure 21.30: Scleroderma.

a) Autoimmune disorder of unknown etiology
b) Systemic features of scleroderma
   i) Painful and refractory wounds usually over bony prominences
   ii) Proliferation of fibroblasts
   iii) Excessive collagen proteins
c) 35% develop skin ulcers during course of disease
d) CREST—scleroderma that is characterized by
   i) Calcinosis (calcium deposits), usually in the fingers
   ii) Raynaud's disease
   iii) Esophageal dysmotility—loss of muscle control, which can cause difficulty swallowing
   iv) Sclerodactyly—a tapering deformity of the bones of the fingers
   v) Telangiectasias—small, red spots on the skin of the fingers, face, or inside of the mouth
e) Autolytic debridement or collagenase is usually the treatment of choice for local wound care.
11. Necrobiosis lipoidica diabeticorum
   a) Usually on tibial surface
   b) Usually bilateral, but asymmetric
   c) Reddish-brown lesion
   d) Raised purple edges, often with good granulation tissue but no epithelialization
   e) Steroids are usually the treatment of choice.

III. Summary

A. Most unusual wounds can be diagnosed correctly with good history and a physical.
B. In some cases, wound biopsy may be needed to make a diagnosis.
C. Appropriate wound management starts with a correct wound diagnosis.

RESOURCES

1. Shah JB. Approach to commonly misdiagnosed wounds and unusual leg ulcers. In: Sheffield PJ, Fife CE, editors. *Wound Care Practice.* 2nd ed. North Palm Beach: Best Publishing Company; 2007: 579-602.

2. Ikeda C, Slade JB Jr. Thermal injury. In: Sheffield PJ, Fife CE, editors. *Wound Care Practice.* 2nd ed. North Palm Beach: Best Publishing Company; 2007: 485-510.

3. Hagood CO, Wilson JR. Necrotic wounds produced by spider bites. In: Sheffield PJ, Fife CE, editors. *Wound Care Practice.* 2nd ed. North Palm Beach: Best Publishing Company; 2007: 561-78.

4. Shah JB, Hamm R. Atypical wounds. In: Hamm R. *Atlas of Wounds and Integumentary Disease.* Philadelphia: Lippincott Williams & Wilkins; 2015.

5. Weinstein D, et al. Atypical wounds. In: Baronoski S, Ayello EA. *Wound Care Essentials: Practice Principles.* 3rd ed. Philadelphia: Lippincott William & Wilkins; 2012.

SAMPLE QUESTIONS

1. The wound of the brown recluse spider can be:
   a) Rather insignificant
   b) Large with a rash, nausea, and fever
   c) Accompanied by the patient having "Coca-Cola" urine
   d) All of the above

2. In which of the following situations should malignancy be suspected?
   a) History of repeated trauma
   b) Exuberant granulation tissue
   c) Ulcer with rolled-out edges
   d) Purple-red color around the ulcer
   e) All of the above

3. Pathergy is a clinical sign that is common in which of the following conditions?
   a) Diabetic foot ulcer
   b) Ulcers due to vasculitis
   c) Pyoderma gangrenosum
   d) Vasculitic ulcers

4. Dermatologic side effects of hydroxyurea include all of the following except:
   a) Hyperpigmentation
   b) Scaling
   c) Erythema
   d) Lipodermatosclerosis
   e) Desquamation of the face and hands and partial alopecia
   f) Leg ulcers

5. Scleroderma ulcers are characterized by:
   a) The presence of excessive collagen
   b) The presence of a low amount of collagen
   c) Spontaneous healing
   d) Occurrence in 90% of scleroderma patients over the course of the disease

6. All of the following statements about pyoderma gangrenosum are true except:
   a) It is associated with gastrointestinal diseases like Crohn's disease and ulcerative colitis.
   b) It is associated with hematologic malignancies like multiple myeloma and lymphoma.
   c) It is associated with rheumatologic diseases like lupus and rheumatoid arthritis.
   d) It is associated with respiratory granulomatous diseases like sarcoidosis and tuberculosis.

7. Which of the following statements about keloids is true?
   a) A histological exam shows dermal fibrosis within the scar.
   b) They grow beyond the margin of original wound.
   c) They grow within the margin of original wound.
   d) A histological exam shows the absence of keloidal collagen.

8. A histological exam of a hypertrophic scar is characterized by:
   a) Dermal fibrosis within the scar
   b) Dermal hypertrophy within the scar
   c) Presence of keloidal collagen
   d) Presence of dermal collagen within the scar

9. All of the following statements about allergic contact dermatitis are true except:
   a) It is clinically characterized by red papulovesicular oozing and crusted lesions that, with persistence, develop into raised, scaling plaques with poorly defined scaling.
   b) Patch testing remains the gold standard for diagnosis in allergic contact dermatitis.
   c) It is associated with multiple systemic diseases.
   d) Topical corticosteroids are often the first line of treatment.

10. Necrobiosis lipoidica diabeticorum:
    a) Is usually called pyoderma gangrenosum
    b) Is usually present in morbidly obese diabetic female patients with a family history of diabetes
    c) Usually occurs because of subclinical community-acquired MRSA infections
    d) Usually presents as bilateral and symmetrical lesions

See answers on page 189.

NOTES

ANSWER KEY

1. d) The wound of the brown recluse spider can be rather insignificant, as only 10% of patients will develop necrosis. However, wounds can also be large depending on host immune response and the amount of toxin released, which can cause the patient to develop rash, nausea, and fever. Patients with spider bites who develop myonecrosis may have "Coca-Cola" urine.

2. e) Malignancy should be suspected if there is a history of repeated trauma, exuberant granulation tissue, rolled-out edges, and purple-red color around the ulcer.

3. c) Pathergy is a clinical sign where a patient develops more necrosis after trauma. This is typically seen in patients with pyoderma gangrenosum.

4. d) Dermatologic side effects of hydroxyurea include hyperpigmentation, scaling, erythema, desquamation of the face and hands and partial alopecia, and leg ulcers. Lipodermatosclerosis is a late finding in patients with venous disease, but it is not found as a dermatologic side effect of hydroxyurea.

5. a) Ulcers in patients with scleroderma have excessive collagen and are refractory and difficult to heal. Only 35% of scleroderma patients develop ulcers.

6. d) Pyoderma gangrenosum is associated with gastrointestinal diseases like Crohn's disease and ulcerative colitis, hematologic malignancies like multiple myeloma and lymphoma, and rheumatologic diseases like lupus and rheumatoid arthritis. Pyoderma gangrenosum is usually not associated with respiratory granulomatous diseases like sarcoidosis and tuberculosis.

7. b) Keloids grow beyond the margin of the original wound and on histology show keloidal collagen.

8. a) A histological exam of a hypertrophic scar is characterized by dermal fibrosis within the scar.

9. c) Allergic contact dermatitis is clinically characterized by red papulovesicular oozing and crusted lesions that, with persistence, develop into raised, scaling plaques with ill-defined scaling. Patch testing remains the gold standard for diagnosis in allergic contact dermatitis and removal of allergens and application of topical corticosteroids are often the first line of treatment.

10. b) Necrobiosis lipoidica diabeticorum occurs in morbidly obese diabetic female patients with a family history of diabetes. Usually those patients have ulcers that are bilateral and asymmetric. Community-acquired MRSA infections do cause necrotic abscesses, but not necrobiosis lipoidica diabeticorum. This condition is different from pyoderma gangrenosum.

MANAGING THE WOUND PATIENT: SURGERY, DEBRIDEMENT, GRAFTS & FLAPS

22

Richard Simman, MD, FACS, FACCWS
Caroline E. Fife, MD, CWSP, FAAFP, FUHM

INTRODUCTION

Managing the wound patient begins with a proper assessment of the wound, followed by preparation of the wound bed. The purpose of this chapter is to focus on the principles of wound bed preparation, the principles of primary and secondary healing, the use of grafts, flaps, and wound closure, and the reconstructive ladder in plastic surgery. Debridement options include autolytic, enzymatic, mechanical, sharp, surgical, ultrasonic, electrosurgical, and biosurgical. Plastic surgical closure options include direct closure, split-thickness and full-thickness skin grafts, cutaneous flaps, fasciocutaneous flaps, musculocutaneous flaps, and free flaps.

OBJECTIVES

Participants should be able to describe each type of debridement as it relates to wound care, discuss types of plastic surgical closure, and discuss the issues relating to plastic surgical closure.

I. Debridement
A. A wound is debrided to remove nonviable material that inhibits granulation and epithelialization and to remove bioburden that enhances bacterial growth and decreases resistance to infection. Debridement converts chronic wounds into acute wounds.
B. Debridement—evidence-based clinical data
   1. Diabetic foot ulcers (n=118):
      a) The extent of debridement improves wound healing in both the placebo and treatment arm of clinical study. (13)
   2. Diabetic, venous, arterial, pressure ulcers (n=432):
      a) When other factors are controlled, sharp debridement significantly increases healing in a variety of chronic wounds. (14)
   3. Diabetic foot ulcers (n=143):
      a) Adequacy of debridement (debridement performance index) is an independent predictor of wound healing. (15)

C. Debridement principles
   1. Clean the wound base of all devitalized tissue.
   2. Chronic non-healing wounds will likely need multiple debridement procedures of different types.
   3. Type of debridement is determined by the needs of the wound and experience of the provider.
D. Debridement types from a clinical viewpoint—mechanical, autolytic, chemical (enzymatic), biological, surgical/sharp
   1. Mechanical debridement
      a) Does not discriminate between viable and nonviable tissue (non-selective)
      b) Examples: wet to dry and pulse lavage
      c) Wet to dry (Figures 22.1a and 22.1b)

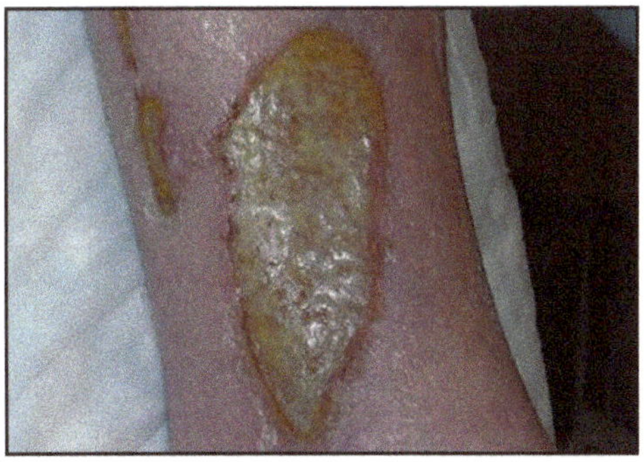

Figure 22.1a: An 80-year-old woman with COPD and active lung cancer on prednisone presents with multiple skin tears treated with saline wet to dry for 16 weeks with no improvement.

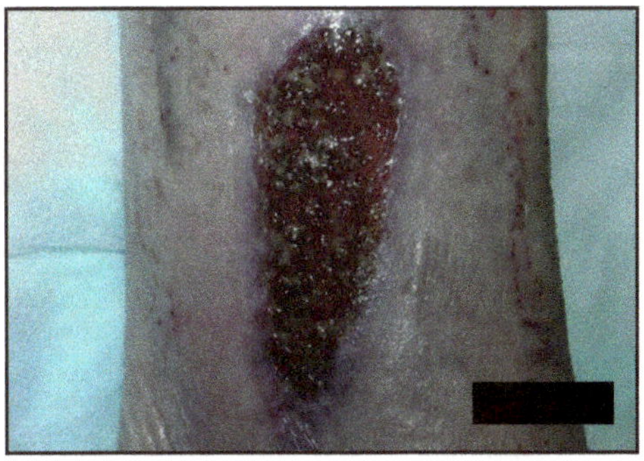

Figure 22.1b: The debrided and healing wound after 14 weeks of moist wound care using a hydrocolloid.

i) Inexpensive
ii) Various interpretations of what wet to dry means
iii) Various gauze types used; most common open weave, woven
iv) Issues of linting and pain
v) Gauze dressings and infection (8-11)
   (1) There is still the general misconception that gauze dressings protect against infection, but studies have shown saline gauze to be a fertile culture media.

2. Autolytic debridement
   a) Necrotic tissue is liquefied using the body's natural enzymes (phagocytic cells, proteolytic enzymes)
   b) Accomplished by keeping the wound moist with occlusive or semi-occlusive dressings
   c) Only works if wound stays moist
   d) Slow, painless
   e) Can be used when the patient is stable from medical and nutritional standpoints and is not a candidate for sharp debridement
   f) Should not be used when the wound is infected

3. Chemical (enzymatic) debridement
   a) Application of topical agents that disrupt or digest extracellular proteins
   b) Collagenase is derived from the fermentation of *Clostridium histolyticum*. It possesses the unique ability to digest collagen in necrotic tissue.
   c) Papain is a proteolytic enzyme from the fruit of *Carica papaya*, a potent digestant of nonviable protein matter but harmless to viable tissue.
      i) Relatively ineffective when used alone
      ii) Usually combined with urea, a substance that denatures proteins
      iii) Urea makes the proteins more susceptible to enzymatic digestion
   d) Example of enzymatic debridement (Figures 22.2a and 22.2b)

4. Biological debridement (maggot therapy) (Figures 22.3a-22.3c)

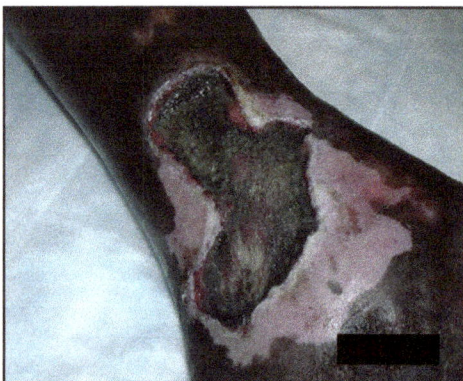

Figure 22.2a: A 54-year-old man with painful mixed arterial and venous disease ulcer.

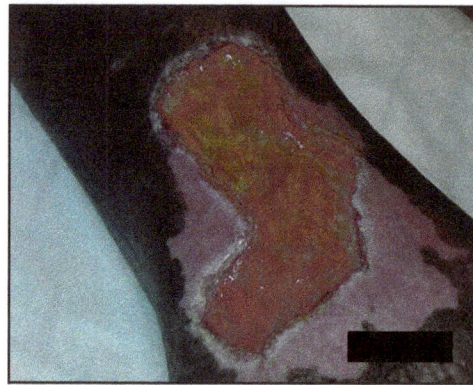

Figure 22.2b: Patient applied papain and urea daily for five weeks.

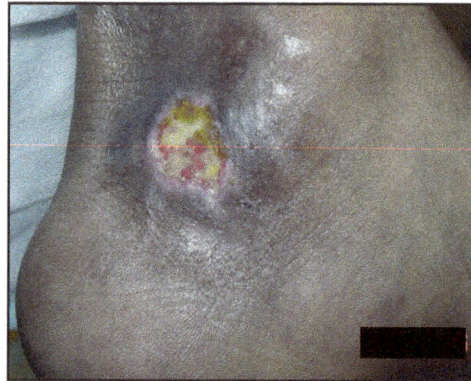

Figure 22.3a: Wound before debridement.

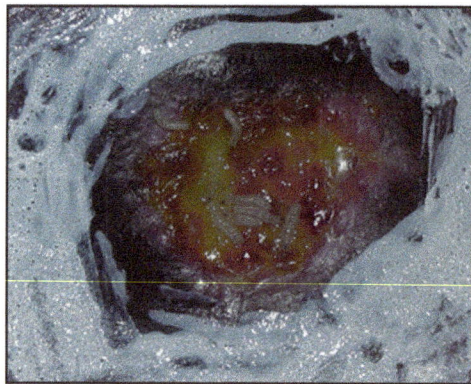

Figure 22.3b: Maggot therapy.

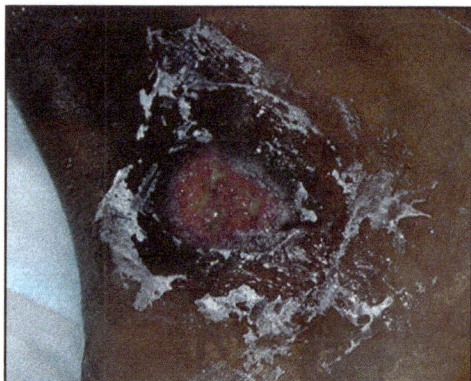

Figure 22.3c: 48 hours after biological debridement.

a) Debrides wounds
   i) Necrotic material is liquefied by proteolytic enzymes secreted during digestion
   ii) Does not damage healthy tissue (selective)
   iii) Painless
   iv) Requires staff training
b) Disinfects by killing bacteria
   i) Secretions possess broad-spectrum antimicrobial activity
   ii) Also ingests and lyses bacteria
   iii) Destroys MRSA, group A and B streptococci, and gram-positive aerobic and anaerobic strains
c) Stimulates wound healing
   i) Secretions amplify healing effects of host epidermal growth factor and IL-6
   ii) Stimulates growth of human fibroblasts and type II collagen
   iii) Secretions contain allantoin (found in shaving gels), which has a soothing effect on the skin
5. Sharp non-selective debridement (Figure 22.4)

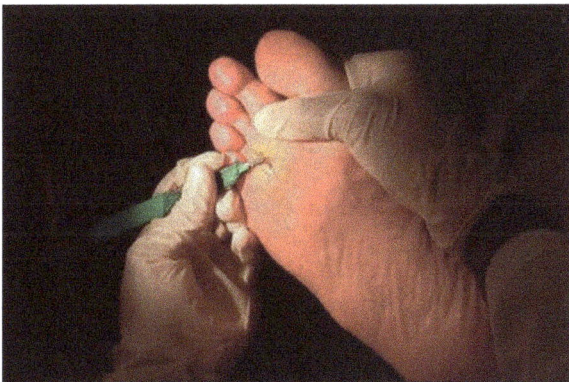

Figure 22.4: Sharp debridement with scalpel.

a) Usually done with a scalpel, scissors, curette, ultrasonic debridement, or diathermy electrosurgery.
   i) Ultrasonic debridement—tip vibrates at a frequency of 22.5 kHz, which results in the formation and collapse of thousands of vapor bubbles at the radiating surface of the probe, referred to as cavitation.
   ii) Diathermy electrosurgery:
      (1) Involves the use of high frequency electrical alternating current (AC) as either a cutting modality or to cauterize small blood vessels to stop bleeding.
      (2) This technique induces localized tissue burning and damage, the zone of which is controlled by the frequency and power of the device.
      (3) Some insist that electrosurgery be accomplished by high frequency AC cutting and that electrocautery be used

only for the practice of cauterization with heated nichrome wires powered by DC current, as in the handheld battery-operated portable cautery tools. After surgical/sharp debridement another form may be continued.
b) Sharp selective debridement
   i) CPT codes 97579 and 97598 are used for the removal of devitalized skin and debris (may use high-pressure waterjets, scalpels, scissors, or forceps); code 11042 is used for the first 20 cm^2 of skin and subcutaneous tissue; 11043 is used for the first 20 cm^2 of skin, subcutaneous, and muscle tissue; and 11044 is used for the first 20 cm^2 of bone debridement.
   ii It is determined by the tissue removed, not what is visible afterward.
   iii) CPT codes 11042-11044 can be performed and billed only by doctors of medicine, doctors of osteopathy, and doctors of podiatry.
   iv) Allied health professionals can perform and bill these services only if they are adequately trained and if these services are within the scope of practice of their state license act.
   v) Often requires anesthesia (conscious sedation, local, regional, or general).

II. Plastic surgical closures
A. Primary and secondary healing
   1. Primary wound healing or healing by first intention occurs within hours of repairing a full-thickness surgical incision primary closure (excision of skin lesion or skin cancer and closure).
      a) Surgical insult with a minimum mortality of cellular constituents
   2. Healing by secondary intention: wound is allowed to close and heal by granulation, contraction, and epithelization.
      a) Inflammatory response is more intense than with primary wound healing
      b) Larger quantity of granulation tissue is needed
      c) May result in significant wound contraction and scarring
B. Surgical options
   1. Direct closure, primary closure, secondary closure (delayed primary closure of open wound)
   2. Full-thickness and split-thickness skin grafts (Figure 22.5a)
   3. Flaps (Figure 22.5b)
      a) Cutaneous flaps
      b) Fasciocutaneous flaps
      c) Myocutaneous flaps
      d) Free flaps
C. Sutured wounds
   1. Absorbable sutures are made of materials that are

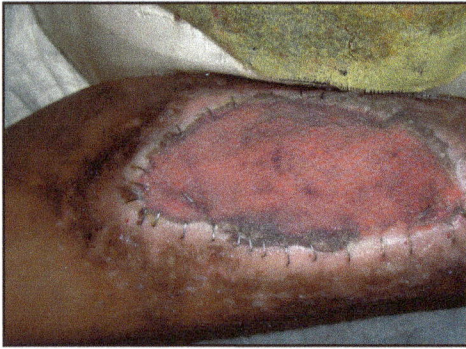

Figure 22.5a: Split-thickness skin graft.
Photo courtesy of Julio Ortiz, MD.

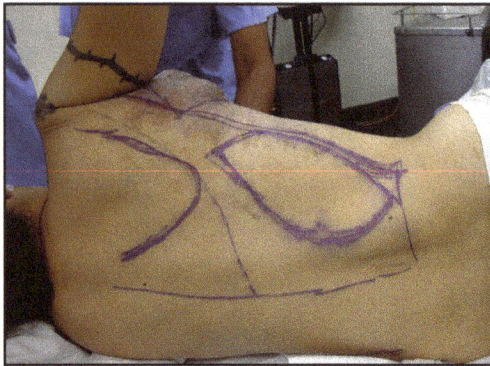

Figure 22.5b: Preparation for a myocutaneous flap.
Photo courtesy of Julio Ortiz, MD.

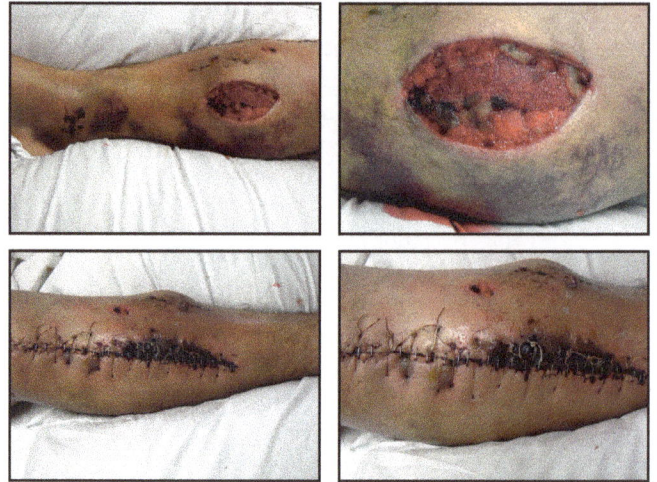

Figures 22.6a-d: Delayed primary wound closure.
Photos courtesy of Julio Ortiz, MD.

broken down in tissue after a given period of time (from ten days to four weeks or more, depending on the suture); they are used in many of the inner tissues of the body.

2. Non-absorbable sutures are made of materials that are not metabolized by the body and are used either on skin wound closures, where the sutures can be removed after a few days to weeks, or in some inner tissues where absorbable sutures are not adequate; for example, in the heart and in blood vessels where sutures are left forever.

D. Closure methods
1. Suturing is the oldest and most commonly used method of wound closure.
2. Alternative techniques—including skin staples, skin-closure tapes, and tissue adhesives—can be used in selected patients.
3. The short-term goal of any closure method is to hold tissue in apposition until the tensile strength of the wound is sufficient to withstand stress. Closed wounds will only achieve up to 80% of their original strength.

E. Primary wound closure
1. Closing of the wound near the time of injury.
   a) Almost always possible with clean wounds seen within hours after injury.
   b) The incidence of bacterial contamination and the risk of infection increase with injuries more than four hours old after injury.

2. For clean wounds in highly vascular areas (e.g., scalp, face, neck), the incidence of infection is so low that primary closure may be possible up to 24 hours after injury.

F. Delayed primary wound closure (Figures 22.6a–22.6d)
1. Delayed primary closure (secondary closure) is the approach of cleaning the wound, leaving the wound open under a moist dressing for approximately four to five days, and then suturing the wound if there is no evidence of infection.
   a) Heavily contaminated wounds, wounds resulting from high-energy missile injuries, or large wounds due to animal bites are ideal for delayed primary closure.
   b) Wounds contaminated by pus, vaginal discharge, feces, or saliva, as well as those where treatment is delayed longer than 12 hours, should also be considered for open wound management.
   c) The first step in delayed primary closure is through cleaning and removal of debris and devitalized tissue.
   d) Prophylactic antibiotics should be considered.

G. Secondary intention
1. Closure by secondary intention is allowing the wound to heal without mechanical closure.
   a) Over a period of time, the tissue slowly granulates, contracts, and epithelializes.
   b) Scar is larger than if a primary closure had been possible.

III. Grafts and flaps

A. Types of grafts
1. Autologous: the donor and recipient are the same (also known as an autograft)
2. Isogeneic: the donor and recipient are genetically identical (e.g., monozygotic twins, animals of a single inbred strain; isograft or syngraft)
3. Allogeneic: the donor and recipient are of the same species (human to human, dog to dog; allograft)

4. Xenogeneic: the donor and recipient are of different species (e.g., bovine cartilage; xenograft or hetero-graft). Example: pig skin in human burns
5. Prosthetic: lost tissue is replaced with synthetic materials such as metal, plastic, or ceramic (prosthetic implants)
6. Heterografts and xenografts
   a) By definition, these are temporary biologic dressings that the body will reject within days to a few weeks.
   b) They are useful in reducing the bacterial concentration of an open wound as well as reducing fluid loss. They serve as biologic dressings
   c) A xenograft is only a temporary covering
7. Alloderm® (LifeCell Corporation, an Acelity company) and TheraSkin® (Soluble Systems, Newport News, VA)
   a) Processed allogenic dermis and/or epidermis approved for use in acute burn resurfacing and reconstruction or in chronic wounds.
      i) Obtained from cadavers screened for transmissible disease.
   b) Alloderm® is used at the time of initial wound closure together with a thin epithelial autograft.
      i) The epithelium is removed and the remaining dermis treated with detergent to create a nonantigenic scaffold with the basement membrane (particularly laminin and collagen types IV and VII) intact.
   c) TheraSkin® can be used on virtually any type of chronic wound, including those with exposed muscle, tendon, and bone. However, Medicare may limit its use among outpatients to only certain types of wounds according to local coverage determinations (LCDs).
      i) Has cryopreserved fibroblasts and keratinocytes, and a fully developed extra cellular matrix (ECM) in its epidermis and dermis layers.
   d) By three months, the Alloderm® is repopulated with the patient's own cells while fibroblasts continue to lay down autologous collagen; the epithelial layer of TheraSkin® sloughs and collagen is incorporated into the wound bed.
8. Split-thickness skin grafts (STSG) (Figures 22.7a-c, 22.8a-c)
   a) Include the entire epidermis and part of the dermis.
   b) Meshing expands the area that can be covered and allows drainage through graft.
   c) Sewn or stapled into place and covered with compression dressings or negative pressure wound therapy (NPWT).
   d) Recipient bed must be well granulated to supply the skin with nutrients.
   e) Most skin grafts are successful, but some do not

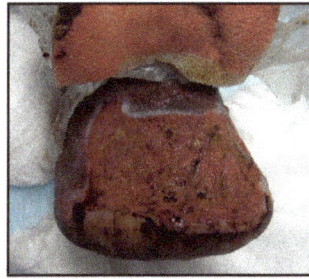
Figure 22.7a: Wound after negative pressure wound therapy and debridement.

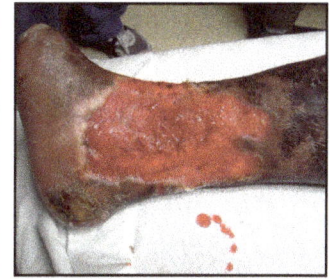
Figure 22.7b: Wound on medial side after debridement and NPWT.

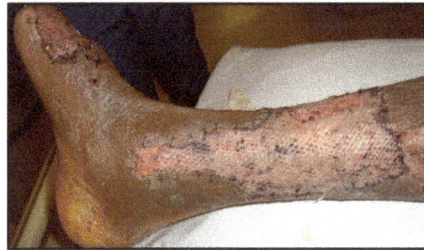
Figure 22.7c: Wound after split thickness skin graft.
Photos courtesy of Julio Ortiz, MD.

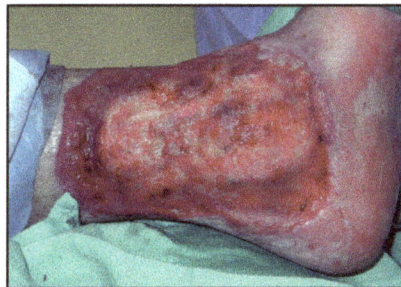
Figure 22.8a: Intraoperative view of left ankle venous ulcer after debridement.

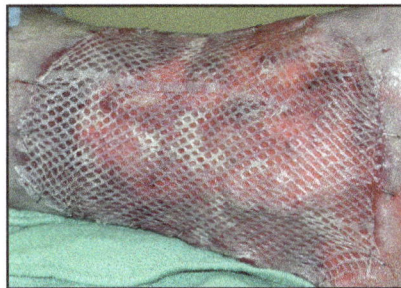
Figure 22.8b: Intraoperative view of meshed skin graft.

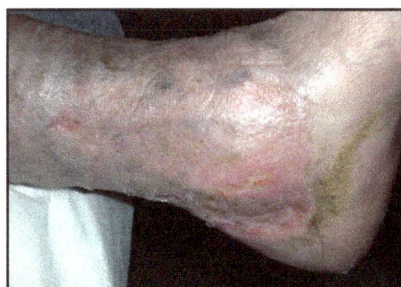
Figure 22.8c: Skin graft three months later.

heal well and require repeat grafting. Graft failure is due to infection, hematoma, mobility, and unprepared wound beds.

f) The recovery from surgery is usually rapid after split thickness skin grafting.

g) The skin graft must be protected from trauma or significant stretching for two to three weeks.

h) Depending on the location of the graft, a dressing may be necessary for one or two weeks.

i) STSG sites heal in 10-14 days and will often require moisturizers forever since they may never have sufficient oil production and may be vulnerable to abrasion.

j) Used for coverage of tissue defects.

k) NPWT may be used as bolster for protection dressing.

   i) STSG cannot be used when deep structures are exposed, there is a significant volume deficit, or if granulation tissue bed is inadequate. In these cases flaps should be considered.

   ii) In such cases, muscle tissue must be mobilized with or without the skin as a covering (flap).

   iii) Unlike skin, which can be provided with nutrients by diffusion from the granulating bed, the flap lives off a native vascular supply (pedicle).

B. Types of flaps—flaps can be classified by blood supply (axilla and random), tissue types, and mobilization and geometrical shapes.

  1. Pedicle flap types—rotation flap, advancement flap, transpositional flap. Example: rotation flap (Figures 22.9a–c, 22.10a–c, 22.11a–c, 22.12, 22.13a–c, 22.14a–b)

   a) A semicircular skin flap that is rotated into the defect on a fulcrum point.

   b) The flap must be adequately large, and a large base is necessary if a back-cut will be needed to lengthen the flap.

   c) If the flap is too small, the residual defect of the donor site can be closed primarily by mobilizing the surrounding tissue.

   d) A drawback of rotation flaps is the extended cutting and undermining needed to create the flap, which increases the risk of bleeding, nerve damage, and partial flap loss.

   e) They provide the ability to mobilize large areas of tissue with a wide vascular base for reconstruction.

   f) The name "rotation flap" refers to the vector of motion of the flap.

    i) Particularly useful when the proposed donor site of the flap is the lateral aspect of the face

   g) Advantageous because they have a particularly wide base and thus an excellent blood supply.

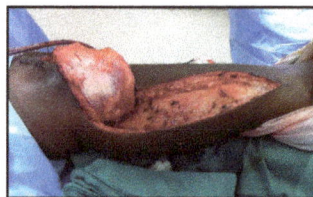

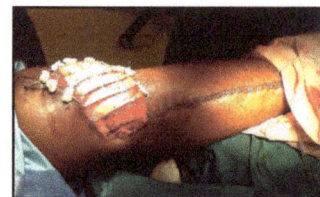

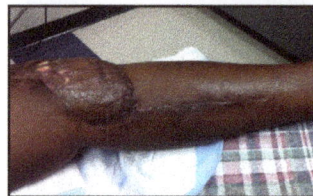

Figure 22.9a-c: Gastrocnemius flap during surgery and healed.
Photos courtesy of Julio Ortiz, MD.

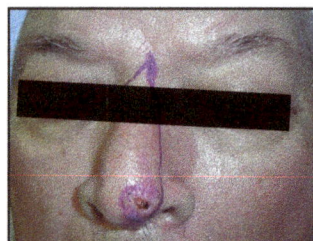

Figure 22.10a: Basal cell cancer to be treated with glabellar and nasal dorsum advancement flap.

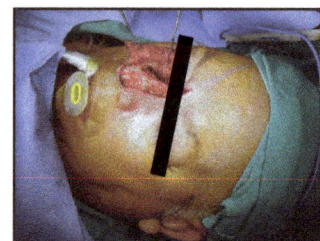

Figure 22.10b: Glabellar flap during surgery.

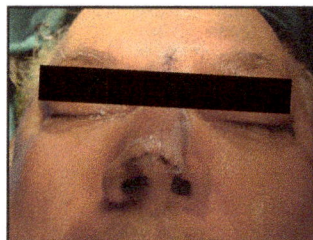

Figure 22.10c: Healed glabellar flap.
Photos courtesy of Julio Ortiz, MD.

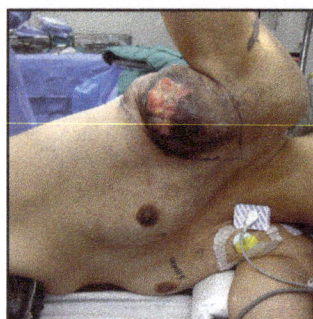

Figure 22.11a: Soft tissue tumor on right chest.

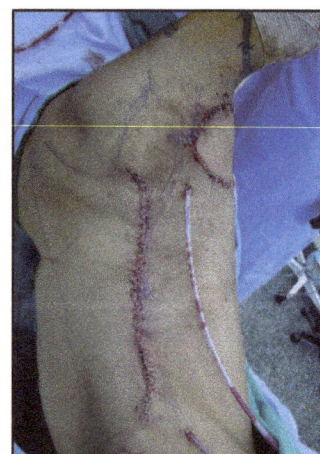

Figure 22.11b: Latissimus dorsi flap.

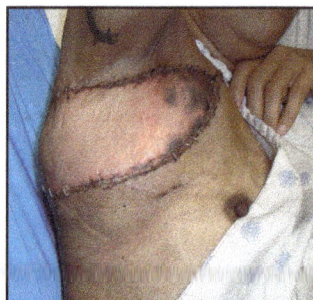

Figure 22.11c: Resection and flap closure.
Photos courtesy of Julio Ortiz, MD.

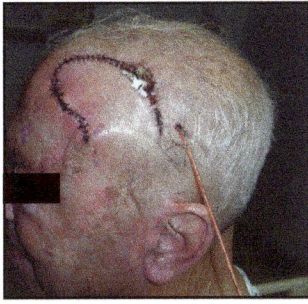

Figure 22.12: Rotation scalp flap. Photo courtesy of Julio Ortiz, MD.

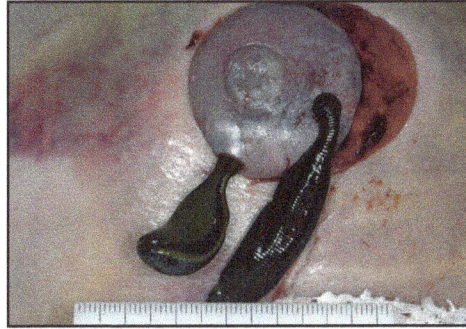

Figure 22.13a: Malignant ulcer of scalp.

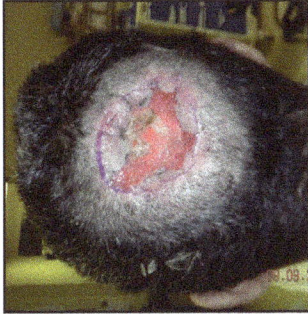

Figure 22.13b: Subsequent to resection of ulcer.

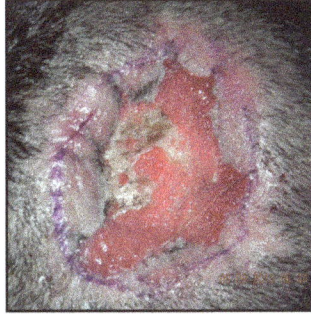

Figure 22.13c: Orticochea flap.

Photos courtesy of Julio Ortiz, MD.

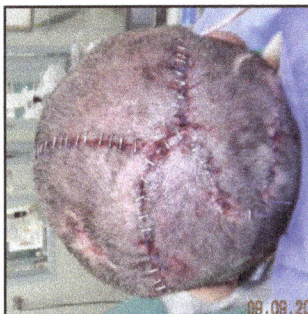

Figure 22.14a: Stage IV sacral pressure ulcer.

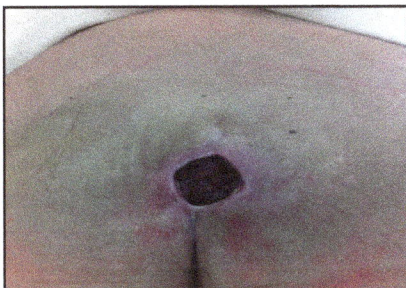

Figure 22.14b: Reconstruction with rotational left gluteal fasciocutaneous flap.

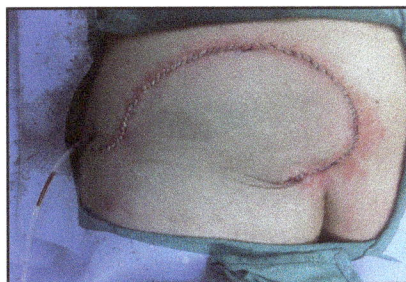

Figure 22.15: Leeches used for venous engorgement of pedicle flap after breast reduction.

h) The disadvantage is that they require relatively extensive cutting beyond the defect to develop the flap, increasing the risk of morbidity of the donor site.

i) The pedicle (blood supply) to the flap is not severed as with a free flap.

j) Pedicle is dissected so that the flap can be moved directly or through a tunnel created under the skin to the defect area.

k) Faster to perform than free flaps, but depending on the defect and anatomy, are not always possible.

l) Complications are similar to those of free flaps (may have partial necrosis); free flap is all or nothing.

m) Examples:
   i) Leeches used for venous engorgement of pedicle flap after breast reduction (Figure 22.15)
   ii) A 34-year-old male with DM after necrotizing infection (Figures 22.16a–22.16i)

2. Free flaps/tissue transfer
   a) "Free" implies that the tissue, along with its blood supply, is detached from the original location (donor site) and transferred to another location (recipient site) and anastomosed to vessels at recipient site.
   b) Various types of tissue may be transferred as a free flap, including skin and fat, skin with fascia, muscle, nerve, bone, or any combination of these depending on tissue needing replacement.
   c) For all free flaps, the blood supply is reconstituted using microsurgery to reconnect the artery and vein.
   d) Indications for free flaps when local flaps are not available:
      i) Cosmetic reconstruction
         (1) Most commonly creating a breast after a mastectomy
         (2) Usually only done if a transverse rectus abdominis myocutaneous (TRAM) pedicle flap is not possible

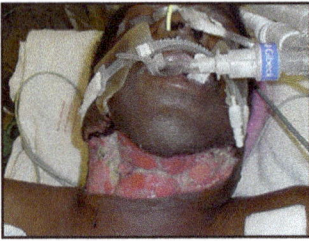

Figure 22.16a: A 34-year-old male with DM after necrotizing infection of neck on initial presentation.

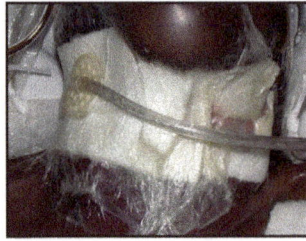

Figure 22.16b: Patient treated with NPWT.

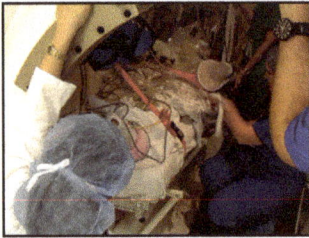

Figure 22.16c: Use of HBOT to prepare recipient wound bed for free flap.

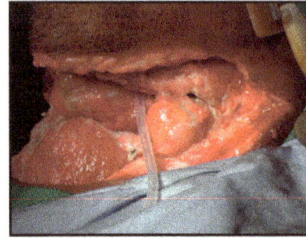

Figure 22.16d: Recipient site on neck prepared for flap transfer.

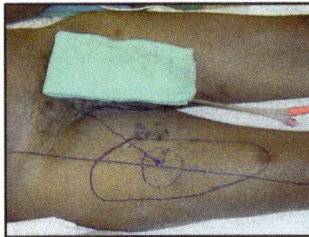

Figure 22.16e: Donor site selected on thigh for harvesting free flap.

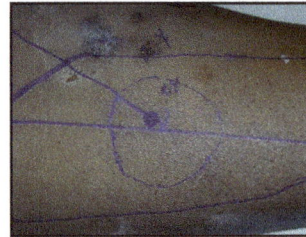

Figure 22.16f: Close-up of donor site.

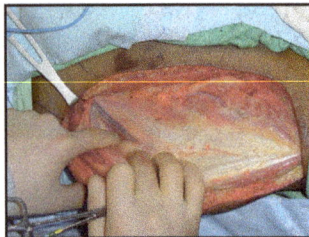

Figure 22.16g: Free flap excised from donor site.

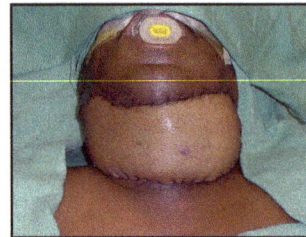

Figure 22.16h: Free flap positioned to recipient site on neck.

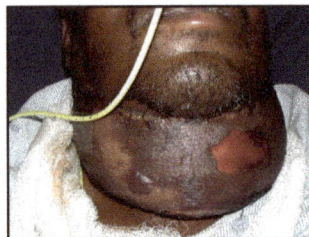

Figure 22.16i: Results.

ii) Traumatic reconstruction
  (1) Tissue is missing, often bone is exposed
iii) Removal of cancer of the mouth, jaw, or neck
  (1) Tumor excision has left a large defect.
e) Steps in creating a free flap:
  i) The flap is dissected and freed from the surrounding tissue.
  ii) Vascular pedicle is created and separated from the body.
  iii) A recipient artery and vein are identified to which the free flap's vascular pedicle can be attached.
  iv) The free flap is anastomosed to the recipient bed using microsurgery.
  v) The donor site area is sutured closed or skin grafted.
  vi) STSG may be placed on top of muscle flap site.
f) Complications of free flaps:
  i) Most common serious complication is flap loss due to venous (congestion) outflow issues caused by pedicle twist, tight closure, or clotted anastomosis.
  ii) Loss of arterial supply will also cause total necrosis.
  iii) Close post-op monitoring is performed.
  iv) Usually donor sites are selected that cause the least amount of disability, but some disability may occur.
g) HBOT can prevent ischemia/reperfusion (IR) injury (16) and is indicated in compromised flaps. Example: free transverse rectus abdominis myocutaneous (TRAM) flap.
  i) A portion of the abdomen tissue group, including skin, adipose tissues, rectus muscles and connective tissues, is taken from the patient's abdomen and transplanted onto the breast site.
  ii) Combines a mastectomy with an abdominoplasty
  (1) Allows the breast to be reconstructed with one's own tissues instead of a foreign implant.
  (2) Is contraindicated for patients who need abdominal strength since the muscle removal weakens the abdomen.

RESOURCES

1. Dolan RW. *Facial, Plastic, Reconstructive, and Trauma Surgery.* New York: CRC Press; 2003.
2. Ip D. *Orthopedic Traumatology - A Resident's Guide.* Berlin: Springer; 2008.
3. Myers EN, Smith MR, Myers J, Hanna E. *Cancer of the Head and Neck.* Philadelphia: Saunders; 2003.
4. Baker SR. *Local Flaps in Facial Reconstruction.* 2nd ed. St. Louis: Mosby; 2007.
5. Wolff KD, Hölzle F. *Raising of Microvascular Flaps: A Systematic Approach.* Berlin: Springer; 2005.
6. Simman R, Phavixay L. Split-thickness skin grafts remain the gold standard for the closure of large acute and chronic wounds. *J Am Col Certif Wound Spec.* 2011; 3(3):55-9.
7. Simman R. Wound closure and the reconstructive ladder in plastic surgery. *J Am Col Certif Wound Spec.* 2009; 1(1):6-11.
8. Lee CK, Chua YP, Saw A. Antimicrobial gauze as a dressing reduces pin site infection: a randomized controlled trial. *Clin Orthop Relat Res.* 2012 Feb; 470(2):610-5.
9. Ovington LG. Hanging wet-to-dry dressings out to dry. *Adv Skin Wound Care.* 2002; 15(2):79-84.
10. Lawrence JC, et al. Dressings and wound infection. *Am J Surg.* 1994 Jan; 167(1 Supp):21S–24S.
11. Spear M. Wet-to-dry dressings—evaluating the evidence. *Plast Surg Nurs.* 2008 Apr-Jun; 28(2):92-5.
12. Jones AM, San Miguel L. Are modern wound dressings a clinical and cost-effective alternative to the use of gauze? *J Wound Care.* 2006 Feb; 15(2):65-9. Published online September 29, 2013. Accessed at: http://dx.doi.org/10.12968/jowc.2006.15.2.26886.
13. Steed DL, Donohoe D, Webster MW, Lindsley L. Effect of extensive debridement and treatment on the healing of diabetic foot ulcers. Diabetic Ulcer Study Group. *J Am Coll Surg.* 1996; 183:61-4.
14. Ennis WJ, Meneses P. Managing wounds in a managed care environment: the integration concept. *Ostomy Wound Manage.* 1998; 44(11):22-6, 28-31, 34-6, passim.
15. Saap LJ, Donohue K, Falanga V. Clinical classification of bioengineered skin use and its correlation with healing of diabetic and venous ulcers. *Dermatol Surg.* 2004; 30:1095–1100.
16. Thom SR. Hyperbaric oxygen: its mechanisms and efficacy. *Plast Reconstr Surg.* 2011 Jan; 127(Suppl 1):131S-41S.

SAMPLE QUESTIONS

1. Which of the following statements about enzymatic debridement is true?
    a) Collagenase can digest collagen in necrotic tissue.
    b) Papain is relatively ineffective when used alone.
    c) Urea makes proteins more susceptible to enzymatic digestion.
    d) Enzymatic agents can cause a burning sensation.
    e) All of the above statements are true.

2. Which statement about biological debridement is false?
    a) Maggots secrete proteolytic enzymes.
    b) Maggots are a form of selective debridement.
    c) Maggots can increase the risk of infection.
    d) Maggots can stimulate wound healing.

3. Which statement about sharp debridement is false?
    a) It can be performed with hydrocolloid dressings.
    b) Only trained professionals can perform it.
    c) It may require anesthesia.
    d) Very specific documentation, billing, and coding rules apply.

4. Which of the following statements about split-thickness skin grafts is false?
    a) They can be used to cover exposed tendons.
    b) They are a form of xenograft.
    c) They are supplied with blood via the anastomosis of an artery at surgery.
    d) None of the above statements are true.

5. What is the most common complication of a free flap?
    a) Compromise of the arterial anastomosis
    b) Compromise of the venous anastomosis
    c) Ischemia reperfusion injury
    d) Infection

6. A flap is likely to be chosen when:
    a) There has been significant subcutaneous tissue loss.
    b) Cosmetic reconstruction is needed.
    c) Deep structures are exposed (e.g., bone, tendon).
    d) All of the above

7. During the first day of application, the skin graft remains viable through:
    a) Capillary formation
    b) Serum absorption
    c) Lymphatic channels formation
    d) Direct oxygenation from the surrounding air

8. All of the following may lead to graft failure except:
    a) Infection
    b) Hematoma
    c) Drug interactions
    d) Unprepared wound beds

9. Which of the following is the most durable in closing a stage IV pressure wound?
    a) Cutaneous flap
    b) Fasciocutaneous flap
    c) Myocutaneous flap
    d) Osteocutaneous flap

10. Paraplegic patients are most likely to develop pressure wounds on their:
    a) Heels
    b) Sacrum
    c) Coccyx
    d) Ischium

See answers on page 202.

NOTES

ANSWER KEY

1. e) All of the statements about enzymatic debridement are true: collagenase can digest collagen in necrotic tissue, papain is relatively ineffective when used alone, urea makes proteins more susceptible to enzymatic digestion, and enzymatic agents can cause a burning sensation.

2. c) Maggots secrete proteolytic enzymes and are a form of selective debridement that stimulates wound healing. Medicinal maggots are sterile larvae and do not increase the risk of infection.

3. a) Sharp debridement is only performed by trained professionals, and it may require anesthesia. Sharp debridement requires very specific documentation, billing, and coding rules. Debridement performed by hydrocolloid dressings (occlusive dressing) is called autolytic debridement.

4. d) None of the statements listed about split-thickness skin grafts are true: STSGs cannot be used to cover exposed tendon—the flap is needed to cover exposed tendons. The flap is not supplied with blood via the anastomosis of an artery at surgery, and an STSG is not a form of xenograft.

5. b) The most common complication of a free flap is compromise of the venous anastomosis.

6. d) A flap is likely to be chosen when there has been significant subcutaneous tissue loss, when cosmetic reconstruction is needed, or when deep structures are exposed.

7. b) After the application of a skin graft, the first 24-hour viability of the graft depends on serum absorption. On the second day inosculation takes place, which is the alignment of microvessels between the graft and the underlying wound bed to establish blood supply needed by the graft to continue to live and take.

8. c) Graft failure is due to infection, hematoma, mobility, and unprepared wound beds.

9. c) Myocutaneous flaps are the most reliable flaps to cover stage IV pressure wounds because they include muscle, fascia, subcutaneous fatty tissue, and skin.

10. d) Paraplegic patients sitting in wheelchairs are most likely to develop ischial pressure wounds. This results from permanent capillary occlusion in tissue compressed between the ischial bony prominence and the chair's hard surface.

PAIN MANAGEMENT, PALLIATIVE CARE, AND PSYCHOSOCIAL ISSUES 23

Jayesh B. Shah, MD, CWSP, FAPWCA, FACCWS

INTRODUCTION

This chapter discusses psychosocial issues in wound care such as dealing with pain, depression, quality of life issues, compliance, body image, and palliative care. Pain assessment and management is also discussed.

OBJECTIVES

Participants should be able to describe how to conduct a pain assessment, explain the goals and objectives of a palliative wound care plan, describe techniques for controlling wound odors, and describe a Kennedy ulcer.

I. Pain

A. Definition: pain is whatever the patient experiencing it says it is, and it exists whenever the patient experiencing it says it does. (1)

B. Types of pain
1. Nociceptive pain results from the ongoing activation of primary afferent neurons by noxious stimuli, with an intact nervous system.
   a) Somatic pain arises from bone, skin, muscle, or connective tissue.
   b) Visceral pain arises from visceral organs.
2. Neuropathic pain is caused by primary lesions or dysfunction of the nervous system.

C. Pain assessment (PQRST)
1. Palliative/provocative factors
2. Quality of pain
3. Region and radiation of pain
4. Severity of pain
5. Temporal aspects of pain

D. Principles of wound management: the chronic wound pain experience model (suffering)

E. Causes of wound pain (Table 23.1)
1. Background pain (chronic wound pain)
   a) Persistent underlying pain due to wound etiology, local wound factors (e.g., ischemia, infection)

Table 23.1: Types of wound pain.
From Krasner D. Caring for the person experiencing chronic wound pain. In: Krasner DL, Rodeheaver GT, Sibbald GR. *Chronic Wound Care: A Clinical Source Book for Healthcare Professionals.* 3rd ed. Wayne: HMP Communications; 2001.

PAIN TYPE	NONCYCLIC ACUTE WOUND PAIN	CYCLIC ACUTE WOUND PAIN	CHRONIC WOUND PAIN
Pharmacologic interventions	Local anesthesia Systemic anesthesia	Local anesthesia Systemic analgesia	Systemic analgesia Antidepressants Anticonvulsants
Non-pharmacologic interventions	Pain-reducing wound care products and techniques	Pain-reducing wound care products and techniques; patient empowerment	Relaxation strategies; transcutaneous electrical nerve stimulation
Reevaluation	Frequently	Frequently	Frequently
Examples	Debridement	Dressing changes Movement-related activities	Secondary to ischemia, vasculitis, infection, and/or malignancy

2. Psychosocial factors: age, gender, culture, education, mental state
3. Environmental factors: timing of procedure, setting (e.g., level of noise), positioning of patient, resources
4. Operative: debridement (noncyclic acute wound pain)
5. Procedural: dressing changes (cyclic acute wound pain)
6. Incident: movement related activities (cyclic acute wound pain)

F. Interventions for noncyclic wound pain
1. Administer topical or local anesthetics.
2. Consider operating room procedure under general anesthesia rather than bedside debridement.

3. Administer opioids and nonsteroidal anti-inflammatory drugs before and after procedures.
4. Avoid wet-to-dry dressings.
5. Consider alternatives to sharp debridement (refer to Table 13.4, page 99).

G. Interventions for cyclic wound pain
1. Avoid using cytotoxic agents.
2. Avoid aggressive packing.
3. Minimize the number of daily dressing changes.
4. Utilize pressure reducing devices in beds or chairs.
5. Provide analgesia, as needed, to allow positioning of the patient.
6. Avoid trauma (shearing and tear injuries) to fragile skin when transferring, positioning, or holding the patient.

H. Interventions for persistent (chronic) wound pain
1. Utilize all the interventions listed for noncyclic and cyclic wound pain.
2. Control edema.
3. Control infection.
4. Monitor wound pain while the patient is resting.
5. Provide regularly scheduled analgesia.
6. Attend to non-wound pain.
7. Address the emotional component of the pain.
8. Recommended steps for analgesia in wound pain (Figure 23.1):
   a) Nonsteroidal anti-inflammatory drug (NSAID)
   b) Opioids

I. Evaluating one's knowledge of pain—which of the following are true, and which are false? (2)
1. Observable changes in vital signs must be relied upon to verify a patient's report of severe pain.
2. Pain intensity should be rated by the clinician, not the patient.
3. A patient who can sleep is not having moderate to severe pain.
4. Intramuscular meperidine is the drug of choice for prolonged pain.
5. Analgesics for chronic pain are more effective when administered as needed rather than around the clock.

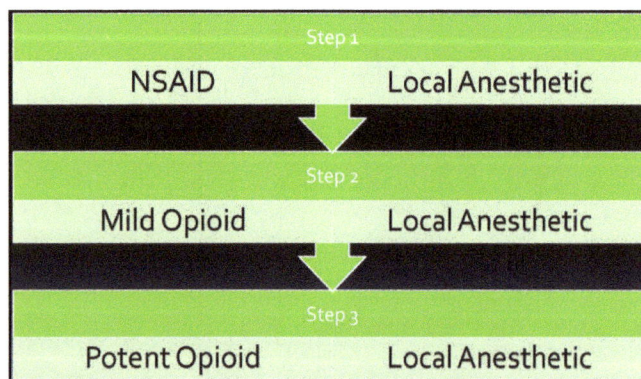

Figure 23.1: Recommended steps for analgesia for wound pain. Adapted from Senecal SJ. Pain management of wound care. *Nurs Clin North Am.* 1999; 34(4):847–60.

6. If the patient can be distracted from the pain, he has less pain than he reports.
7. The patient in pain should be encouraged to endure as much pain as possible before resorting to a pain relief measure.
8. Respirator depression (less than 7 breaths per minute) probably occurs in at least 10% of patients who receive one or more doses of an opioid for relief of pain.
9. Vicodin (5/500) is approximately equal to analgesia of one-half of a dose of meperidine 75 mg IM.
10. If a patient's pain is relieved by a placebo, the pain isn't real.
11. Beyond a certain dose, increasing the dosage of an opioid, such as morphine, will not increase pain relief.
12. When opioids are used for pain relief for more than three to six months, there is a high chance of addiction.
   a) All of the above statements are FALSE.

J. Wound pain myths
1. Wet-to-dry dressings are still the gold standard for wound care.
2. Transparent films are the best dressings for treating and reducing the pain of skin tears.
3. Using paper tape is the least painful way to secure a dressing.
4. Pulling a dressing off faster rather than slower reduces pain at dressing changes.
5. People with diabetic foot wounds do not experience pain.

K. Pain management
1. The majority of patients experience pain during dressing changes and wound bed treatments.
   a) Removing dry and adherent dressing
   b) Cleansing procedures
   c) Turning the patient for wound care
2. The end of life patient may have persistent pain occurring, even when wound is not manipulated. This pain is called chronic pain, and the following should be done for pain management:
   a) Be aware of the current status of pain.
   b) Know and avoid pain triggers, where possible.
   c) Know and use pain reducers, where possible.
   d) Avoid the unnecessary manipulation of wounds.
   e) Explore simple patient-controlled techniques such as counting up and down, focusing on the breath entering and leaving the lungs, or listening to music.
   f) Observe the wound and surrounding skin for evidence of infection, necrosis, maceration, etc.
   g) Use topicals that contain local anesthetic agents, e.g., lidocaine gel, EMLA cream, Regenecare®.
   h) Use minimal mechanical force, e.g., 4-15 psi irrigation force.
   i) Use warmed products such as normal saline or gauze pads.

j)   Avoid antiseptic and cytotoxic agents.
k)   Pre-medicating the patient with pain medication 20-30 minutes prior to changing the dressing should be a standard of care for patients with palliative wounds.
l)   Ongoing evaluation and modification of the management plan and treatment intervention is essential as wounds change over time.
m)   More advanced non-pharmacological techniques that require specialized training or skilled personnel, such as the use of hypnosis or therapeutic touch, can be considered.

II. Palliative care

A.   Definition: palliative care is care that affirms life and views death and dying as part of a normal process that neither speeds nor delays death, provides relief from pain and other symptoms, and offers support to the patient and family. Palliative care focuses on holistically supporting the individual for comfort rather than cure.
B.   Extent of the problem
1.   By 2030, 20% of the US population will be >65.
2.   Significant increase in number of frail, elderly patients for whom cure may not be the goal.
3.   Wounds affect more than one-third of nearly 1 million hospice patients.
C.   Issues related to palliative care (3)
1.   Palliative care is not synonymous with the absence of care.
2.   Wounds treated appropriately can improve in 50% of palliative cases, even when the goal is not healing or when patients are in hospice units.
3.   Moving a patient from curative to palliative treatment requires a determination that the patient's wound is non-healing, not under-treated.
D.   Goals of palliative care
1.   Control pain
2.   Control odor
3.   Control exudates
4.   Control bleeding
5.   Preserve self-image
6.   Preserve dignity
7.   Maximize quality of life
E.   Skin care needs in palliative care patient
1.   A low pH skin cleanser is useful, along with a moisture barrier, to minimize the effects of excess moisture (gently cleanse the skin).
2.   Avoid massage over a reddened area.
3.   Manage incontinence.
4.   Individualize the patient's turning and positioning schedule based on his pain tolerance and comfort level.
5.   Protect the skin.
a)   To protect the buttocks and sacral areas, use a lift sheet or an overhead trapeze.

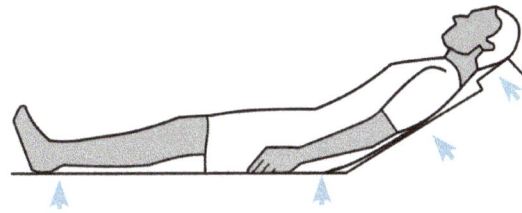

Figure 23.2a: Elevating 30 degrees or less.[13]

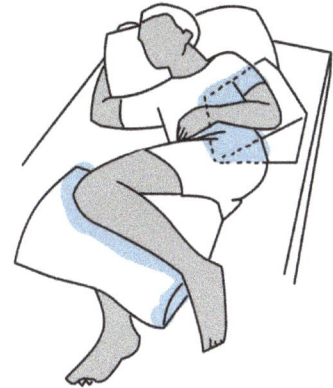

Figure 23.2b: Protecting pressure areas.[13]

b)   Keep the bed at the lowest possible elevation, preferably 30 degrees or lower to minimize friction and shear to the sacrum and buttocks.
c)   When turning the patient side to side, the angle should only be 30 degrees.
F.   Positioning the palliative care patient (Figures 23.2a and 22.3b)
G.   Nutrition and hydration in the palliative care patient
1.   Fluid and food requirement generally decrease at end of life.
2.   Lessening of oral intake can occur weeks to months before death.
3.   Nutrition and hydration status worsens because of draining wounds.
4.   Swallow reflex decreases, which increases the risk of aspiration.
H.   Wound dressings for a palliative wound care patient
1.   Dressings that can stay for several days
2.   Dressings that can protect the wound from incontinence
3.   Non-adherent dressings are best
4.   For minimal or no drainage:
a)   Hydrogel
b)   Transparent film
c)   Hydrocolloid
d)   Composite dressings
5.   For moderate exudates:
a)   Hydrogel
b)   Hydrocolloid
c)   Foam
d)   Calcium alginate
e)   Cadexomer iodine
f)   Silver dressings
g)   Silver foam dressings

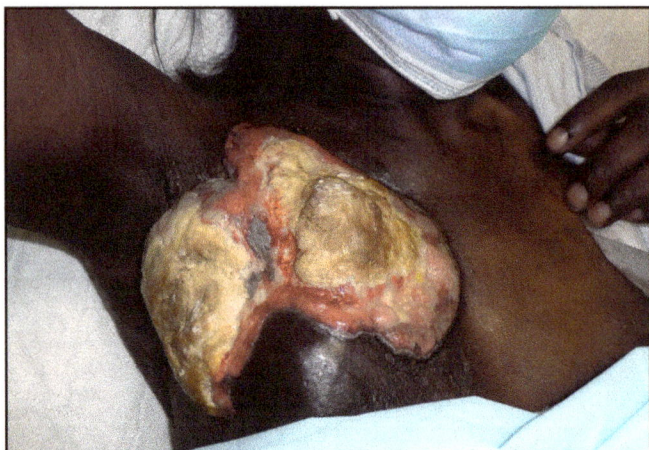

Figure 23.3: Breast cancer with fungating wound.

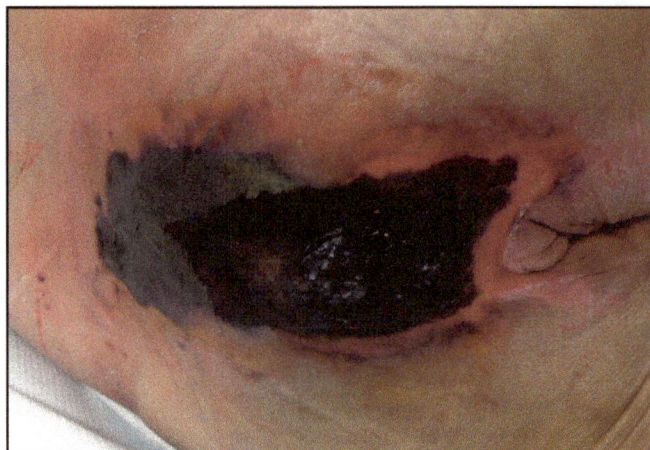

Figure 23.4: Kennedy ulcer in the sacrococcygeal area.

6. For severe exudates:
   a) Composite foam
   b) Calcium alginate dressings
   c) Combination of calcium alginate and silver
   d) Combination of calcium alginate and honey
I. Debridement in the palliative care patient
   1. Nonsurgical
   2. Autolytic/enzymatic debridement is preferred to prevent "seeding" of malignant cells in fungating and radiation wounds
J. Topical dressings for odor control
   1. Topical metronidazole
   2. Activated charcoal dressings
   3. Sugar paste and honey
   4. Room deodorizer
   5. Frequent dressing changes
K. Fungating wounds (Figure 23.3)
   1. Do not forget that families need help when viewing patients with fungating growth.
   2. Non-adherent dressings are ideal.
   3. Alginate dressings with high seaweed content exchange sodium ions for calcium ions in the wound bed and encourage the clotting cascade.
L. Kennedy ulcer (Figure 23.4)
   1. Terminal ulcer that develops as the patient is dying
   2. Pear shaped, usually on sacrum, and borders of ulcer are irregular
   3. Sudden onset
   4. Rapid progression
   5. Often appears as little black spots
   6. Most patients die within 8–24 hours
M. Summary of palliative care issues
   1. Cure is not always realistic, but symptom relieving and compassionate care is always possible.
   2. Controlling pain, odor, exudates, and bleeding are the main goals of palliative wound care.
   3. Preserving patient dignity and self-esteem and maximizing quality of life are the main goals of palliative care.

III. Psychosocial issues

A. Ulcers are the source of severe physical dysfunction, emotional distress, and poor quality of life.
B. Foot ulceration is not predictive of depressive symptoms.
C. Foot ulceration is a source of ulcer-specific emotional responses, which either facilitate (fear of potential consequences) or inhibit (anger at heathcare providers) patient compliance and eventual healing.
D. Factors that shape a patient's emotional response to his or her wounds include:
   1. Etiology of wound
   2. Gender
   3. Age
   4. Social support
   5. Spirituality
   6. Visibility
   7. Pain
   8. Odor, leakage
   9. Impact on activities of daily living
   10. Coping patterns
E. Quality of life treatment decisions should be based on the patient's perception of well-being.
F. Wounds that are hidden under clothing or beneath dressings can still cause emotional pain when exposed to family members or healthcare personnel.
G. Wound care professionals should work with patients on the challenge of balancing physical wound healing and psychological and emotional healing.

RESOURCES

1. McCaffery M. *Nursing Practice Theories Related to Cognition, Bodily Pain, and Man-Environment Interactions.* Los Angeles: University of California at Los Angeles Students' Store; 1968.

2. McCaffery M, Robinson ES. Your patient is in pain, here's how you respond. *Nursing.* 2002; 32(10):36-45.

3. Tippet AW. Wounds at the end of life. *Wounds.* 2005; 17(4):91-8.

4. Soto LL, Sheffield KM. Comforting the patient. In: Sheffield PJ, Fife CE, editors. *Wound Care Practice.* 2nd ed. North Palm Beach: Best Publishing Company; 2007: 1035-54.

5. Wells LT. Acute and chronic pain management. In: Sheffield PJ, Fife CE, editors. *Wound Care Practice.* 2nd ed. North Palm Beach: Best Publishing Company; 2007: 799-826.

6. Krasner DL. Wound pain management: a wound care specialist's perspective. In: Sheffield PJ, Fife CE, editors. *Wound Care Practice.* 2nd ed. North Palm Beach: Best Publishing Company; 2007: 827-44.

7. The Support Principal Investigators. A controlled trial to improve care for seriously ill hospitalized patients. The study to understand prognosis and preferences for outcomes and risks of treatments. *JAMA.* 1995 Nov 22-29; 274(20):1591-8.

8. Dallum LE, et al. Pain management and wounds. In: Baranoski S, Ayello EA, editors. *Wound Care Essentials: Practice Principles.* Philadelphia: Lippincott Williams & Wilkins; 2004: 217-38.

9. Baranoski S, Ayello EA, editors. *Wound Care Essentials.* 3rd ed. Philadelphia: Lippincott Williams & Wilkins; 2013.

10. Vileikyte L, Gonzalez JS. Psychosocial aspects of diabetic foot complications. In: Bowker JH, Pfeifer MA, editors. *Levin and O' Neal's The Diabetic Foot.* 7th ed. Amsterdam: Mosby Elsevier; 2008: 573-83.

11. Senecal SJ. Pain management of wound care. *Nurs Clin North Am.* 1999; 34(4):847–60.

12. Krasner D. Caring for the person experiencing chronic wound pain. In: Krasner DL, Rodeheaver GT, Sibbald GR. *Chronic Wound Care: A Clinical Source Book for Healthcare Professionals.* 3rd ed. Wayne: HMP Communications; 2001.

13. Defloor T. The effect of position and mattress on interface pressure. Appl Nurs Res. 200:13(1):2–11. From Sussman & Bates-Jensen Wound Care 4th Edition.

SAMPLE QUESTIONS

1. Implementing a palliative wound care plan would be most appropriate for which of the following patients?
   a) A 65-year-old venous stasis ulcer patient with a 10-year history of recurrent ulcerations
   b) A 45-year-old osteoradionecrosis patient undergoing hyperbaric oxygen therapy
   c) A 50-year-old terminal cancer patient with a granulating pressure ulcer
   d) A 92-year-old nursing home resident with a stage IV sacral pressure ulcer losing weight and muscle mass and on tube feedings

2. For palliative wounds, which of the following is not a key objective?
   a) Healing
   b) Pain management
   c) Infection prevention
   d) Wound deterioration prevention

3. Which of the following is a goal of palliative care?
   a) Preserving patient self-image
   b) Preserving patient quality of life
   c) Decreasing wound odor
   d) All of the above

4. All of the following can help with odor control except:
   a) Topical metronidazole
   b) Activated charcoal dressings
   c) Hydrogel dressing
   d) Sugar paste and honey

5. An 80-year-old female is admitted to the ICU with adult respiratory distress, sepsis, and terminal cancer. The patient developed a sudden onset pear-shaped ulcer with irregular edges on her sacrum. This patient most likely has a:
   a) Stage IV pressure ulcer
   b) Unstageable ulcer
   c) Deep tissue injury
   d) Kennedy ulcer

6. The emotional response by a patient to his or her wound is dependent on all of the following except:
   a) Visibility of wound
   b) Odor and amount of exudate
   c) Etiology of wound
   d) Alcohol use

7. Quality of life treatment decisions should be based on:
   a) The family members' perception of the patient's well-being
   b) The patient's perception of his or her own well-being
   c) The nurse's perception of the patient's well-being
   d) The physician's perception of the patient's well-being

8. Which of the following would constitute a palliative wound care plan for a 72-year-old female with a fungating wound on her left hand?
   a) A hydrogel-based sheet to be placed on the wound every three days and as needed
   b) Negative pressure wound therapy every other day to control exudate
   c) Wet-to-dry dressing changes every four hours around the clock
   d) Enzymatic debridement applied to the wound twice a day

9. A home health wound care nurse is requesting approval for the following orders in the care of a 90-year-old hospice patient with a large stage IV ulceration. Which one of the orders may not be appropriate for this patient?
   a) Irrigate the wound with cold normal saline
   b) Apply a mixture of morphine and silver hydrogel
   c) Cover the wound with 4 × 4/fluffs and Kerlix gauze (secondary dressing)
   d) Dressing changes every three days and on PRN basis

10. Of the following choices, which is the most preferred way of debriding a palliative wound care patient?
    a) Mechanical debridement
    b) Surgical debridement
    c) Autolytic debridement
    d) Biosurgical debridement

See answers on page 210.

NOTES

ANSWER KEY

1. d) A palliative wound care plan is most appropriate in the 92-year-old nursing home patient with a stage IV pressure ulcer and severe malnutrition. The 50-year-old terminal cancer patient has a granulating wound, which could heal with appropriate wound care. The 45-year-old osteoradionecrosis patient is already receiving HBOT and needs an aggressive treatment plan to heal the wound, which is also true of the 65-year-old venous stasis patient who has not healed for the last 10 years.

2. a) The goals for palliative wound care plans involve managing pain, preventing infection, and preventing wound deterioration. Healing the wound is not usually the goal in the non-healable palliative wound care patient.

3. d) The goals of palliative care include preserving patient self-image and quality of life and decreasing wound odor.

4. c) Topical metronidazole, activated charcoal dressings, and sugar paste and honey can all decrease wound odor. Hydrogel dressings will keep the wound moist but will not decrease odor.

5. d) This terminal patient in ICU has developed a Kennedy ulcer, which is usually a sudden onset, pear-shaped wound with an irregular edge that occurs in the sacral region. Its presence indicates multiorgan failure, including that of the skin, and patients have an extremely poor prognosis.

6. d) The emotional response by a patient to his or her wound is dependent on the size, location, drainage, visibility, odor, and etiology of the wound. It is not dependent on the patient's alcohol use.

7. b) Quality of life treatment decisions should be based on the patient's perception of his or her own.

8. a) A 72-year-old female with a fungating wound on her left hand will benefit from using a hydrogel-based sheet, which can keep the wound moist for three days. Decreasing the frequency of dressing changes and keeping the wound moist will help decrease the pain associated with dressing changes. Negative pressure wound therapy is not indicated in a fungating malignant wound. Wet-to-dry dressing changes every four hours and enzymatic debridement will increase pain to this palliative wound care patient and are not the best choices of wound management.

9. a) Warm rather than cold saline is recommended when irrigating wounds in palliative wound care patients. A mixture of morphine and silver hydrogel will keep the wound moist and also decrease pain. The use of a secondary dressing will help with the absorption of exudate and protect the wound. Changing the dressing every three days will also help to decrease pain in this patient.

10. c) The most preferred way of debriding a palliative wound care patient is with autolytic debridement, which is, comparatively, the least painful way of debriding the wound.

WOUND DRESSINGS 24

Dianne Rudolph, RN, DNP, APRN-BC, CWOCN
Jesse Cantu, RN, BSN, CWS, FACCWS

INTRODUCTION

This chapter will introduce the various categories of wound dressings, describe their uses, and discuss the decision-making processes involved in choosing an appropriate wound dressing from the large selection available.

OBJECTIVES

Participants should be able to describe the major categories of wound dressings and compression bandages, state the indications for each type of dressing, and contrast the advantages of various wound dressings.

I. Wound dressings
A. Factors influencing dressing choice include anatomical site, amount of exudates, dead space, surrounding skin, caregiver ability, wound status, aggressive therapy vs. palliative care, cost, and reimbursement.
B. Dressing categories
 1. Cleansers
 2. Gauze
 3. Transparent films
 4. Hydrocolloids
 5. Hydrogels
 6. Alginates
 7. Foams
 8. Wound fillers/absorbers
 9. Collagen
 10. Silicone gel sheets
 11. Antimicrobials
  a) Antiseptics
  b) Enzymatic agents (collagenase)
 12. Composite dressings
 13. Compression dressings
C. Wound cleansers
 1. Purpose: cleansing is an important first step in preparing the pressure ulcer wound bed to heal. Cleansing removes surface debris and dressing remnants and allows better wound visualization for assessment. Apply cleansing solution with sufficient pressure to

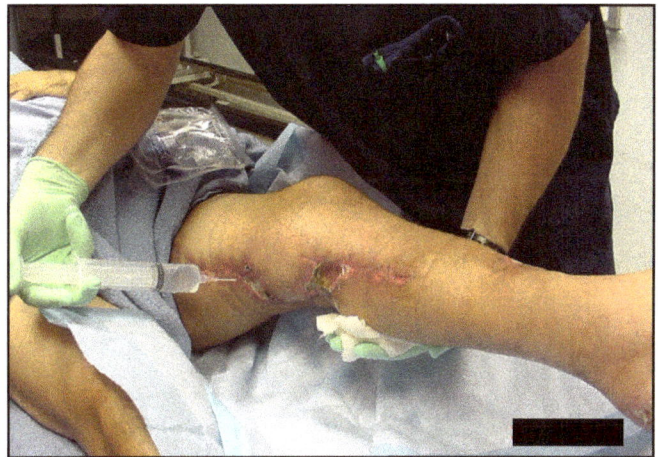
Figure 24.1: Wound cleansing with normal saline.

cleanse the wound without damaging tissue or driving bacteria into the wound.
 2. Normal saline: most physiologically compatible and widely used (Figure 24.1)
  a) Use 19 gauge catheter/30-35 ml syringe to deliver 8 psi (between 4-15 psi recommended)
  b) Advantages: cheap, readily available, no hypersensitivities
  c) Disadvantages: short shelf life, requires mechanism to apply, need to avoid cross-contamination with use
 3. Commercial wound cleansers (pH balanced surfactants)
  a) Advantages: effective, noncytotoxic, longer shelf life, easy to apply
  b) Disadvantages: availability
D. Gauze dressings
 1. Types
  a) All purpose (woven and non-woven)
  b) Impregnated (PHMB, oil emulsion, bismuth, etc.)
  c) Non-adherent
  d) Packing
  e) Debriding

      f) Rolls for wrapping

      g) Absorbent wraps

  2. Indications

      a) Primary dressing

      b) Secondary dressing

      c) Filler for dead space

      d) Absorber

      e) Cleansing material

      f) Mechanical debridement

      g) Carrier for medication

  3. Advantages

      a) Widely available

      b) Inexpensive, but not necessarily cost effective

      c) Used wet or dry

      d) Variety of sizes

  4. Disadvantages

      a) Frequent changes are costly in nursing time and money

      b) Minimal absorption

      c) Painful removal

      d) Difficulty maintaining moist wound bed

      e) No barrier to contamination by urine and feces

      f) Overpacking can impede wound healing

E. Transparent film dressings (Figure 24.2)

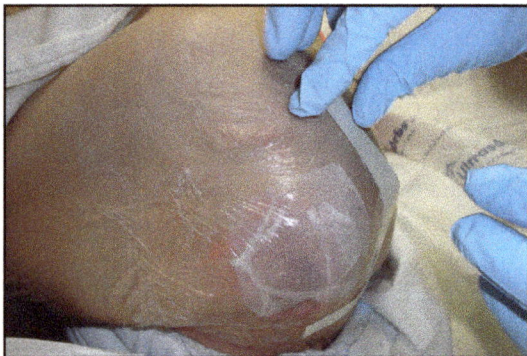

Figure 24.2: Application of a transparent dressing.

  1. Types

      a) Polyurethane

      b) Polyethylene

      c) Copolyester

  2. Indications

      a) Acts as a covering to maintain a moist wound bed in shallow wounds

      b) Waterproofs site

      c) May protect from friction and shear

      d) Promotes autolytic debridement

      e) Occlusion may reduce pain by keeping nerve endings in a moist state

      f) Neuropathic pain management

  3. Advantages

      a) Acts as cover dressing and may be left in place for several days

      b) Apply over gauze dressings to act as a waterproof covering

      c) One-piece dressing, no need for tape

      d) Creates a moist wound environment that softens thin areas of eschar and/or slough

      e) Covers recently epithelialized areas

      f) Protects against external contamination from bacteria, urine, and stool

  4. Disadvantages

      a) Not an absorptive dressing; may cause maceration if left too long over exudate

      b) When wrinkled it may lift and allow leakage of fluid

      c) Traumatic on removal

      d) Contraindicated in cavity wounds, undermining, or tunneling, unless wound is filled with packing material

      e) Do not use if clinical signs of infection are present

F. Hydrocolloid dressings (Figure 24.3)

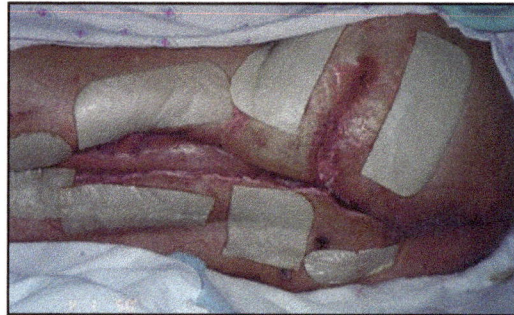

Figure 24.3: Hydrocolloids used as a taping platform.

  1. Types

      a) Gelatin

      b) Pectin

      c) Colloids

      d) Carboxymethylcellulose

      e) Considered occlusive dressings

      f) Various forms: wafers, granules, pastes, powders

  2. Indications

      a) Shallow wounds with minimal to moderate exudates

      b) Use as a secondary dressing with alginates or hydrofiber

      c) Facilitates the creation of a moist wound environment to increase fibrinolysis

      d) Moisture may also reduce pain to nerves.

      e) May prevent contamination

      f) Facilitates autolytic debridement

      g) May serve as a taping platform to minimize damage to periwound tissue

  3. Advantages

      a) Occlusive, waterproof, and may prevent contamination

      b) Absorptive

      c) Flexible

      d) Long wear time

      e) Ease of use

4. Disadvantages
   a) Risk of hypergranulation tissue
   b) Melting down
   c) Occlusion and odor
   d) Can be dislodged in the presence of heavy exudates
   e) May damage fragile periwound skin
   f) Not for wounds with undermining or tunneling
   g) Not for heavily draining wounds

G. Hydrogel dressings (Figure 24.4)

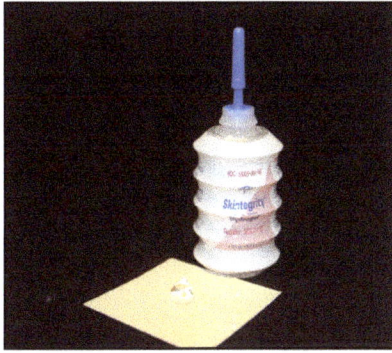

Figure 24.4: Example of a hydrogel.

1. Description
   a) Water or glycerin based
   b) Available in impregnated gauze, amorphous gels, and in sheets
   c) Limited absorptive capacity
   d) Considered hydrators
   e) Viscosity varies by manufacturer
   f) Available in sterile one-time use or multi-application forms
2. Indications
   a) Assist in maintaining a moist wound environment
   b) Insulators
   c) Moist wound environment may promote autolytic debridement
   d) Limited absorptive capability
3. Advantages
   a) Rehydrate the wound bed
   b) Soothing (refrigerate hydrogel sheets)
   c) Longer wear time than damp gauze
   d) Easy to apply and remove
   e) In gauze form, can be used to fill wounds
   f) Do not leave residue in wounds
   g) Facilitate autolytic debridement
4. Disadvantages
   a) May break down in wound bed—will depend on viscosity for wear time
   b) Limited absorption
   c) May cause maceration if exudate increases
   d) Usually require a secondary dressing

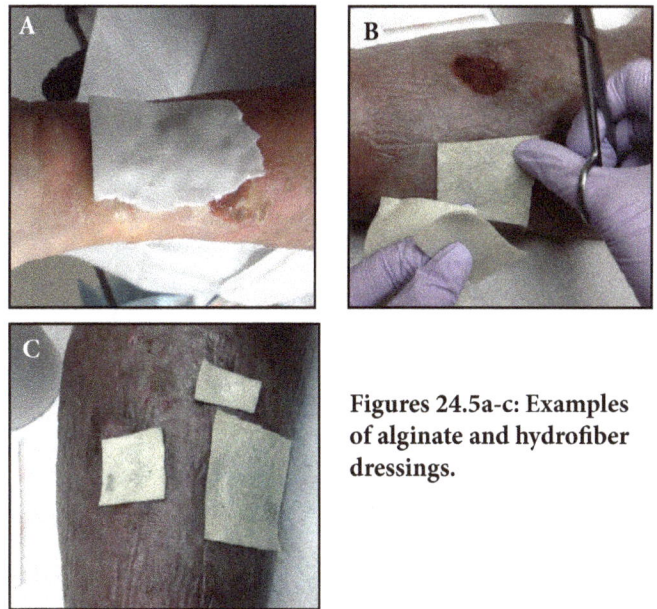

Figures 24.5a-c: Examples of alginate and hydrofiber dressings.

H. Alginate (Figure 24.5a) and hydrofiber dressings
   1. Description
      a) Derived from the calcium salt of alginic acid (seaweed)
      b) Soft, non-woven fibers of a cellulose-like polysaccharide
      c) Hydrofiber: carboxymethylcellulose
      d) Available in flat pads (Figure 24.5b) for open wounds and ropes (Figure 24.5c) for filling
      e) Weaving techniques vary among manufacturers
   2. Indications
      a) Wounds with moderate to heavy drainage
      b) Wound filling
      c) May use in infected wounds
      d) Interacts with wound fluid to form a gel that creates a moist wound environment
      e) Leg ulcers, non-healing surgical wounds, full-thickness wounds
   3. Advantages
      a) High capacity for absorption
      b) Easy to apply and remove
      c) May be used under compression
      d) May be used with a variety of wound types
   4. Disadvantages
      a) May desiccate a wound bed if used inappropriately
      b) May cause maceration to periwound skin
      c) May leave residual fibers in wound bed (alginates)

I. Foam dressings (Figure 24.6)
   1. Description
      a) Composed of polyurethane foam
      b) Hydrophilic properties
      c) Vary in thickness
      d) May have a film backing on outer surface
      e) Available in adhesive or non-adhesive sheets, pillows, or wafers, with or without borders

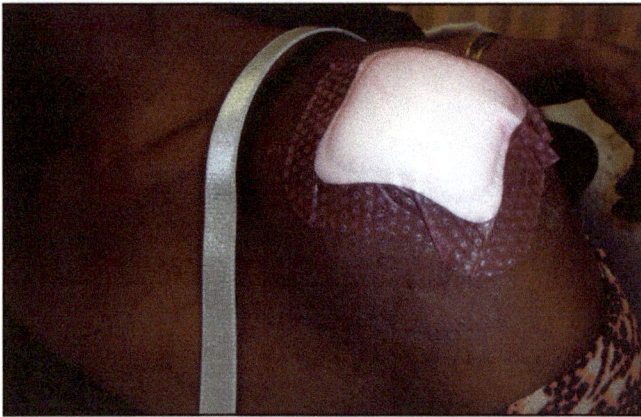

Figure 24.6: Example of an applied foam dressing.

2. Indications
   a) Able to absorb light to heavy amounts of exudate (less absorbent than alginates)
   b) Semi-occlusive
   c) Filler in dead space
   d) Maintain moist wound environment
   e) May retard hypergranulation tissue
   f) Use for percutaneous endoscopic gastronomy (PEG)/trach tubes

3. Advantages
   a) Absorb under compression
   b) Insulator for wound
   c) Easy to apply
   d) Adhesive foams leave no residue
   e) Gentle on friable skin
   f) Do not adhere to wound bed
   g) Padding benefit

4. Disadvantages
   a) If used inappropriately, may dry out wound bed
   b) May lead to maceration of periwound skin if left in place too long
   c) Some foams may require a secondary dressing
   d) Ineffective for dry wounds (e.g., eschar)

J. Wound fillers/absorbers
1. Description
   a) Various compositions as gels, strands, beads, powders, granules, and pastes
   b) Varying levels of absorption

2. Indications
   a) May fill in dead space
   b) Some forms may promote autolytic debridement

3. Advantages
   a) Autolytic debridement
   b) Easy to apply and remove
   c) Absorbent
   d) May be used in combination with other products

4. Disadvantages
   a) Require secondary dressing
   b) Not recommended for use in dry wounds (follow manufacturer guidelines for use)

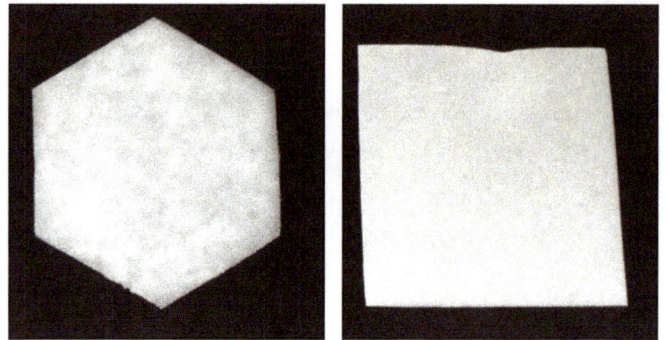

Figure 24.7: Collagen dressings.

K. Collagen dressings (Figure 24.7)
1. Description
   a) Fibrous insoluble protein found in the connective tissue (skin, bone, ligaments, cartilage)
     i) Provide an exogenous source of protein for healing
     ii) Available in gels, pads, particles, powders, sheets, and ribbons/strips
   b) Subintestinal submucosa (SIS): acellular extracellular matrix
     i) May attract cellular components necessary for wound healing i.e., stimulate fibroblasts
     ii) May be composed of bovine or porcine material—watch for sensitivities/cultural issues

2. Indications
   a) Moderate to heavily draining wounds
   b) Vascular wounds
   c) Pressure ulcers
   d) Donor and graft sites
   e) Infected wounds (will need to clarify with manufacturer)
   f) Recalcitrant wounds

3. Advantages
   a) Useful in a variety of wounds
   b) Relatively easy to use
   c) Low risk of allergic/hypersensitivity issues

4. Disadvantages
   a) Costly
   b) Not recommended for necrotic wounds
   c) Require a secondary dressing

L. Silicone gel sheets (Figure 24.8)

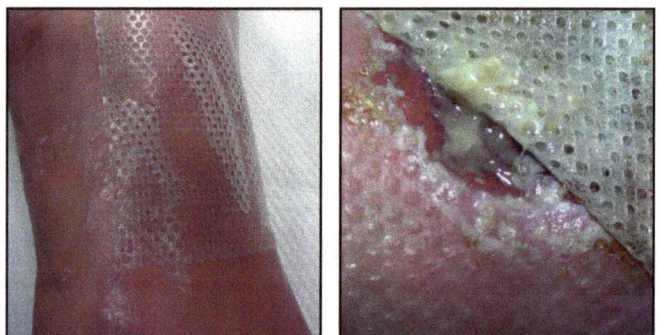

Figure 24.8: Applied silicone gel sheet.

1. Description
   a) Soft semiocclusive adhesive sheets: screen or fenestrated to allow exudates to exit wounds
   b) Composed of medical grade silicone reinforced with a silicone membrane backing
   c) The adhesive is a silicone adhesive within the gel itself
   d) Adhesive allows washing with soap and water and resumes a tacky surface upon drying
2. Indications
   a) Manage hypertrophic scars
   b) Prevent keloid formation
   c) Increase scar elasticity (decreases contracture)
   d) Blanche scar color
   e) Use as a primary dressing over friable granulation or grafts
3. Advantages
   a) Ease of use
   b) Pain control
   c) Atraumatic to wound bed
4. Disadvantages
   a) Costly
   b) Accessibility
   c) May cause maceration if exudates increase

M. Antimicrobial dressings (Figure 24.9)

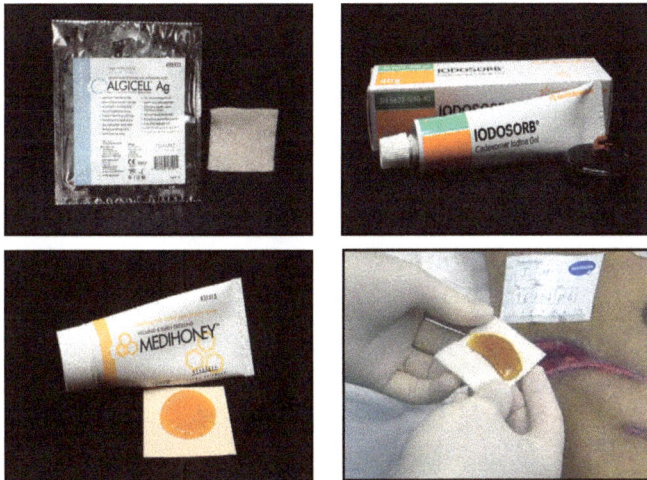

Figure 24.9: Examples of antimicrobial dressings.

1. Types
   a) Silver
   b) Cadexomer iodine
   c) Methylene blue/gentian violet
   d) Honey
   e) Mucipirocin/bacitracin/TAO
   f) Metronidazole (specific uses only)
   g) Maltodextrin
2. Indications
   a) Partial and full thickness wounds
   b) Infected wounds
   c) Wounds at risk for infection
   d) First and second degree burns
   e) Pressure ulcers
   f) Vascular ulcers
   g) Skin tears/traumatic wounds
   h) Donor sites (selected agents)
3. Advantages
   a) Wide variety of uses
   b) Use in wounds with infection/critical colonization
   c) May help with odor control
   d) May assist with debridement (honey)
4. Disadvantages
   a) May require a secondary dressing
   b) Ensure adequate moisture balance
   c) Costly
   d) Infected wounds still require systemic therapy

N. Antiseptics
   1. Types
      a) Dakin's solution
      b) Acetic acid
      c) Povidone iodine
      d) Aluminum acetate
      e) Chlorhexidine
   2. Indications
      a) Vary, for short-term use
   3. Advantages
      a) Inexpensive
      b) Readily available
   4. Disadvantages
      a) Cytotoxic; avoid contact with eyes
      b) May impede wound healing with long-term use

O. Enzymatic agents (collagenase)
   1. Description
      a) Selective proteolytic topical agent
   2. Indications
      a) Chemical (nonsurgical) debridement of wounds with nonviable tissue
   3. Advantages
      a) Non-painful wound debridement
      b) Can be used in any setting
      c) Use in infected or non-infected wounds
   4. Disadvantages
      a) Slower than other forms of debridement
      b) Appropriate application is key
      c) Require secondary dressing with some moisture retention
      d) Contact with periwound tissue may cause irritation

P. Composite dressings
   1. Description
      a) May incorporate distinct features of two or more products with different activities (gel and alginate, silver and hydrofiber, charcoal and alginate, etc.)
      b) Provide multiple functions in the wound: absorption, autolysis, odor control
      c) Different sizes and shapes for flexibility

2. Indications
   a) Acute wounds
   b) Abrasions and lacerations
   c) IV sites (peripheral and central)
   d) Surgical incisions
   e) Skin tears
   f) Primary or secondary dressings
3. Advantages
   a) Easy to use
4. Disadvantages
   a) The manufacturer must give the primary indication of the dressing
   b) Reimbursement is determined by indication
   c) May be confusing to caregivers
Q. Hydroconductive dressings
   1. Description
      a) Cross layered fiber dressing that uses a combination of capillary, hydroconductive, and electrostatic actions to move exudate, wound debris, bacteria, and MMPs into the porous material of the dressing
   2. Advantages
      a) Can be used on a variety of wounds and around tubes
   3. Disadvantages
      a) Costly
      b) Availability
R. Compression bandages
   1. Compression: application of external pressure to the lower extremities to promote return from peripheral to central veins
   2. Laplace's law: the formula used to calculate sub-bandage pressure
      a) As it relates to compression bandages, Laplace's law states that sub-bandage pressure (P) is directly proportional to bandage tension (T) and inversely proportional to the radius (r) of the limb to which it is applied, so:

$$P = T/r$$

Where: P = sub-bandage pressure; T = bandage tension; r = radius of curvature of limb

      b) As the radius of the limb increases, the pressure decreases. In practice the radius is not easily measured, so the circumference is used instead. This means that, when even bandage tension is applied throughout, the pressure is greater at the smaller circumferences of the limb (wrist/ankle) than at the larger circumferences (thigh/upper arm). It is also important to consider the number of bandage layers applied (N) and the width of the bandage (W). The pressure is expressed in mmHg, which gives the final equation:

$$P = T \times N \times constant\ 4630/C \times W$$

Limb Circumference (cm)	Bandage Tension (Kgf)									
	0.2	0.4	0.6	0.8	1.0	1.2	1.4	1.6	1.8	2.0
18	10.3	20.5	30.8	41.1	51.3	61.6	71.9	82.1	92.4	102.7
20	9.2	18.5	27.7	37.0	46.2	55.4	64.7	73.9	83.2	92.4
22	8.4	16.8	25.2	33.6	42.0	50.4	58.8	67.2	75.6	84.0
24	7.7	15.4	23.1	30.8	38.5	46.2	53.9	61.6	69.3	77.0
26	7.1	14.2	21.3	28.4	35.5	42.6	49.8	56.9	64.0	71.1
28	6.6	13.2	19.8	26.4	33.0	39.6	46.2	52.8	59.4	66.0
30	6.2	12.3	18.5	24.6	30.8	37.0	43.1	49.3	55.4	61.6
32	5.8	11.6	17.3	23.1	28.9	37.4	40.4	46.2	52.0	57.8
34	5.4	10.9	16.3	21.7	27.2	32.6	38.0	43.5	48.9	54.4
36	5.1	10.3	15.4	20.5	25.7	30.8	35.9	41.1	46.2	51.3

Figure 24.10: Relationship between limb circumference and sub-bandage pressure. From Thomas S, Fram P. An evaluation of a new type of compression bandaging system. World Wide Wounds; 2003.

Where: P = the interface pressure under the bandage (mmHg), also called the compression force; T = the tension of the bandage (or kilogram force [Kgf]), which depends on the material and its % stretch; N = the number of layers (defined by the level of overlap and the number of bandages); Constant 4630 = kilogram force (Kgf) for single layer bandage; C = the circumference at the measurement point (cm); W = the bandage width (cm)

3. Goal: 30-40 mmHg at the ankle
4. Indications: chronic venous insufficiency (CVI) and CVI with ulceration
5. Limb circumference and bandage tension (Figure 24.10)

II. Types of compression

A. Types
   1. Unna's boot
   2. Short stretch
   3. Long stretch
   4. Multilayered (2, 3, 4 layers) (Figure 24.11)
   5. Gradient compression stockings
   6. Sequential pneumatic compression pumps (also indicated for lymphedema)

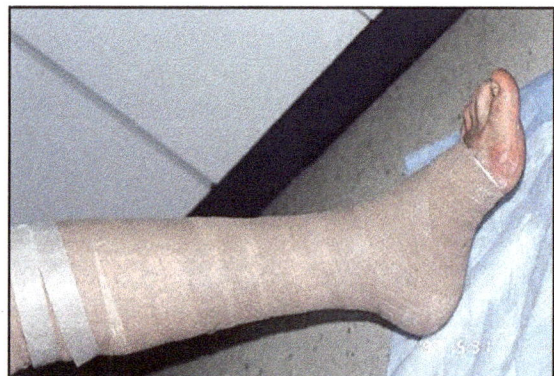

Figure 24.11: Multilayered compression dressing.

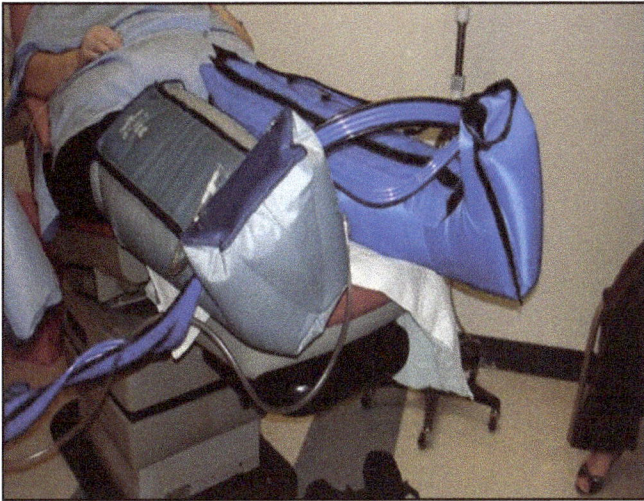

Figure 24.12: Pneumatic compression device.

   7. ACE® wraps and T.E.D.™ hose (thromboembolic deterrent anti-embolism stockings) are ineffective and should be avoided

B. Pneumatic compression devices (PCD) (Figure 24.12)

C. Considerations for compression
   1. Assess ABI prior to application (0.08 or better)
   2. Should only be applied by a trained professional
   3. Pad bony prominences
   4. Use caution with congestive heart failure (CHF); may cause exacerbation

III. Considerations for choosing an appropriate dressing

A. What does the wound need?
B. What does the product do?
C. How well does the product do it?
D. What does the patient need?
E. What is available?
F. What is practical?

RESOURCES

1. National Pressure Ulcer Advisory Panel. NPUAP Prevention and Treatment of Pressure Ulcers: 2014 Clinical Practice Guidelines [Internet]. 2014. Accessed at: http://www.npuap.org/resources/educational-and-clinical-resources/prevention-and-treatment-of-pressure-ulcers-clinical-practice-guideline/.
2. Wound, Ostomy and Continence Nurses Society (WOCN) Wound Committee; Association for Professionals in Infection Control and Epidemiology, Inc. (APIC) 2000 Guidelines Committee. Clean versus Sterile Techniques for Management of Chronic Wounds: a fact sheet. *J Wound Ostomy Continence Nurs.* 2012 Mar-Apr; 39(2 Suppl):S30-4.
3. International Consensus. *Appropriate Use of Silver Dressings in Wounds. An expert working group consensus.* London: Wounds International [Internet]. 2012 [cited 2014 Nov 11]. Accessed at: http://www.woundsinternational.com/pdf/content_10381.pdf.
4. The effective use of Hydrofera Blue Bacteriostatic Dressing in difficult-to-heal wounds: an evaluation of six case studies [Internet]. 2012. Accessed at: http://woundcare.org/wp-content/uploads/2012/08/Hydrofera-Blue-Clinical-Monograph-Brochure.pdf.
5. Zieger B. Which topical therapy for which wound? *Consultant.* 2013; 53(9):660-1.
6. Krasner DL, Rodeheaver GT, Sibbald G, editors. *Chronic Wound Care: A Clinical Source Book for Healthcare Professionals.* 4th ed. Malvern: HMP Communications; 2007.
7. Larson-Lohr V, Fleck CA. Modern wound dressings: principles, form and function. In: Sheffield PJ, Fife CE, editors. *Wound Care Practice.* 2nd ed. North Palm Beach: Best Publishing Company; 2007: 921-46.
8. Thomas S, Fram P. An evaluation of a new type of compression bandaging system. World Wide Wounds [Internet]. Updated 2003 Sept. Accessed at: http://www.worldwidewounds.com/2003/September/Thomas/New-Compression-Bandage.html.

SAMPLE QUESTIONS

1. Which dressing would be best suited for a wound with high levels of surface bacterial contamination (bioburden)?
   a) Silver impregnated
   b) Hydrogel
   c) Hydrocolloid
   d) Petroleum gauze

2. Transparent film dressings:
   a) Absorb exudates
   b) Will not tear fragile skin
   c) Are used on infected wounds
   d) Retain moisture in the wound bed

3. Foam dressings:
   a) Adhere to the wound bed
   b) Never require a secondary dressing
   c) Are effective for wounds with dry eschar
   d) May macerate the wound edge if the dressing becomes saturated

4. Alginate dressings:
   a) Are never painful
   b) Are used in dry wounds
   c) Form moist gel in the wound
   d) Do not control exudates

5. Hydrocolloid dressings:
   a) Facilitate autolytic debridement and reduce pain
   b) Can be used in infected wounds
   c) Will not adhere to the skin surrounding the wound
   d) Can be used in heavy exudates

See answers on page 220.

NOTES

ANSWER KEY

1. a)   Silver impregnated dressing would be best suited for a wound with high levels of surface bacterial contamination. Some silver dressings are bacteriostatic while some are bactericidal. Hydrogel, hydrocolloids, and petroleum gauze will not decrease bacterial bioburden.

2. d)   Transparent film dressings retain moisture in the wound bed. They do not absorb exudates and are not used on infected wounds. Transparent film may tear fragile skin upon removal.

3. d)   Foam dressings do not adhere to the wound bed but they may require a secondary dressing. Foam is not effective for wounds with dry eschar and may macerate the wound edge if the dressing becomes saturated.

4. c)   Alginate dressings form a moist sodium alginate gel in the wound bed and are mainly used in exudative wounds. They aid in autolytic debridement, and dressing removal may be painful.

5. a)   Hydrocolloid dressings are occlusive dressings that facilitate autolytic debridement. The moisture may reduce pain to nerves.

THE ROLE OF PHYSICAL THERAPY IN WOUND CARE 25

Rose L. Hamm, DPT, CWS, FACCWS

INTRODUCTION

The role of physical therapy in caring for patients with wounds involves the identification of both physical and medical factors that contribute to wound formation and failure to heal, the debridement of necrotic tissue as part of wound bed preparation, the use of biophysical technologies that facilitate wound healing, compression therapy, and exercise and functional training to address impairments that contribute to or result from wounds. This chapter presents the background for each of the physical therapy interventions, including the following technologies: negative pressure wound therapy, electrical stimulation, ultrasound, ultraviolet C, and pulsed lavage with suction.

OBJECTIVES

Participants should be able to identify factors that contribute to wound formation or impede wound healing, select the optimal debridement technique for different types of necrotic tissue, discuss the theory of each of the biophysical technologies used by physical therapists for wound management, select the best type of compression for a lower-extremity wound, design an exercise program for a patient with an arterial or venous wound, and select the appropriate biophysical technology for a wound based on healing phase and tissue present in the wound bed.

I. Role of physical therapy in wound care
A. Overview
  1. Evaluation of the patient with a wound
  2. Sharp/selective debridement of necrotic tissue
  3. Hydrotherapy
    a) Pulsed lavage with suction
    b) Whirlpool
  4. Electrical stimulation
  5. Ultrasound
  6. Ultraviolet C
  7. Negative pressure wound therapy
  8. Edema management with compression
  9. Exercise and gait training

B. Evaluation of the patient with a wound
  1. The evaluation of a patient with a wound, when performed by a physical therapist, includes all of the subjective and objective information that has been discussed in previous chapters, as well as the following:
    a) Strength and range of motion measurements of the involved extremity, especially for patients with diabetic foot wounds, chronic venous insufficiency wounds, lymphedema, and arterial wounds
    b) Assessment of gait and need for assistive devices, e.g., to help off-load foot wounds
    c) Assessment of footwear and need for orthotics, braces, and foot positioners
    d) Functional assessment, e.g., transfers of a patient with spinal cord injury or cerebrovascular accident (CVA)
    e) Wheelchair and cushion assessment
    f) In-depth discussion of factors that impede wound healing, e.g., diet, medications, social habits (smoking and alcohol use), family support, and work requirements
  2. The information gained from the comprehensive evaluation is then used to establish a care plan for both the wound and any functional impairments that are identified.
C. Sharp/selective debridement of necrotic tissue
    a) Wound evaluation includes tissue identification and need for debridement or removal of devitalized tissue.
    b) State practice acts allow physical therapists to remove devitalized tissue (not viable tissue, as in surgical debridement).
    c) CMS billing codes define sharp debridement as removal of devitalized tissue with scalpel, forceps, scissors, or high-powered irrigation devices.
    d) Contact low-frequency ultrasound is also used by physical therapists to remove devitalized tissue.
    e) Therapist competency is guided by facility policies and procedures.

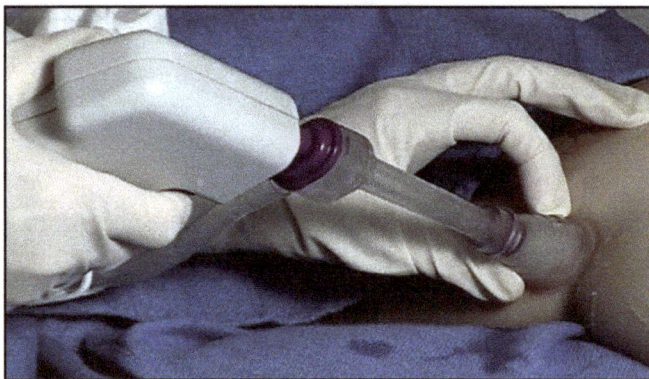

Figure 25.1: Pulsed lavage consists of a handpiece that controls the psi of the irrigation fluid as it is pulsed into the wound bed, a tip that directs the fluid into the wound bed, tubing that carries the sterile irrigation fluid from the bag to the handpiece, and tubing that carries the contaminated fluid from the wound to the suction canister.

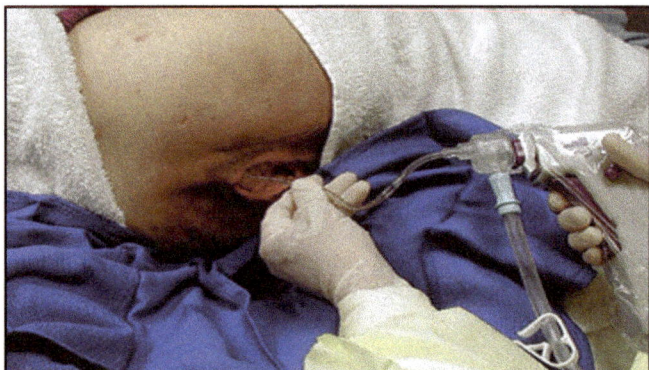

Figure 25.2: Pulsed lavage with suction using a tracking tip to irrigate a sinus or tunneling of a sacral wound.

D. Hydrotherapy
  a) Pulsed lavage with suction (PLWS)
      i) PLWS is the recommended method of cleansing a wound with hydrotherapy.
      ii) The two components of PLWS are:
          (1) Pulsing an irrigation solution, usually normal saline, into a wound bed with controlled force (defined as pounds per square inch or psi)
          (2) Suction of the contaminated fluids and exudate with negative pressure (Figures 25.1 and 25.2)
      iii) Recommended psi for treatment:
          (1) 4-8 psi provides effective irrigation that removes bacteria and exudate and is usually comfortable for the patient
              (a) 9-15 psi is effective in removing bacteria and exudate, softening necrotic tissue, and facilitating debridement
              (b) <4 psi is not effective in removing bacteria
              (c) >15 psi may cause tissue trauma,

pain, and drive bacteria into the tissue
      iv) Indications
          (1) Critically colonized wounds
          (2) Infected or necrotic wounds
          (3) Draining wounds (with exudate)
          (4) Undermining, tunnels, and tracts
          (5) Open amputation sites (for removal of coagulation and necrotic debris)
          (6) Dehisced surgical incisions
          (7) Traumatic wounds with foreign debris
          (8) Stage III and IV pressure ulcers
      v) Precautions
          (1) Potential or active bleeding (low platelet count)
          (2) Sinuses or tracts that may connect to a body cavity
          (3) Proximity of blood vessels
          (4) Exposed bone or tendon
          (5) Recent bypass grafts or surgical closures
          (6) Facial wounds
          (7) Area around left ventricular assist device (LVAD) drive line
          (8) Impaired or absent sensation
      vi) Contraindications
          (1) No known contraindications
      vii) Recommendations by CDC for infection control with pulsed lavage with suction (PLWS)
          (1) The risk of aerosolization and spread of bacteria has resulted in the following CDC guidelines for application of PLWS to an open wound:
              (a) Clinician wears personal protective equipment (PPE) consisting of waterproof gown, gloves, facial shield with eye cover, and hair cover.
              (b) Treatment occurs only in single-patient rooms or an enclosed room with door (curtain separation of beds or treatment areas is not sufficient).
              (c) Containers of contaminated fluids are placed in biohazard bags after treatment.
              (d) Patient personal belongs and any exposed tubes, lines, etc. are covered with clean towels.
              (e) Family members, visitors, or assisting staff wear PPE.
              (f) Disposable tips are used for only one treatment.
              (g) Battery-operated handpieces are stored in tight bags and labeled with the patient's name and date first used.

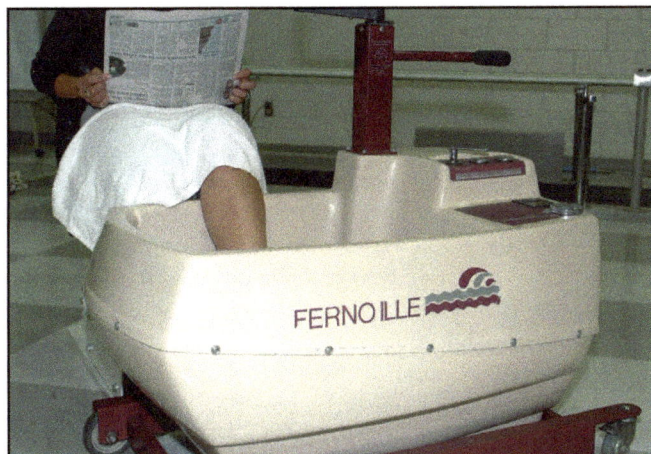

Figure 25.3: Whirlpool.

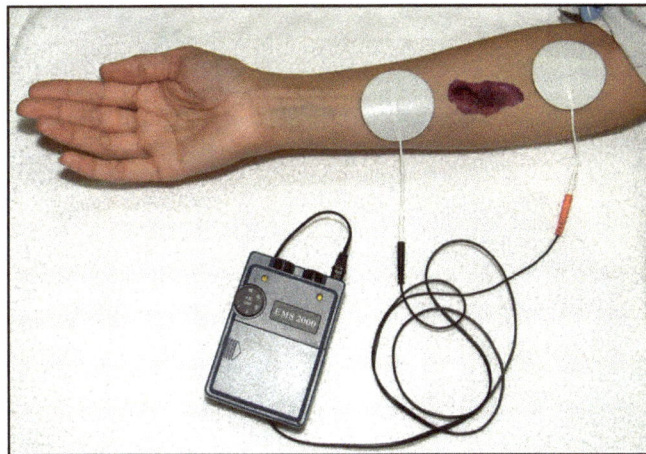

Figure 25.4: Electrical stimulation.

(h) Environmental surfaces are cleansed after treatment.

2. Whirlpool (Figure 25.3)
   a) It is very seldom indicated for a patient with an open wound.
   b) Exceptions are diffuse or full body skin disorders that result in large areas of crusty or scaling necrotic epidermis and dermis, such as pemphigus, as well as disorders that would benefit from vasodilation, such as sickle cell disease or cryoglobulinemia.
   c) Whirlpool is contraindicated in the following conditions:
      i) Lower extremity edema
      ii) Lethargy
      iii) Unresponsiveness
      iv) Skin maceration
      v) Febrile conditions
      vi) Acute phlebitis
      vii) Renal failure
      viii) Dry gangrene
      ix) Incontinence (for full body immersion)
      x) Diabetic neuropathy

E. Electrical stimulation (ES)
   1. Electrical stimulation for wound healing uses the principle of electrotaxis (or galvanotaxis), defined as the attraction of cells to an electrical field of the opposite charge.
   2. Electrodes are placed in or around the wound bed to facilitate the endogenous flow of sodium ions to the negatively charged skin surface after injury (termed the current of injury). This signals that the repair process needs to take place or attracts the cells needed for a particular phase of wound healing.
   3. The process of electrotaxis is present throughout the repair process; therefore, electrical stimulation can be beneficial at any phase of wound healing (Figure 25.4).
   4. Certain cells have been determined to have a negative charge (epithelial cells, macrophages, neutrophils,

mast cells), while some have a positive charge (fibroblasts, infected neutrophils).
   a) One protocol is to use an active electrode (the one over or around the wound bed) with the opposite charge of the cells needed, depending on the healing phase of the tissue.
      i) E.g., to attract fibroblasts (positively charged) for granulation formation, the active electrode would need a negative charge.
   b) Another protocol is to alternate the polarity every two to three treatments or when wound healing plateaus.
   5. Ideally, treatment would be provided daily; however, in the outpatient setting treatment may only be feasible two to three times per week.
   6. Several types of electrical stimulation devices are available to produce specific combinations of current, polarity, waveform, and voltage to elicit the desired therapeutic effects; however, the most commonly used type of current is high voltage pulsed current.
   7. Indications
   a) CMS has approved the use of electrical stimulation for arterial, venous, neuropathic, and pressure ulcers that have not responded to 30 days of standard care for the etiology.
   b) Other wound types that have stalled in the healing process may respond positively to electrical stimulation, e.g., a surgical incision that is failing to epithelialize.
   8. Contraindications
   a) The presence of squamous or basal cell carcinoma or any other neoplasm in or around the wound because of possible mitogenic activity of the cancer cells
   b) The presence of untreated or non-resolving osteomyelitis in underlying bony structures
   c) The presence of metal ions, e.g., silver from topical medications
   d) The presence of any electronic implant that would be affected by the electrical current,

including a pacemaker and internal defibrillator device
- e) The presence of any reflex center (carotid sinus, phrenic nerve, heart, or laryngeal muscles) that would be sensitive to ES. In other words, ES is not recommended on the chest or anterior neck.
- f) Any transcerebral application
9. Precautions
- a) Children under three years old
- b) Skin irritation or burns under the electrodes
- c) Areas of impaired or absent sensation

F. Ultrasound
1. Ultrasound (US) uses a piezoelectric crystal to convert electrical energy into sound waves that emanate from the US head, travel through a conductive medium, and penetrate the tissue, where they produce cellular changes that can facilitate healing.
2. Traditionally US was used for wound healing by using 3 MHz pulsed sound at 20% duty cycle and 0.5 w/cm^2; however, the treatment required that the sound head be in contact with the conducting medium directly on the wound base.
3. Low-frequency (20-50 KHz) US
- a) It can be either contact or noncontact and is now the standard delivery mode for treating wounds.
- b) Contact low-frequency US, utilized for selective debridement, uses 20-50 KHz with a sound head that is shaped much like a mini ice cream scoop.
- c) Using sterile saline as the conducting medium, the sound head is moved across the wound bed to remove adhered fibrous nonviable tissue.
4. Noncontact low-frequency US (40 KHz)
- a) Uses a disposable applicator over the sound head that prevents direct contact with the wound bed (Figure 25.5)
- b) Normal saline is dispersed from an attached bottle to serve as the conducting medium.
- c) The sound waves penetrate the wound bed and, through the mechanisms of cavitation and microstreaming, create changes at the cellular level that facilitate wound healing.

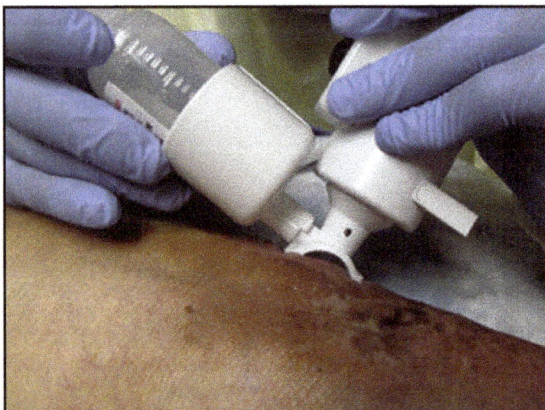

Figure 25.5: Noncontact low-frequency ultrasound applied to a lower extremity wound.

- d) These changes include:
  - i) Increased fluid movement in the interstitial spaces, which results in a decrease in edema
  - ii) Increased attraction of neutrophils, fibroblasts, and endothelial cells to the wound, which facilitates autolysis and results in granulation formation
  - iii) Improved scar formation with stronger tensile strength of remodeling tissue
- d) Indications include acute and chronic wounds of the following etiologies:
  - i) Trauma
  - ii) Burn and friction injuries
  - iii) Pressure wounds, especially deep tissue injury
  - iv) Venous insufficiency
  - v) Inflammation, e.g., vasculitis
  - vi) Diabetes
- e) Contraindications (for general ultrasound)
  - i) Presence of neoplasm
  - ii) Over epiphyseal plates of growing children
  - iii) Over breast implants
  - iv) Pregnancy
  - v) Joint replacement cement
  - vi) Plastics used for prosthetics
  - vii) Proximity to pacemaker
  - viii) Eyes
  - ix) Over the heart
- f) Contraindications (for wound care)
  - i) Untreated osteomyelitis
  - ii) Tendency to bleed
  - iii) Arterial insufficiency
  - iv) Deep vein thrombosis

G. Ultraviolet C
1. Ultraviolet (UV) light is a component of sunlight that encompasses nonvisible wavelengths between 180-400 nm of the electromagnetic spectrum (visible light is between 400-800 nm).
2. There are three spectral bands of UV light
- a) UVA (320-400 nm)—nonionizing, produces most of the tanning effects
- b) UVB (290-320 nm)—nonionizing, produces erythema and blistering
- c) UVC (180-290 nm)—ionizing, bactericidal, virucidal
3. UVA and UVB are both known to be carcinogenic.
4. UVC
- a) UVC is delivered with lamps that use the specific wavelength of 254 nm, which is at the upper range of being bactericidal, and contain filters that reduce the risk of being carcinogenic (Figure 25.6).
- b) UVC has been shown to alter the DNA of the bacteria, leading to cell death without harming the host tissue.

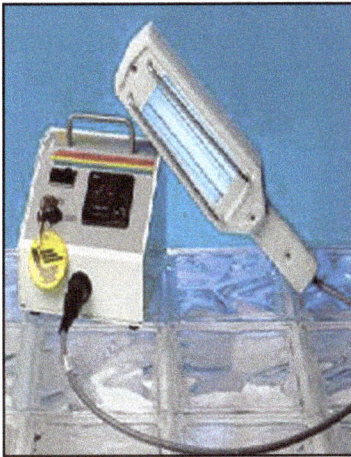

Figure 25.6: UVC device for treating wounds.

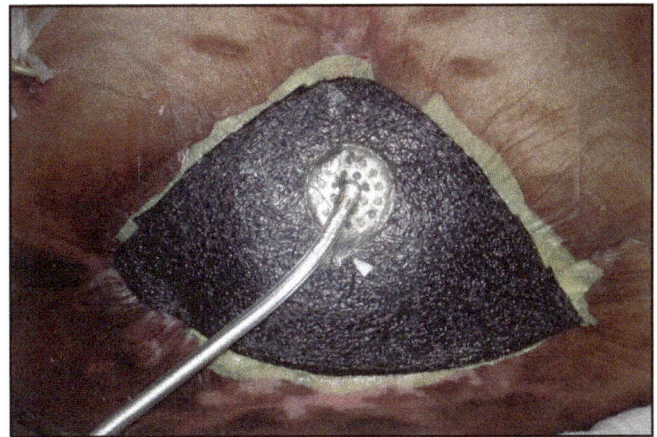

Figure 25.7: Negative pressure dressing on an abdominal wound.

c) Treatments, usually 30-90 seconds and according to manufacturer recommendations for equipment, are provided five to six times daily.

d) UVC can be safely used on a colonized or infected wound of any etiology with care to observe for adverse effects such as burning, itching, or pain.

5. Contraindications
   a) Acute eczema, dermatitis, psoriasis
   b) Neoplasm
   c) Around the eyes
   d) Diabetes
   e) Hepatic or renal disease
   f) Cardiac disease
   g) Herpes simplex
   h) Hyperthyroidism
   i) Pulmonary tuberculosis
   j) Systemic lupus erythematosus

6. Precautions
   a) Photosensitivity
   b) Recent x-ray or radiation
   c) History of skin cancer
   d) Generalized fever

H. Negative pressure wound therapy (NPWT) (Figure 25.7)
   1. NPWT consists of a sterile wound filler (usually polyurethane reticulated foam or a sterile drape of transparent film), tubing that connects to a collection canister, and a pump that provides the negative pressure.
   2. NPWT is discussed in Chapter 13 on advanced technologies in wound care; however, physical therapists who provide wound care are proficient in determining if and when NPWT is indicated, the safe parameters for its use in different wounds, and the application and removal of the dressings.

I. Edema management
   1. Edema is known to be an impeding factor in wound healing, especially in the extremities.
   2. Physical therapists provide noninvasive vascular screening (e.g., palpation of pulses, Doppler assessment, ankle-brachial index, rubor of dependency) during the evaluation process and determine the safe

yet efficacious method of compression when treating lower extremity wounds.

3. Multi-layer compression systems (high working and resting pressure), short-stretch bandages (high working pressure and low resting pressure), compression garments, and intermittent compression pumps are considered standard methods of compression used by physical therapists to reduce and manage edema due to trauma, lymphedema, venous insufficiency, systemic disorders (e.g., renal and hepatic insufficiency, congestive heart failure), and medications.

J. Gait training and exercise
   1. Gait is assessed for patients with lower extremity wounds to determine if gait impairments are contributing to the wound formation or if the wound is causing gait impairments. Exercises and assistive devices are then recommended to:
      a) Assist in off-loading the plantar diabetic foot ulcer
      b) Improve balance with the use of total contact casts, CROW or CAM walkers, or other devices that create balance impairments
      c) Activate the venous pump in patients with chronic venous insufficiency, especially if there is ankle fusion or hypomobility
      d) Stretch restricted or contracted joints that may be affecting normal gait patterns
      e) Strengthen weakened muscle groups that may be contributing to gait impairments, especially in patients who have diabetes
      f) Assist patients with pressure ulcers in pressure redistribution strategies
      g) Improve lymphatic flow

RESOURCES

1. Bowker JH, Pfeifer MA, editors. *Levin and O'Neal's The Diabetic Foot.* 7th ed. Amsterdam: Mosby Elsevier; 2008.
2. Crosby K. Physical therapy modalities in wound care. In: Shah JB, Sheffield, PJ, Fife CE, editors. *Wound Care Certification Study Guide.* North Palm Beach: Best Publishing Company; 2011: 213-7.
3. Hamm R. *Text and Atlas of Wound Diagnosis and Management.* New York: McGraw Hill Company; 2015.
4. McCulloch JM, Kloth LC. *Wound Healing: Evidence-Based Management.* 4th ed. Philadelphia: F.A. Davis Company; 2010.
5. Sussman C, Bates-Jensen B. *Wound Care: A Collaborative Practice Manual for Health Professionals.* 4th ed. Baltimore: Lippincott Williams & Wilkins; 2012.
6. Unger PG. The physical therapist's role in wound management. In: Krasner DL, Rodeheaver GT, Sibbald RG. *Chronic Wound Care: A Clinical Source Book for Healthcare Professionals.* 4th ed. Malvern: HMP Communications; 2007: 381-8.
7. Vaughn MM. Physical therapy modalities in wound healing. In: Sheffield PJ, Fife CE, editors. *Wound Care Practice.* 2nd ed. North Palm Beach: Best Publishing Company; 2007: 869-900.

SAMPLE QUESTIONS

1. A patient is referred with a chronic venous insufficiency wound that shows signs of infection, including purulent drainage, erythema, and odor. Which of the modalities is most indicated for initial treatment?
    a) Whirlpool
    b) Electrical stimulation
    c) Ultraviolet C
    d) Negative pressure wound therapy

2. Low-frequency ultrasound assists with wound healing by microstreaming, which:
    a) Increases MMPs
    b) Increases fluid movement and circulation in close proximity to the cellular membranes
    c) Causes implosion of stable gas bubbles and the destruction of tissues
    d) Has antibacterial effects at the cellular level

3. For a wound with adhered fibrous tissue and bioburden, which modality would be most effective for debridement?
    a) Electrical stimulation
    b) Low-frequency contact ultrasound
    c) Low-frequency noncontact ultrasound
    d) Ultraviolet light

4. An important component of treating a patient with a history of chronic venous insufficiency and an ankle fusion is exercise to strengthen the gastrocnemius/soleus muscle group.
    a) True
    b) False

5. Electrical stimulation uses the principle of electrotaxis to:
    a) Change the DNA of bacteria to decrease bacteria burden
    b) Decrease the pain associated with chronic wounds
    c) Stimulate muscle action around the wounded tissue
    d) Attract cells of opposite charge that are needed to facilitate wound healing

6. A patient with venous insufficiency and bilateral venous leg ulcers is referred to physical therapy. The patient cannot tolerate sharp debridement of the necrotic tissue in the wounds. Which is the ideal treatment option to address the necrotic tissue?
    a) Whirlpool
    b) Pulsed lavage

7. Ultrasound can be used for bacteriocidal effects.
    a) True
    b) False

8. In which band of UV radiation is the bacteriocidal range found?
    a) UVA
    b) UVB
    c) UVC
    d) UVD

9. Which type of electrical current is most frequently used for wound healing?
    a) Interferential
    b) Direct current
    c) High voltage pulsed current
    d) Low voltage microcurrent

10. Whirlpool treatment may cause all of the following except:
    a) *Pseudomonas* infections of wounds
    b) Decreased circulation to wound bed
    c) Impeded venous blood flow in legs
    d) Maceration of periwound skin

See answers on page 229.

NOTES

ANSWER KEY

1. c) UVC can safely be used on a colonized or infected wound of any etiology. UVC has been shown to alter the DNA of the bacteria, leading to cell death without harming the host tissue.

2. b) Low-frequency ultrasound assists with wound healing by microstreaming, which increases fluid movement and circulation in close proximity to the cellular membranes. UVC has antibacterial effects at the cellular level. MMPs usually decrease as a wound heals. Low-frequency ultrasound causes the implosion of stable gas bubbles and the destruction of tissues, which is called unstable cavitation.

3. b) Of the modalities listed, low-frequency contact ultrasound would be the most appropriate for debriding a wound with adhered fibrous tissue and bioburden. Low-frequency noncontact ultrasound does not help with debridement, but it may help facilitate wound healing. UVC is bactericidal and is indicated for use in infectious wounds. While electrical stimulation helps with wound healing, it does not help with debridement.

4. a) An important component of treating a patient with a history of chronic venous insufficiency and an ankle fusion is exercise to strengthen the gastrocnemius/ soleus muscle group.

5. d) Electrical stimulation uses the principle of electrotaxis to attract cells of the opposite charge needed to facilitate wound healing. UVC changes the DNA of bacteria, which decreases bacteria burden. Electrical stimulation has not proven to decrease pain in chronic wounds; however, transcutaneous electrical nerve stimulation (TENS) is used in pain management.

6. b) Pulse lavage at 9-15 psi pressure is effective in removing bacteria and exudate, softening necrotic tissue, and facilitating debridement. Whirlpool is also helpful in debridement; however, as the patient described above has venous stasis, whirlpool may worsen the venous edema.

7. b) Ultrasound does not have bactericidal effects.

8. c) UVC is bactericidal.

9. c) High voltage pulse current is most frequently used for wound healing.

10. b) Whirlpool treatment may cause *Pseudomonas* infections of wounds, impeded venous blood flow in legs, and maceration of periwound skin. It does not, however, cause arterial insufficiency.

HYPERBARIC OXYGEN THERAPY 26

E. Patricia Rios, RN, MSN, CHRN-C
Yvette Ponce-Hall, CHT
Jayesh B. Shah, MD, CWSP, FAPWCA, FACCWS

INTRODUCTION

This chapter discusses the use of hyperbaric oxygen therapy (HBOT) as an advanced wound care modality for specific wound types. Included will be the definition of HBOT, indications for treatment, contraindications for receiving HBOT, dressings allowed/prohibited in the hyperbaric chamber, patient preparation, monitoring for side effects, chamber operations, equipment and safety, and emergency protocols.

OBJECTIVES

Participants should be able to describe how HBOT works, identify approved indications or contraindications to therapy, recognize any potential side effects from receiving therapy, and understand the importance of safety and emergency protocols.

I. Hyperbaric oxygen therapy

A. UHMS definition: the patient breathes 100% oxygen while the treatment chamber is pressurized to a pressure greater than 1.0 atmosphere absolute (ATA) (sea level). Current information indicates that pressurization should be at least 1.4 ATA.

B. Mechanisms of action
1. Increases the generation of oxygen free radicals, which inhibit bacterial metabolic functions
2. Improves oxygen-dependent transport of some antibiotics across bacterial cell walls
3. Reduces adherence of leukocytes to ischemic tissue, which prevents vasoconstriction and reperfusion injury
4. Limits post-ischemic reductions in ATP production, which decreases lactate accumulation in ischemic tissue

C. Indications
1. Wound-related indications
   a) Acute thermal burn injury
   b) Acute traumatic ischemia
      i) Crush injury
      ii) Compartment syndrome
   c) Arterial insufficiencies
      i) Enhancement of healing in selected problem wounds

d) Clostridial myositis and gas gangrene
e) Compromised grafts and flaps
f) Delayed radiation injury (soft tissue and bony necrosis)
g) Intracranial abscess
h) Necrotizing soft tissue infections
i) Osteomyelitis (refractory)
2. Non-wound indications
   a) Air or gas embolism
   b) Carbon monoxide poisoning
      i) Carbon monoxide poisoning complicated by cyanide poisoning
   c) Decompression sickness
   d) Idiopathic sudden sensorineural hearing loss
   e) Severe anemia
   f) Central retinal artery occlusion

D. Absolute contraindication
1. Untreated pneumothorax
   a) Can further damage the lung and cause a life-threatening event

E. Contraindications if recently or currently receiving the following medications:
1. Bleomycin—antineoplastic antibiotic
   a) Lung fibrosis
2. Doxorubicin (Adriamycin®)—chemotherapy drug
   a) Cardiotoxicity may occur
3. Cisplatinum
   a) Wound healing may be impaired
4. Disulfiram (Antabuse®)
   a) Blocks the production of superoxide dismutase, which protects against oxygen toxicity
5. Mafenide acetate (Sulfamylon®)
   a) Wound healing may be impaired

F. Relative contraindications
1. Asthma
   a) May result in a pneumothorax
2. Chronic sinusitis
   a) May lead to possible barotrauma
3. Congenital spherocytosis
   a) Hemolysis may occur due to fragile red blood cells

4. Claustrophobia
   a) May lead to increased anxiety
5. Emphysema with CO_2 retention
   a) May present a risk of pneumothorax
   b) May lead to CO_2 narcosis secondary to decreased respiratory drive
6. High fever
   a) Could potentially lower the threshold for seizures
7. History of ear surgery
   a) Patients may not be able to clear their ears; forced clearing increases the risk of trauma to the ear
8. History of seizures
   a) Lowers the threshold for seizures
9. Optic neuritis
   a) Rare cases of worsening vision and blindness have occurred
10. Pacemaker/defibrillator
    a) There is a possibly of malfunction of the device.
       i) Ensure the device manufacturer has cleared the device for hyperbaric treatment
11. Pregnancy
    a) Potential complications for the fetus
12. Thorax surgery
    a) There is a small risk of air trapped in scarring caused during surgery
13. Upper respiratory infections
    a) Patients may have trouble with ear clearing, which can result in trauma to the ear

G. Dressings allowed in the hyperbaric therapy chamber
1. Adaptic®
2. Adhesive tape
3. Alginate
4. Altrazeal™ powder dressing
5. Apligraf®
6. Betadine® Antiseptics
7. Bacitracin
8. Cast
   a) Fiberglass or plaster has set for more than 10 hours
9. Collagen matrix dressing
10. Compression wraps
11. Cotton gauze
12. Dakin's solution
13. Dressings for negative pressure wound therapy (NPWT)
    a) Does not apply to the NPWT device/unit
14. Dry gauzes, pads, foams, and sponges
15. Hydrocolloid
16. Hydrating dermal wound gel
17. Hydrofera Blue®
18. Iodosorb™
19. Iodoflex™
20. Lidocaine gel
21. Medihoney®
22. Mepitel®

23. Nystatin
24. OASIS® Wound Matrix
25. Other jellies, gels, and pastes that do not contain alcohol or other potentially flammable material
26. Pads, foams, and sponges containing water-based hydrating gels
    a) NPWT foam dressing is permitted but the NPWT unit/device is prohibited
27. Regranex® Gel
28. Silicone dressings
29. Silver-impregnated dressings
30. Transparent film
31. Transdermal patches
32. Tubular net bandage, tube gauze
33. Unna's boot (unless visibly soiled)
34. Vaseline® petrolatum gauze
    a) Covered with a clean cotton gauze
35. Xenaderm®
    a) Covered with a clean cotton gauze
36. Xeroform™ petrolatum dressing

H. Dressings prohibited in the hyperbaric therapy chamber
1. Any dressing/device/material that employs the use of Velcro® fasteners
   a) If unable to exclude the use of a Velcro® fastener, it must be inactivated by completely wrapping each area of closure with tape
2. Dressings that utilize metal prong fasteners
3. Dressings that contain mineral oil

I. Patient preparation
1. Prior to first treatment
   a) Obtain a physician order that includes the indication for treatment, number of treatments, duration of each treatment, and air breaks, if utilized.
   b) Hyperbaric risk assessment should be completed by hyperbaric-trained nurse.
   c) Hyperbaric-specific instruction should be given.
   d) Consents to treat should be obtained.
2. First and subsequent treatments
   a) Pretreatment: vital signs, temperature, blood pressure, pulse, respirations, and pain level should be obtained.
      i) Temperature
         (1) For oral temperature greater than 101°F, consider an antipyretic prior to therapy.
         (2) Patients with increased temperature are at increased risk for oxygen toxicity seizure.
      ii) Blood pressure
         (1) Consult treating physician when:
             (a) Systolic blood pressure (SBP): <100 or >180
             (b) Diastolic blood pressure (DBP): <60 or >100
             (c) SBP >180 mmHg or DBP >100 mmHg

iii) Pulse
  (1) Consult treating physician when:
    (a) Symptomatic bradycardia (<60 bpm)
    (b) Symptomatic tachycardia (>100 bpm)
    (c) New incidence of irregular heartbeat
iv) Respirations
  (1) Consult treating physician when:
    (a) Breathing is labored or irregular
    (b) Breathing is abnormal from the patient's normal cycle
v) Blood glucose
  (1) Consult treating physician when:
    (a) Blood glucose is <110
    (b) Blood glucose is >280
vi) Lung auscultation
  (1) Ensure that all lung fields are clear and patient is free from rales or rhonchi
vii) Ear evaluation
  (1) Examine the tympanic membrane.
  (2) Educate patient on methods for ear clearing during treatment.
  (3) Patients with signs and symptoms of a cold, sinusitis, or seasonal allergies may have increased difficulty in clearing ears during treatment.
viii) Patient attire for treatment
  (1) No street clothes, including undergarments.
  (2) Patient must change into hospital-supplied gown or scrubs.
    (a) Gown or scrubs are 100% cotton or greater than or equal to 50% cotton/polyester blend.
ix) Patient grounding device is utilized
  (1) Ensures static electricity is dispersed
x) Patient is placed in the chamber.
  (1) Monitor patient throughout treatment
  (2) Reassure patient and instruct on ear clearing as needed
xi) Post-treatment
  (1) Assess patient vital signs, blood glucose, and pain level
J. Monitoring for side effects
  1. Pressure injuries
    a) Ear barotrauma
    b) Inner ear barotrauma (round window blowout)
    c) Sinus squeeze
    d) Dental problems
  2. Decrease in blood glucose
    a) Typically, blood sugar drops 50 points during a 90 minute treatment.
    b) Always obtain blood glucose levels on diabetic patients prior to hyperbaric treatment.

3. Visual refractive changes
  a) Most common in older patients receiving more than 20 treatments
  b) Myopia (distance vision) deteriorates further, presbyopia (close vision) improves
  c) Visual changes usually reverse upon completion of hyperbaric treatments
  d) Eyewear prescriptions should not be adjusted for at least two months after completing hyperbaric treatments
4. Cataract formation
  a) Potential for faster growth of existing cataracts in individuals receiving HBOT
5. Claustrophobia
  a) Educate the patient prior to the first treatment; offer a mock run of the treatment experience.
  b) Make sure the patient understands he/she is in control and will be observed by trained hyperbaric staff at all times while receiving treatment.
  c) Consider pretreatment medication with benzodiazepine.
6. Pulmonary oxygen toxicity
  a) Oxygen toxicity in lung tissue typically happens in patients receiving BID or TID treatments or in patients who require ongoing O_2 support (e.g., on ventilators or oxygen dependent).
  b) Patient may experience:
    i) Substernal chest pain
    ii) Dry cough
    iii) Decrease in vital capacity
  c) Consider a pulmonologist consult
7. Central nervous system (CNS) oxygen toxicity
  a) Seizure during hyperbaric treatment
    i) Low risk: 0.7 in 10,000 treatments
    ii) Chamber decompression must not occur while the patient is in the tonic phase
    iii) Patient is at risk for increased injury from flailing or aspiration
    iv) Consider utilizing air breaks to reduce risk of seizure
  b) Post-seizure
    i) Assess vital signs and blood glucose.
    ii) Reassure patient and assess for injury.
K. Chamber operation
  1. Chamber types
    a) Class A (multiplace) (Figure 26.1)
      i) Multiple human occupancy chambers
      ii) Maintain less than 23.5% oxygen inside
      iii) Chambers are pressurized with air; the patient wears a hood that delivers 100% oxygen during the prescribed treatment
    b) Class B (monoplace) (Figure 26.2)
      i) Single human occupancy chambers
      ii) Compressed with 100% oxygen
      iii) Air breaks are delivered via demand-flow mask or free-flow mask

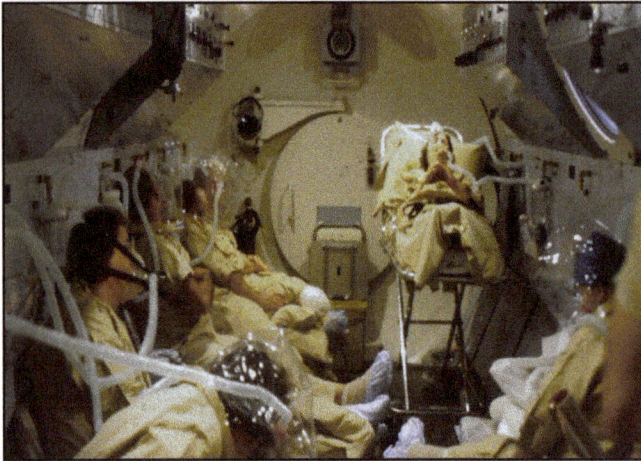

Figure 26.1: Class A (multiplace) hyperbaric chamber.

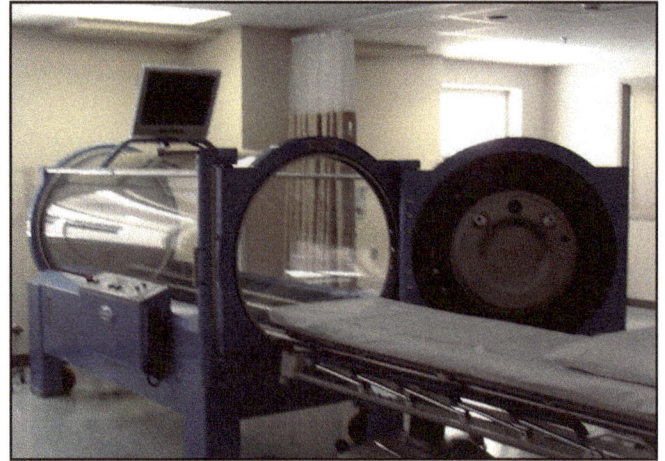

Figure 26.2: Class B (monoplace) hyperbaric chamber.

c) Class C (animal)
   i) Not for human use
L. Equipment and safety
   1. Multiplace chambers
      a) Typically, approved medical devices may be taken in the chamber
      b) Require a fire suppression system
      c) Attendant is present inside the chamber during the treatment
   2. Monoplace chambers
      a) Approved medical devices are passed into the chamber via penetrator ports
      b) Attendant is chamber side to observe the patient throughout treatment
   3. Fire safety
      a) Prevention is always the focus
         i) Anything that goes into the chamber is a risk
         ii) Limit the number of combustibles taken into the chamber
         iii) Grounding
            (1) Chamber is grounded to the building
            (2) In monoplace chambers a grounding strap or wrist strap is worn by the patient
         iv) Signs detailing prohibited items are required
M. Emergency protocols
   1. Patient seizure
      a) Chamber operator
         i) Stop travel or maintain chamber at constant pressure
         ii) Notify physician and nurse
         iii) Ascend (decompress) the chamber under the direction of the supervising physician and upon verification that the patient is breathing
      b) Nurse
         i) Prepare to assist with patient as necessary
            (1) Upon patient exit from chamber

         (a) Vital signs
         (b) Blood sugar
         (2) Provide recovery actions as necessary
      ii) Document actions
   2. Suspected pneumothorax
      a) Chamber operator
         i) Stop travel or keep pressure stable
         ii) Notify physician and nurse
         iii) Maintain constant depth until directed to terminate treatment by the supervising physician
         iv) Ascend (decompress) the chamber slowly under the direction of the supervising physician
      b) Nurse
         i) Prepare to assist with patient as necessary
         ii) Notify code team or EMS as applicable
         iii) Provide recovery actions as necessary
   3. Unresponsive patient/cardiac arrest
      a) Chamber operator
         i) Stop travel or keep pressure stable
         ii) Maintain constant chamber depth
         iii) Notify physician and nurse
         iv) Ascend (decompress) the chamber at a rate of 5 psi/min once directed to terminate treatment by the supervising physician
      b) Nurse
         i) Initiate code as per hospital policy
         ii) Assist with CPR
            (1) Ensure patient is clear of the chamber prior to defibrillation
               (a) Linen, gurney, and mattress will be oxygen saturated
         iii) Prepare to transfer patient to ED or for EMS evacuation
   4. Loss of chamber pressure
      a) Chamber operator
         i) Adjust rate of depressurization
            (1) Lower ventilation control valve

    ii) Notify supervising physician
    iii) Notify patient of unexpected chamber ascent
    iv) Determine reason for uncontrollable decrease in chamber pressure prior to resuming chamber operation
       (1) Monoplace chambers are designed to self-decompress at a low rate when a chamber gas supply is suddenly lost
  b) Nurse
    i) Prepare to assist with patient as necessary
    ii) Reassure patient as needed

5. Uncontrollable increase in chamber pressure
  a) Chamber operator
    i) Secure gas supply
    ii) Notify physician
    iii) Notify patient of need to end treatment
    iv) Determine reason for uncontrollable increase in chamber pressure prior to resuming chamber operation
  b) Nurse
    i) Prepare to assist with patient as necessary
    ii) Reassure patient as needed

6. Oxygen leak
  a) Chamber operator
    i) Determine leak source and correct if possible
    ii) Notify physician
    iii) Notify patient of need to end treatment
    iv) Determine reason for oxygen leak prior to resuming chamber operation
  b) Nurse
    i) Prepare to assist with patient as necessary
    ii) Reassure patient as needed

7. Loss of communication/power
  a) Chamber operator
    i) Stop travel or keep pressure stable
    ii) Switch to battery power
    iii) Determine the cause of power loss and correct if possible
    iv) Notify physician
    v) Communicate with patient by use of flash cards
    vi) Inform patient of need to end treatment
    vii) Determine reason for loss of communication power prior to resuming chamber operation
  b) Nurse
    i) Prepare to assist with patient as necessary
    ii) Reassure patient as needed

8. Patient complaint
  a) Chamber operator
    i) Stop travel or keep pressure stable
    ii) Communicate with patient to determine nature of complaint
    iii) Notify physician
    iv) Complete treatment if complaint has been resolved
    v) If complaint is related to severe anxiety or claustrophobia:
       (1) Reassure patient and terminate treatment as directed by supervising physician
    vi) If complaint is related to any sign or systems of oxygen toxicity:
       (1) Reassure patient and prepare to terminate treatment as directed by supervising physician
       (2) Be aware patient first sign/complaint in oxygen toxicity is "not feeling right"
  b) Nurse
    i) Prepare to assist with patient as necessary
       (1) If oxygen toxicity is suspected, prepare for necessary emergency response
    ii) Reassure patient as needed

9. Prohibited items in the chamber
  a) Chamber operator
    i) Notify physician
    ii) Stop travel. If in descent phase of treatment, begin ascent at a safe control rate. If at treatment pressure, begin ascent at a safe controlled rate. Remove patient and item from chamber once at surface pressure
    iii) Chamber emergency vent should only be used if risk of fire is present

10. Fire in the chamber room
  a) Chamber operator
    i) Stop travel if ascending or descending
    ii) Activate fire alarm/call code as per hospital policy
    iii) Don smoke mask
    iv) Extinguish fire if possible
       (1) Fire extinguisher: PASS
         (a) Pull pin
         (b) Aim at base
         (c) Squeeze handle
         (d) Sweep from side to side
    v) Start patient evacuation
       (1) Decompress the chamber
       (2) Remove the patient
  b) Nurse
    i) Prepare to assist with patient as necessary
    ii) Reassure patient as needed

11. Fire in the chamber
  a) Chamber operator
    i) Start patient evacuation
       (1) Decompress the chamber at its fastest rate
       (2) If possible have patient don air break mask
    ii) Activate fire alarm/call code as per hospital policy

     iii) Begin emergency termination for other chambers in the room

     iv) Once chamber is depressurized:
- (1) Stand by with handheld fire extinguisher to spray into chamber when the chamber door opens (if needed to extinguish fire)
- (2) Remove patient
- (3) Evacuate to safe area

     v) Evacuate from chamber room

     vi) Shut off main chamber room oxygen

  b) Nurse
- i) Prepare to assist with patient as necessary
- ii) Notify code team or EMS as applicable
- iii) Provide recovery actions as necessary
- iv) Evaluate/prepare for need to transfer patient to ED or for EMS evacuation

12. Earthquake
  a) Chamber operator
- i) Stop travel or maintain constant depth
- ii) Move away from space between chambers
- iii) When tremor has stopped
  - (1) Remove patient from chamber at a quick rate of travel
- iv) Perform chamber shut down procedure
- v) Inspect chamber for damage
- vi) Inspect gas systems for damage

  b) Nurse
- i) Prepare to assist with patient as necessary
- ii) Evaluate patient to determine if transfer to backup facility is required

RESOURCES

1. Kindwall EP, Whelan H, editors. *Hyperbaric Medicine Practice.* 3rd ed. North Palm Beach: Best Publishing Company; 2008.
2. Larson-Lohr V, Norvell H, Josefsen L, Wilcox JR, editors. *Hyperbaric Nursing and Wound Care.* North Palm Beach: Best Publishing Company; 2011.
3. Neuman TS, Thom SR. *Physiology and Medicine of Hyperbaric Oxygen Therapy.* Philadelphia: Saunders Elsevier; 2008.
4. Sheffield DA , Sheffield RB (authors). CHT and CHRN Certification Exam Review Course. [DVD]. 2nd ed. San Antonio: International ATMO; 2013. 4 DVD set.
5. Sheffield DA , Sheffield RB. *CHT and CHRN Certification Exam Practice Book.* 2nd ed (rev). San Antonio: International ATMO; 2013.
6. Workman WT, editor. *Hyperbaric Facility Safety: A Practical Guide.* North Palm Beach: Best Publishing Company; 2000.

SAMPLE QUESTIONS

1. A febrile patient is at the greater risk of which of the following while in the chamber?
   a) Nitrogen narcosis
   b) Oxygen toxicity
   c) Anemia
   d) Barotrauma

2. Which item must be completed prior to the start of a hyperbaric treatment?
   a) Hyperbaric risk assessment
   b) Patient orientation and instruction
   c) Physician orders specifying hyperbaric treatment protocol
   d) All of the above

3. When it comes to fire safety, which of the following is always the main priority?
   a) Patient diagnosis
   b) Hyperbaric risk assessment
   c) Prevention
   d) Navy diving protocols

4. In the case of a seizure in the chamber, the chamber should be decompressed once the patient is in the tonic phase.
   a) True
   b) False

5. A class B chamber is classified as a hyperbaric chamber that is meant for:
   a) Animal use only
   b) Multiple human occupancy
   c) Single human occupancy
   d) Commercial divers

6. When a suspected pneumothorax occurs, the chamber operator should:
   a) Stop travel, ascend slowly, notify physician, and assess the patient
   b) Notify physician and nurse, stop travel, maintain depth until directed to terminate treatment, and ascend slowly under supervising physician direction
   c) Stop travel, maintain depth until directed to terminate treatment, notify physician and nurse, and ascend slowly under supervising physician direction
   d) Stop travel, notify physician and nurse, maintain depth until directed to terminate treatment, and ascend slowly under supervising physician direction

7. In the case of an earthquake, the chamber operator should quickly remove the patient from the chamber after the tremor has stopped.
   a) True
   b) False

8. Blood glucose will typically drop how many points during a standard 90-minute hyperbaric oxygen treatment?
   a) 200
   b) 50
   c) 30
   d) 10

9. All of the following are UHMS accepted hyperbaric oxygen therapy indications except:
   a) Compromised grafts and flaps
   b) Cerebral palsy
   c) Osteomyelitis (refractory)
   d) Necrotizing soft tissue infections

10. An absolute contraindication to hyperbaric oxygen therapy is an untreated pneumothorax, because it can further damage the lung and cause a life-threatening event.
    a) True
    b) False

See answers on page 239.

NOTES

ANSWER KEY

1. b) Vital signs should be taken prior to hyperbaric treatment to determine the patient's stability. Patients with a temperature greater than 101°F are at greater risk of having a seizure in the hyperbaric chamber. The supervising physician should consider an antipyretic prior to treatment.

2. d) All of the above apply to an initial start of hyperbaric treatment. Patients should be informed of the risks and benefits of the treatment. An orientation should consist of a description of the chamber's environment as well as a clear list of approved and prohibited items in the chamber. Patients should have a basic understanding of how the hyperbaric oxygen treatments assist with accelerated healing. A hyperbaric risk assessment should be completed by the RN or hyperbaric physician. Any contraindications should be addressed by the hyperbaric physician prior to the start of treatment. Finally, there should be clear and concise physician orders that specify the indication for treatment, the treatment protocol, and the number of treatments ordered.

3. c) Prevention is the main priority in fire safety. A safety checklist should be completed prior to the patient's entrance into the chamber. All potentially hazardous items should be prohibited from entering the chamber. If there is ever a doubt about an item, it is best to prohibit it from entering the chamber. Remember, "if in doubt, leave it out."

4. b) Never decompress a patient while they are in the tonic phase. The chamber operator, under the supervision of the attending physician, must wait until the patient resumes normal breathing and completes the tonic phase of seizure before starting the ascent (decompression) of the chamber. Due to Boyle's law, barotrauma can occur from the increase of volume within the lungs during the decompression of the chamber.

5. c) A class B chamber is commonly referred to as a monoplace chamber. These chambers are meant for single human occupancy only.

6. d) In the case of a suspected pneumothorax, the chamber operator should first stop travel. While the chamber pressure idles, the hyperbaric physician and nurse may be notified. The chamber operator must maintain depth until directed by the physician to terminate the treatment. This time could be used to prepare for the removal of the patient. A code team, crash cart, and chest tube cart can be retrieved during this time. Once the physician gives the order, slowly decompress the chamber.

7. a) Do not attempt to decompress a chamber during a tremor. Decompression of the chamber on an unstable surface can be hazardous for the patient and the chamber operator. The chamber operator should remove themselves from between the chambers for his/her safety. Once the tremor has passed, the chamber should be decompressed quickly and the patient removed from danger.

8. b) Blood glucose typically drops about 50 points during a standard treatment. Diabetic patients should eat an adequate meal before treatment. Dietary supplements should be provided for patients who have not eaten before their treatment. Follow blood glucose parameters of >110mg/dL and <280mg/dL for minimizing complications during HBOT.

9. b) Although hyperbaric oxygen studies have been performed on cerebral palsy patients, it is currently not a UHMS approved indication.

10. a) During the hyperbaric risk assessment, the patient should be asked if they have an unresolved or untreated pneumothorax. Decompressing a patient with an untreated pneumothorax can further injure the lung and cause arterial gas embolism (AGE), which can complicate and compromise the patient's condition. This process can lead to a life-threatening event.

WOUND DOCUMENTATION AND LEGAL/ETHICAL ISSUES IN WOUND CARE 27

Dianne Rudolph, RN, GNP-BC, DNP, CWOCN

INTRODUCTION

The purpose of this chapter is to discuss legal and ethical issues in wound care. Millions of dollars have recently been awarded by juries or settled in cases involving pressure ulcers. The elements of a lawsuit and the plaintiff's attorney's perceptions will be discussed. Medical malpractice is prevented through caring, communication, competence, and charting. Common sense tips for protecting oneself from lawsuits will be presented.

OBJECTIVES

Participants should be able to list the four essential elements of a lawsuit, discuss the ethical issues pertaining to off-label application of a medical treatment, and discuss how to limit exposure to legal liability.

I. Legal and ethical issues
A. Doing what is right for the patient
  1. Because of advanced technologies and life and limb salvaging procedures that generate revenue, physicians and clinicians are finding themselves in a dilemma of whether or not to proceed.
B. Informed consent
  1. Are there any alternative treatments?
  2. What level and type of scientific data supports the potential therapeutic use of HBOT?
  3. Does the potential benefit outweigh the risk, and can the facility handle complications?
  4. Does the patient understand he/she is responsible for cost even if no benefits occur?
  5. Is there a protocol or registry? This could be offered and would require a separate consent form.
  6. Informed consent should include any financial issues that could affect the patient-provider relationship.
C. Awareness
  1. Increased public awareness
  2. Concerns over nosocomial ulcers in healthcare facilities

  3. Concerns over inappropriate therapies or treatments
  4. Increased litigation with multimillion dollar settlements
D. Why people initiate lawsuits
  1. Grief, guilt, anger, money, expectations, ignorance
  2. Compensation/awards
    a) Texas (2002): $312.8 million; Alabama (1993): $65 million; Florida (2000): $19.9 million
    b) Recent awards and settlements in cases involving pressure ulcers: Illinois: $1.5 million, $2.5 million, $350,000, $45,000; Georgia: $5.3 million; New Jersey: $450,000
    c) 17,000 lawsuits are related to pressure ulcers yearly. It is the second most common claim after wrongful death, surpassing even the number of suits related to falls or emotional distress.
    d) The plaintiff's attorney's perceptions:
      i) All pressure ulcers are preventable.
      ii) Pressure ulcers progress through the "stages."
      iii) Higher stage pressure ulcers have progressed from lower stage pressure ulcers.
      iv) Pressure ulcers form from the outside-in. (Stage II, which represent friction and sheer, form outside-in, but deep pressure sores like III/IV and DTI form from the inside-out.)
      v) All wounds should heal.
      vi) Pressure ulcers are proof of bad care.
      vii) Wounds are proof of neglect.
      viii) Ischemic lower extremity ulcers are pressure ulcers.
      ix) These are all incorrect!
E. Elements of a lawsuit
  1. Duty
    a) Did the individual/institution have a duty to the individual?
  2. Breach of duty
    a) Was there a breach of duty that fell below the standard of care?
    b) Standard of care
      i) Assessing risk (Braden scale, Norton scale)
      ii) Preventive measures

        iii) Pressure-relieving support surface
        iv) Devices for off-loading
        v)   Debridement as indicated
        vi) Treatment of s/s infection
        vii) Nutritional assessment/interventions
        viii) Specialist consults
        ix) Documentation of treatment and its effectiveness
        x)   Providing moist healing as indicated
        xi) Proper use of topical therapies/treatments
        xii) Documentation of pain assessment
        xiii) Evidence of communication
        xiv) Evidence of competencies/credentials

3. Injury/damages
   a) Was there an injury (damages)?
      i) Pressure ulcer, wound dehiscence, infection, amputation, wrongful death
   b) Is there a link between the injury and the breach of duty? (Proximate cause, causal connection)

4. Causation
   a) Was the injury related to the care?
   b) Does the injury speak for itself? (E.g., leaving a surgical sponge or instrument inside the patient, performing surgery on the wrong body part or person.)
   c) Was the injury related to the underlying condition?

F. Case presentations

1. Case 1
   a) A 90-year-old female with peripheral vascular disease, mild dementia, and hypertension presented to a primary care physician's office with a one-month history of a non-healing ulcer of the right lower extremity (RLE) (Figure 27.1a).
   b) She was placed in an Unna's boot from below the tibial prominence to just about the ankle with instructions to return in two weeks.
   c) A lower-extremity ulcer developed (Figure 27.1b).

2. Case 2
   a) A 68-year-old male with a history of coronary artery disease, peripheral vascular disease, hypertension, and type 2 diabetes was admitted as an inpatient for an elective coronary artery bypass graft. The post-op course was complicated by AFib with RVR, respiratory failure, and hypotension requiring Levophed®. On post-operative day (POD) three he developed ecchymotic areas on his sacrum. On POD six he developed spinal cord infarct with subsequent paralysis. On POD 14 he had eschar on the sacral area.
   b) A critical care ulcer developed (Figure 27.2).

3. Case 3
   a) A 59-year-old female with a history of mild obesity, hypertension, and hypothyroidism was admitted as an inpatient for a routine lap cholecystectomy, complications required open

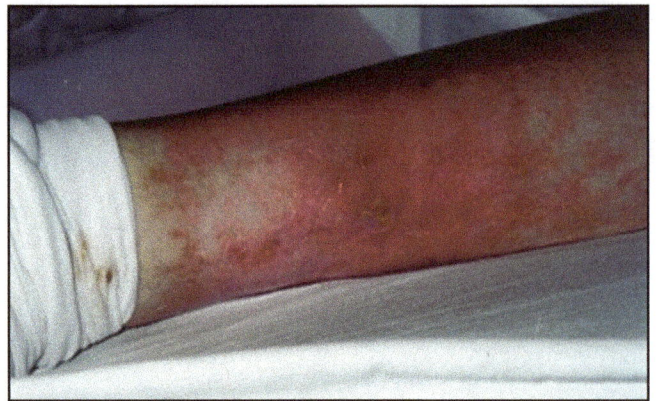

Figure 27.1a: Lower extremity ulcer on initial presentation.

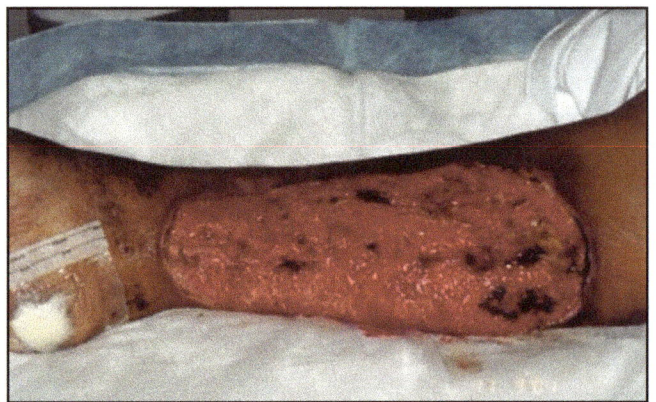

Figure 27.1b: Ulcer two weeks after the patient was placed in an Unna's boot.

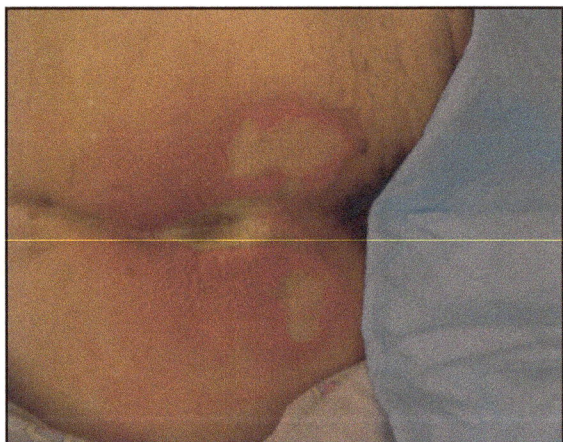

Figure 27.2: Critical care ulcer.

cholecystectomy. The patient postoperatively developed hypotension and required dopamine. Her IV subsequently infiltrated and was discontinued and restarted at another site.
   b) An ulcer occurred at the site of infiltration (Figure 27.3).

4. Case 4
   a) A 42-year-old female with type 2 diabetes, hypertension, morbid obesity, and end stage renal disease on hemodialysis underwent TAH/BSO

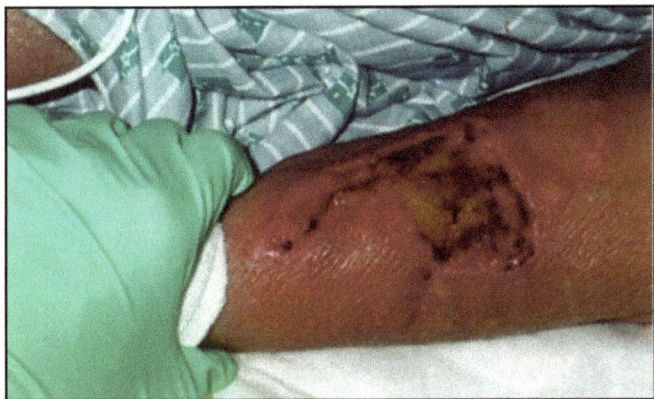

Figure 27.3: Ulcer at IV infiltration site.

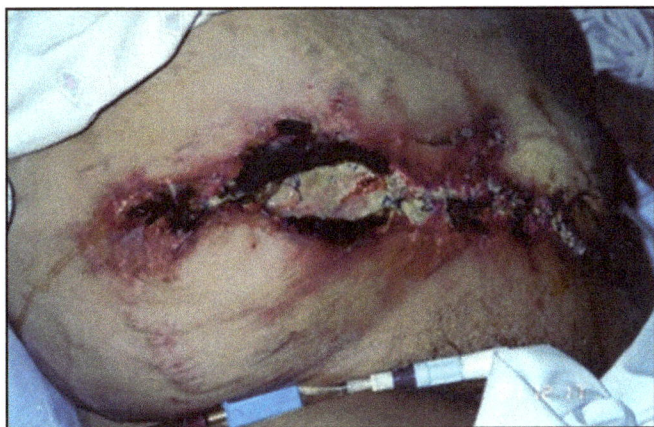

Figure 27.4: Wound dehiscence subsequent to total abdominal hysterectomy.

with panniculectomy. She developed subsequent wound dehiscence.

b) Total abdominal hysterectomy/bilateral salpingo-oophorectomy (TAH/BSO) (Figure 27.4).

G. The issue of pressure ulcers

1. Are all pressure ulcers preventable?

a) "Unavoidability" is a CMS payment term defined as "The resident developed a pressure ulcer even though the facility had evaluated the resident's clinical condition and pressure ulcer risk factors: defined and implemented interventions that are consistent with resident needs, resident goals, and recognized standards of practice; monitored and evaluated the impact of the interventions; and revised the approaches as appropriate." This defines "unavoidability" according to the care that is provided, not the status of the patient.

b) There are medically unpreventable pressure ulcers.

i) An unpreventable ulcer is one that occurs despite evidence of appropriate care. In some circumstances a patient can have multiple comorbidities that may lead to the development of a pressure ulcer, even when appropriate care is provided.

c) Pressure ulcers are not CMS Never Events (refer to Chapter 28, page 251). In the Federal Register, pressure ulcers are found under subpart (F)(b) "Hospital Acquired Conditions" (HACs) but not under subpart (F)(c) "Serious Preventable Events." (9)

H. Long-term care issues

1. F314: Pressure Ulcer Investigative Protocol: addresses avoidable vs. unavoidable pressure ulcers

2. Concerned with Medicare compliance, not medical determinations

a) Did the facility evaluate the resident's condition and pressure ulcer risk factors?

b) Are interventions implemented that are consistent with resident needs, goals, and recognized standard of care?

c) Are interventions monitored, re-evaluated, and revised as appropriate?

d) Were all evaluations and interventions documented in a timely fashion?

I. Acute care issues

1. NPUAP statements on avoidable vs. unavoidable pressure ulcers in acute care

2. Similar to CMS statements on long term care

3. Unanimous agreement that there are some clinical situations when pressure ulcers may be unavoidable

a) Critical patients with hemodynamic instability and/or when patient turning and repositioning may not be feasible

b) Patients who refuse to be turned

c) Patients with "skin failure"

II. Protecting yourself from lawsuits

A. The four C's of medical malpractice prevention

1. Caring

2. Communication

3. Competence

4. Charting

III. Wound Documentation

A. Common sense tips

1. Conduct a good admission assessment: document any preexisting areas on admission (POA)

2. Documenting etiology of the wound is critical

3. Conduct PU risk assessment (Braden)

4. Initiate preventive measures

5. Maintain consistency of documentation

6. Follow facility policies and current guidelines (NPUAP, WOCN, AHRQ)

7. Assess/manage comorbidities, nutrition

8. Use a team approach: nursing/MD or NP/PA/specialist/RD/social worker/case manager

B. Dubious documentation pitfalls

1. Gaps in documentation

2. Repetitive and rote

3. "I've never seen this patient before"

4. Inconsistencies in the chart/patterns of behavior
5. Too good to be true
6. Things don't add up
C. Things to be leery of
1. Poorly kept records
2. Constructed after the fact (late entries)
3. Failure to note obvious problems
4. Contradictions between departments
5. Orders not followed
6. MD not notified
7. Records altered
8. Lack of measurements
9. Inaccurate staging
10. Untimely assessments
11. Failure to recognize and treat infection
12. Improper treatment orders
D. The issue of photos
1. Essential to tracking progress; photograph wounds on initial appearance and at least once a week. Ensure photos and written documentation are congruent.

IV. Summary

A. Thoroughly assess and document
B. Provide care according to standards
C. Use consultants and a team approach
D. Maintain competencies and certification
E. Communicate
F. Maintain vigilance

RESOURCES

1. American Board of Wound Management Code of Ethics [Internet]. 2014. Accessed at: http://www.abwmcertified.org/about-us/code-of-ethics/.
2. Kinnunen UM, Saronto K, Ensio A, Livanainen A, Dykes P. Developing the standard wound care documentation model . *J Wound Ostomy Continence Nurs.* 2012; 39(4):397-407.
3. Black JM, Edsberg LE, Baharestani MM, Langemo D, Goldberg M, McNichol L, Cuddigan J. Pressure ulcers: avoidable or unavoidable? Results of the National Pressure Ulcer Advisory Panel Consensus Conference. *Ostomy Wound Manage.* 2011; 57(2):24–37.
4. Moore GP, Plaff JA. Malpractice cases in wound care and a legal concept: special defense. *West J Emerg Med.* Nov 2008; 9(4):238–9.
5. Ferguson H, Harris NG. Legal aspects of wound care and hyperbaric medicine. In: Sheffield PJ, Fife CE, editors. *Wound Care Practice.* 2nd ed. North Palm Beach: Best Publishing Company; 2007: 1073-97.
6. Fife CE. Ethics in wound care and hyperbaric medicine. In: Sheffield PJ, Fife CE, editors. *Wound Care Practice.* 2nd ed. North Palm Beach: Best Publishing Company; 2007: 1057-67.
7. Rios EP, Larson-Lohr V. Documentation: telling the story of care. In: Sheffield PJ, Fife CE, editors. *Wound Care Practice.* 2nd ed. North Palm Beach: Best Publishing Company; 2007: 1161-74.
8. Brandeis GH, Berlowitz DR, Katz P. Are pressure ulcers preventable? A survey of experts. *Adv in Skin and Wound Care.* 2001; 14(5):244-8.
9. Federal Register. Volume 72, Issue 85 (May 3, 2007). Accessed at: http://edocket.access.gpo.gov/2007/pdf/07-1920.pdf.

SAMPLE QUESTIONS

1. The essential elements of a lawsuit include all of the following except:
   a) Duty
   b) Breach of duty
   c) Injury or damages
   d) Causation
   e) Legal counsel

2. All of the following statements concerning a medical malpractice lawsuit are true except:
   a) A malpractice claim is based on the legal concept of negligence.
   b) To prevail, the plaintiff must prove that the healthcare provider's treatment deviated from the accepted standard of care.
   c) The plaintiff does not have to prove injury or damages if the medical provider has deviated from the accepted standard of care.
   d) It is typically necessary for the plaintiff to establish negligence through a medical expert.

3. All of the following are opportunities to limit exposure to legal liability except:
   a) Fully disclosing the risks and benefits of treatment with the patient
   b) Utilizing a commonly available medical product for a novel, untested, or experimental procedure without the patient's consent
   c) Thoroughly examining and documenting the patient's wound
   d) Closely monitoring patient treatment and making appropriate and timely adjustments as necessary

4. Pressure ulcers may be unavoidable in which of the following situations?
   a) Critical patients with hemodynamic instability and/or when patient turning and repositioning may not be feasible
   b) Patients confined to wheelchairs that self-reposition every 15 minutes
   c) Hemodynamically stable, completely conscious patients who present with acute stroke in the first 24 hours of hospitalization
   d) Patients with heart failure

5. The four C's of medical malpractice prevention include all of the following except:
   a) Consulting
   b) Communication
   c) Competence
   d) Charting

See answers on page 247.

NOTES

ANSWER KEY

1. e) The essential elements of a lawsuit include duty, breach of duty, injury or damages, and causation. Legal counsel is not an essential element of a lawsuit; although, it is needed by both the plaintiff and defense.

2. c) A malpractice claim is based on the legal concept of negligence, and, to prevail, the plaintiff must prove that the healthcare provider's treatment deviated from the accepted standard of care. The plaintiff must prove injury or damages if the medical provider has deviated from the accepted standard of care, and it is typically necessary for the plaintiff to establish negligence through a medical expert.

3. b) Legal liability exposure can be limited by fully disclosing risks and benefits of treatment with the patient, thoroughly examining and documenting the patient's wound, closely monitoring treatment, and making appropriate and timely adjustments to treatment. The legal liability exposure usually increases when utilizing a commonly available medical product for a novel, untested, or experimental procedure without the patient's consent.

4. a) There is unanimous agreement that there are some clinical situations when pressure ulcers may be unavoidable, such as in critical patients with hemodynamic instability, when patient turning and repositioning may not be feasible, and in patients who refuse to be turned. There are some patients who have multiorgan failure, including skin failure, where pressure ulcers are unavoidable; however, pressure ulcers developing in conscious, hemodynamically stable patients with acute stroke or congestive heart failure may be avoidable.

5. a) The four C's of medical malpractice prevention are caring, communication, competence, and charting.

REGULATORY AND REIMBURSEMENT ISSUES IN WOUND CARE

28

Dianne Rudolph, RN, GNP-BC, DNP, CWOCN

INTRODUCTION

The purpose of this chapter is to discuss regulatory issues pertaining to documentation, discharge planning, outcome measures, and maintaining patient privacy and confidentiality of protected health information. Also included are reimbursement and cost issues.

OBJECTIVES

Participants should be able to discuss the need for appropriate documentation, understand the rules for informed consent, and contrast Medicare Part A and Part B reimbursement.

I. Regulatory issues related to wound care

A. Regulatory guidance: CMS (Centers for Medicare and Medicaid Services) sets up the system for coding, billing, and collecting based on a payment scheme it has developed. Most other insurance companies use this as a guide to provide coverage. The US Federal Government pays over 50% of all the money spent in healthcare.

B. Medicare Part A—services that require hospitalization as an inpatient or that are provided by a hospital, skilled nursing facility, home health agency, or hospice

C. Medicare Part B—services provided on an outpatient basis or ambulatory basis, physician office visits, durable medical equipment (DME), and medical supplies

D. Health Insurance Portability and Accountability Act (HIPAA)
  1. Enacted by Congress in 1996
  2. The HIPAA Privacy Rule provides federal protections for personal health information held by covered entities and gives patients an array of rights with respect to that information. At the same time, the Privacy Rule is balanced so that it permits the disclosure of personal health information needed for patient care and other important purposes.
  3. Title I of HIPAA protects health insurance coverage for workers and their families when they change or lose their jobs. Title II of HIPAA, known as the Administrative Simplification (AS) Provisions, requires the establishment of national standards for electronic healthcare transactions and national identifiers for providers, health insurance plans, and employers.

II. Consent for treatment

A. The doctrine of informed consent is the cornerstone of modern medical jurisprudence. Although the need for bare consent to treatment is old, informed consent arose after World War II, driven by the Nuremberg doctrine and the rise of technological medicine. It has been one of the most misunderstood principles in medical law, sometimes driving a wedge between patients and their healthcare providers.

B. A number of key principles apply:
  1. Informed consent is the core principle of modern medical practice.
  2. In some very limited circumstances (i.e., emergency situations), care can be provided without consent.
  3. Medical care practitioners must disclose conflicts of interest that may affect their clinical judgment.
  4. There are special laws governing consent for minors and incompetents.
  5. Patients have the right to refuse medical care, even when it means they will die.
  6. Patients do not have a right to improper care.
  7. As of 2015, four US states allow assisted suicide: Oregon, Washington, Vermont, and Montana.

III. Documentation

A. Documentation should always contain the three C's: clarity of plan of care, conciseness or focus of topic, and consistency in documentation. This should include an accurate, legible course of treatment. Documentation should include:
  1. History and symptoms, skin assessment, and risk assessment
  2. Documentation of existing wounds, including staging for pressure ulcers present on admission (POA)
  3. Diagnosis
  4. Clinical findings, observations, test results, and treatment plan
  5. Treatments

6. Treatment alternatives and options
7. Communication with consultants and staff
8. Communication with patient and family
9. Rationale for course of treatment selected
10. Outcomes and reasons for changes in treatment
11. Patient's non-compliance/missed appointments
12. Advice and instructions given

B. Evaluation and management (E/M) service level can be selected by the key components of history, examination, and medical decision making. Time spent with a patient may be the controlling factor in counseling, coordination of care, and the nature of the visit. This must be documented in the chart.

IV. Performance improvement plan

A. Establish indicators: collect information from chart audits and staff surveys
B. Set levels based on amount of improvement necessary for complete documentation
C. Review quarterly or as needed
D. In-service or train in areas that require improvement (toolkits and protocols)
E. Allows for continuous monitoring of documentation and process improvement

V. Reimbursement issues affecting wound care

A. Reimbursement and cost issues: there are a few commonly used CPT codes in wound care and hyperbaric medicine. Becoming familiar with them can decrease coding errors.
B. Proper billing: the medical code that best describes the reason for visit is first; additional codes can be added that describe other disease processes as long as they are addressed at the visit. This can add complexity to the visit and qualify for a higher CPT code, resulting in higher reimbursement. Documentation should reflect such.
C. To help ensure payment of services rendered, close attention should be given to coding, documentation, and pre-authorizations from private insurances.
D. Documentation for consults for HBOT treatments should include patient history, review of systems, physical exam, and testing that indicates the HBOT treatment is reasonable and medically necessary. These steps can save hours of writing medical necessity letters and provide the best chance of receiving reimbursement with minimal requests for additional information.

VI. Other issues related to wound care

A. Photo documentation
1. Essential to tracking wound progress
2. Photo of wound on initial wound appearance and at least once a week
3. Ensure photos and written documentation are congruent
B. Tools (informed consent)

1. Medical-legal principle is defined as consent to treatment obtained after adequate disclosure
2. Diagnosis
    a) Description of purpose and nature of procedure or treatment
3. Risk associated with treatment or procedure
    a) Benefit expected
    b) Reasonable alternatives with risk and benefits
    c) Risk and consequences of no treatment
C. Patient privacy
1. Patient information should never be discussed outside the confines of direct patient to doctor or healthcare provider contact.
2. Protected health information (PHI) requires maintenance of health information in addition to state laws and facility polices.
3. The Health Insurance Portability and Accountability Act of 1996 (1996 HIPAA) imposes an obligation to maintain the confidentially of health information.
4. Health information cannot be released without expressed written consent.
D. Discharge planning
1. Critical component of documentation, but often neglected
2. Consists of short-term and long-term goals
    a) Short-term goal example: maintain compliance with compression wraps for edema control
    b) Long-term goal example: fit for compression hose to maintain edema control
3. Outcome measures are developed from a comprehensive plan of care to identify problem areas, set short- and long-term goals to prevent adverse outcomes, and make adjustments as needed to ensure favorable outcomes.

VII. Multidisciplinary care

A. Outpatient wound healing center
1. Team approach: having a multidisciplinary wound team is important. This can consist of a team of doctors, nurse practitioners, nurses, and other healthcare professionals that work together within a wound care center or by referrals to outside specialists.
B. Specialties that should be involved
1. Vascular surgeons
2. Plastic surgeons
3. Internal medicine specialists
4. Endocrinologists
5. Nurses
6. Physical therapists
7. Technical support staff

VIII. CMS Never Events

A. The Deficit Reduction Act (DRA) of 2005 required that by October 1, 2007, CMS had to identify at least two conditions that were: high cost, high volume, or both; resulted in the assignment of a case to a diagnosis related group (DRG) that had a higher payment due to this secondary diagnosis; and could reasonably have been prevented through the application of evidence-based guidelines.
   1. CMS announced eight hospital-acquired conditions (HACs) deemed preventable. (12)
   2. There are four Serious Preventable Events (these are the Never Events):
      a) Leaving an object in the patient
      b) Performing the wrong surgery (wrong body part, wrong patient, wrong procedure)
      c) Air embolism following surgery
      d) Incompatible blood products
   3. Hospital-acquired conditions (HACs): in the Federal Register, pressure ulcers are found under subpart (F)(b) "Hospital Acquired Conditions" but not under subpart (F)(c) "Serious Preventable Events." (13)
      a) The HACs are:
         i) Stage III and IV pressure ulcers
         ii) Catheter-associated urinary tract infection
         iii) Vascular catheter-associated infection
         iv) Surgical site infections
   4. The bottom line on pressure ulcers per CMS—they are not Never Events.
      a) CMS acknowledges that some pressure ulcers are "unavoidable."
      b) Pressure ulcers are only identified as high-volume and high-cost conditions that may be prevented through the application of evidence-based guidelines

IX. Medical ethics
A. Cost considerations
   1. In the United States, approximately 5 million chronically ill patients have wounds; the aggregate cost of their care has been documented at more than $20 billion annually.
   2. Because individuals with wounds represent varied racial, ethnic, and socioeconomic groups, this large population must be examined in terms of racial/ethnic diversity, poverty, immigration status, and health insurance limitations.
   3. Strategies to reduce costs of wound care have included:
      a) Correct diagnosis
      b) Treatment appropriate to the cause and condition of the wound
      c) Prevention of complications
      d) Prevention of hospitalizations
   4. As a way to coordinate care, the number of wound

care centers has increased throughout the country.
   5. The success of wound care centers is based on:
      a) Multidisciplinary team approach
      b) Use of evidence-based treatment protocols
      c) Efficient clinical structure
      d) A supportive system
B. Level of care
   1. The level of care or patient setting is another factor that must be considered when managing patients with acute or chronic wounds.
   2. Availability of products and services may vary based on:
      a) Levels of reimbursement
      b) Knowledge and skill of the providers
      c) Accessibility of wound specialists and other consultants
   3. It is also important to consider the goals of care
      a) For example, a wound specialist may have different goals for managing a stage IV pressure ulcer in a 95-year-old patient with advanced dementia compared to an active 40-year-old paraplegic patient.
   4. Wound care clinicians must consider the following when making decisions about wound care:
      a) Lack of health insurance
      b) Low income
      c) Language skills
      d) Culture
      e) Literacy
      f) Protocol adherence
      g) Wound care reimbursement

RESOURCES

1. Ferguson H, Harris NG. Legal aspects of wound care and hyperbaric medicine. In: Sheffield PJ, Fife CE, editors. *Wound Care Practice.* 2nd ed. North Palm Beach: Best Publishing Company; 2007: 1073-97.

2. Fife CE. Ethics in wound care and hyperbaric medicine. In: Sheffield PJ, Fife CE, editors. *Wound Care Practice.* 2nd ed. North Palm Beach: Best Publishing Company; 2007: 1057-67.

3. Bangasser RP, Bozzuto TM. Coding, charging, billing and collecting for wound care and hyperbaric medicine services: getting paid for the work you do. In: Sheffield PJ, Fife CE, editors. *Wound Care Practice.* 2nd ed. North Palm Beach: Best Publishing Company; 2007: 1177-92.

4. Rios EP, Larson-Lohr V. Documentation: telling the story of care. In: Sheffield PJ, Fife CE, editors. *Wound Care Practice.* 2nd ed. North Palm Beach: Best Publishing Company; 2007: 1161-74.

5. Pieper B. Vulnerable populations: considerations for wound care. *Ostomy Wound Manage.* 2009; 55(5):24-37.

6. Centers for Medicare & Medicaid Services Regulations & Guidance [Internet]. 2014. Accessed at: https://www.cms.gov/Regulations-and-Guidance/Regulations-and-Guidance.html?redirect=/home/regsguidance.asp.

7. Reinach-Lannen S. Mission possible: Getting Medicare reimbursement for wound care in acute-care settings. Wound Care Advisor [Internet]. 2012. Accessed at: http://woundcareadvisor.com/mission-possible-vol1-no3/.

8. Schaum KD. Medicare resources that you should use. *Adv Wound Care.* 2013 Dec; 2(10):559-62.

9. Carter MJ. Health economics information in wound care: the elephant in the room. *Adv Wound Care.* 2013 Dec; 2(10):563-70.

10. Nusgart M. HCPCS coding: an integral part of your reimbursement strategy. *Adv Wound Care.* 2013 Dec; 2(10):576-82.

11. Dotson P. CPT codes: what are they, why are they necessary, and how are they developed? *Adv Wound Care.* 2013 Dec; 2(10):583-7.

12. Centers for Medicare and Medicaid Services. Medicare Program; Changes to the Hospital Inpatient Prospective payment Systems and Fiscal Year 2008 Rates. Accessed at: http://www.cms.hhs.gov/AcuteInpatientPPS/downloads/CMS-1533-FC.pdf; 311-7.

13. Federal Register. Volume 72, Issue 85 (May 3, 2007). Accessed at: http://edocket.access.gpo.gov/2007/pdf/07-1920.pdf.

SAMPLE QUESTIONS

1. Over 50% of all funds spent on healthcare in the United States are paid by:
   a) Patients
   b) Employers
   c) Private insurance companies
   d) The US Federal Government

2. Documentation should always include which of the following:
   a) Clarity of plan of care
   b) Conciseness or focus of topic
   c) Consistency in documentation
   d) An accurate, legible course of treatment
   e) All of the above

3. Health information can be released with verbal consent of the patient.
   a) True
   b) False

4. Medicare Part B includes all of the following except:
   a) Services that are billed by a hospital during hospitalization as an inpatient
   b) Services provided on an outpatient basis or ambulatory basis by a physician
   c) Physician office visits
   d) Durable medical equipment (DME) and medical supplies

5. Which of the following adverse clinical outcomes will likely not be reimbursed by CMS?
   a) Hypertensive crisis
   b) Cellulitis of the lower extremity
   c) Stage III sacral pressure ulcer
   d) Post-operative pneumonia

6. Which of the following is not a principle of informed consent?
   a) The 90-year-old unresponsive nursing home patient being treated for sepsis who cannot consent to care
   b) The 65-year-old female with malignant melanoma who refuses surgery to remove a large lesion on her back and is not cognitively impaired
   c) The 80-year-old male with metastatic colon cancer requesting medication that will allow him to take his life intentionally
   d) The 45-year-old brain injury patient whose parents request a feeding tube for long-term nutrition

7. Documentation for HBOT services should include which of the following to ensure adequate reimbursement?
   a) Patient history
   b) Review of systems
   c) Physical exam
   d) Recent vascular assessment
   e) All of the above

8. Which of the following issues could be developed into an appropriate a performance improvement project?
   a) Conducting chart reviews to determine average healing rates for venous ulcers
   b) Performing customer satisfaction surveys
   c) Reviewing laboratory microbiology results to determine trends in wound culture results
   d) All of the above

9. Which of the following examples constitutes a HIPAA violation?
   a) Discussing diagnostic results with a patient's family member with the patient's permission
   b) Discussing a clinical issue regarding a patient in the elevator
   c) Mailing a printed copy of laboratory results to a patient
   d) Giving information about a patient to a friend on the phone
   e) All of the above
   f) Both b and d

See answers on page 255.

NOTES

ANSWER KEY

1. d) Over 50% of all funds spent on healthcare in the United States are paid by the US Federal Government.

2. e) Documentation should always contain the 3 C's: clarity of plan of care, conciseness or focus of topic, and consistency in documentation. This should include an accurate, legible course of treatment.

3. b) Health information can be released with written consent of the patient, not verbal consent.

4. a) Medicare Part B does not include services that are billed by the hospital during hospitalization as an inpatient. It does include services provided on an outpatient basis or ambulatory basis by physician, physician office visits, and durable medical equipment (DME) and medical supplies.

5. c) Stage III pressure ulcers, along with several other diagnoses, have been classified by CMS as Never Events, and those adverse outcomes will not be reimbursed. According to CMS, these conditions greatly complicate treatment of the illness or injury that caused the hospitalization and are "reasonably preventable" through proper care.

6. c) The 80-year-old male with metastatic colon cancer requesting medication that will allow him to take his life intentionally is considered euthanasia, which is not a principle of informed consent.

7. e) Documentation for HBOT services should include patient history, review of systems, physical exam, and recent vascular assessment.

8. d) All the choices listed are good examples of performance improvement projects.

9. f) Examples of HIPPA violations include discussing a clinical issue regarding a patient in the elevator and giving information about a patient to a friend on the phone.

EVIDENCE-BASED PRACTICE AND RESEARCH 29

Dianne Rudolph, RN, GNP-BC, DNP, CWOCN

INTRODUCTION

The term evidence-based medicine originated in the early 1990s at McMaster University in Ontario, Canada, and it encouraged clinicians to be aware of the evidence in support of their clinical practices and the strength of that evidence. In 1996, DL Sackett defined it as "the conscientious, explicit, and judicious use of current best evidence in making decisions about the care of individual patients." (1) Evidence hierarchies reflect the relative authority of various types of biomedical research.

Traditional criteria used in selecting wound care interventions is slowly being replaced by an evidence-based practice approach. The value of such an approach for providing optimal care has been established, but the definition of evidence-based care and the process used to generate this evidence continue to evolve. Ultimately, when selecting the best practices for wound care, it is imperative for the clinician to use evidence to ask two key questions—is the product/device effective? Is it safe? (8)

OBJECTIVES

Participants should be able to define evidence-based medicine, discuss seven levels of research evidence, and discuss the quality of evidence on the evidence hierarchy.

I. Evidence-based practice (Figure 29.1)
A. Evidence-based practice: the integration of individual clinical experience and the best evidence to guide decision making and patient preference.
B. Without evidence, practice rapidly becomes out-of-date. Traditions have a place elsewhere.

II. Benefits
A. Validates current practice
B. Validates changes in practice
C. Validates cost effectiveness
D. Validates quality of care
E. Supports lifelong learning

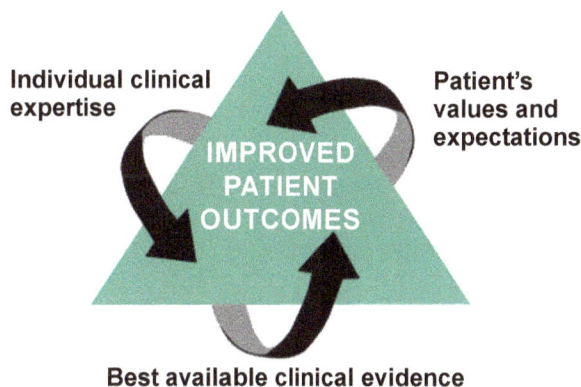

Figure 29.1: Diagram of evidence-based practice.

F. Allows the provider to keep up to date
G. PICO (four components of a well-built clinical question)
   1. Patient or population
   2. Intervention
   3. Comparison intervention
   4. Outcome
H. Process
   1. Ask: what aspect of my clinical practice am I interested in? (PICO)
   2. Gather: collect the best evidence
   3. Assess and appraise: evaluate the quality and strength of the evidence relevant to the question and population of interest
   4. Act: integrate and implement
   5. Evaluate: assess the outcomes
I. Evidence rating
   1. Oxford rating
      a) Levels of evidence: 1a, 1b, 1c, 2a, 2b, 2c, 3a, 3b, 4, 5
      b) Oxford clinical grades of recommendation based on the rating: A = level 1 (provided studies are consistent); B = level 2 or 3 (provided studies are consistent or extrapolations from level 1 studies); C = level 4 (extrapolations from level 2/3)
   2. Agency for Health Care Policy and Research (AHCPR)
      a) Levels of evidence: 1–7

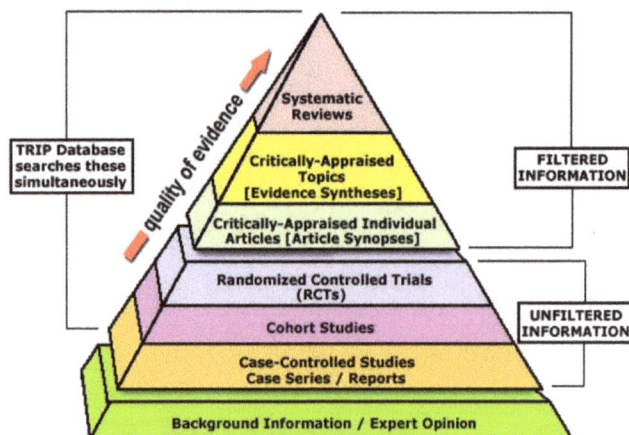

Figure 29.2: Levels of evidence. Courtesy of Janis Glover.

      b)   Clinical recommendations are A (for 1-2), B (for 3-5), C (for 6-7)
   3.   US Preventive Services Task Force (USPSTF)
      a)   Levels: I, II.1, II.2, II.3, III
      b)   Clinical recommendation grades A (good I), B (fair II), C (poor III)
J.   Quality of evidence (Figure 29.2)
K.   Study designs
   1.   Quantitative vs. qualitative
      a)   Quantitative: RCTs, cohort, case control, case series
      b)   Qualitative: field study, survey study, descriptive narratives
   2.   Randomized controlled trials (RCTs) (Figure 29.3)
      a)   Considered the gold standard of research design.
      b)   Classical scientific design involving a treatment group and control group. The treatment group receives the treatment or intervention while the control receives either no treatment (placebo) or the standard treatment. May include multiple arms.
      c)   Patients or subjects are randomly assigned.
      d)   Double blind method: reduces bias and minimizes threats to validity via the placebo effect.
   3.   Cohort studies (Figure 29.4)
      a)   Longitudinal studies involve a comparison of two groups over time, one of which has a certain exposure or treatment and one group that does not have the exposure or treatment.
      b)   May be either prospective or retrospective.
      c)   Good example is the Framingham Heart Study.
      d)   May not be as reliable as RCTs.
      e)   Require large sample sizes, take long periods of time, and are inefficient for studying rare outcomes or conditions.
   4.   Case control studies (Figure 29.5)
      a)   Comparison of patients or subjects who have a certain condition and those who do not.
      b)   Common in epidemiology.
      c)   Designed to estimate the odds (using an odds

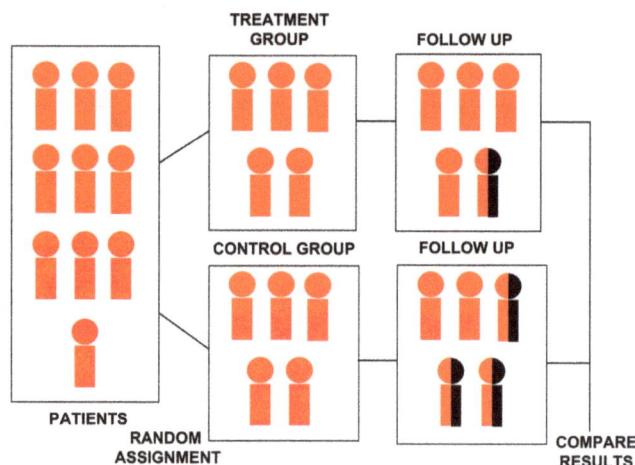

Figure 29.3: Randomized controlled trial.

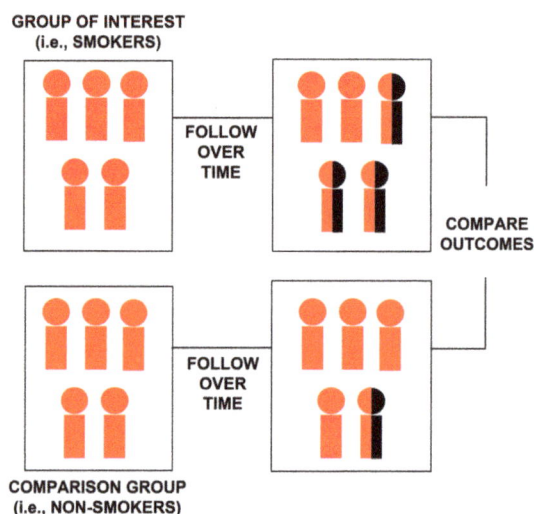

Figure 29.4: Cohort study.

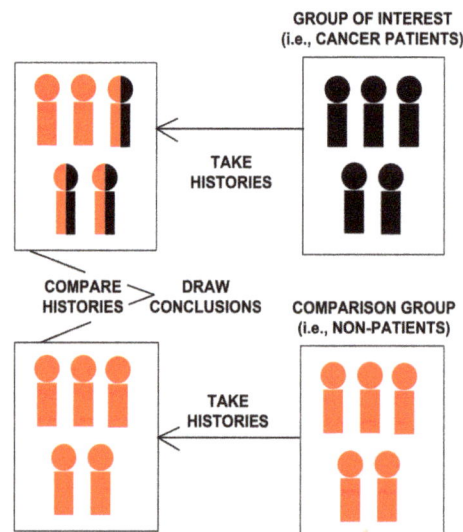

Figure 29.5: Case control study.

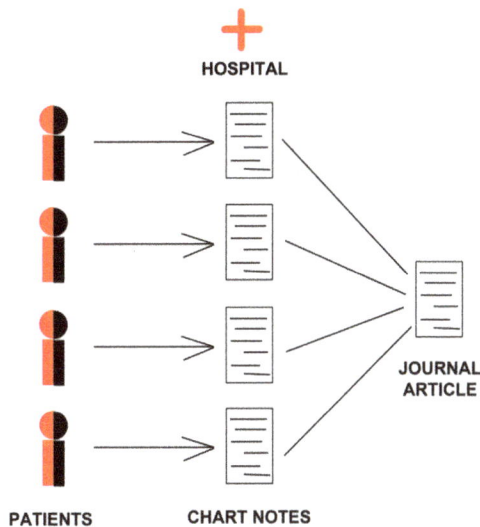

Figure 29.6: Case series.

ratio) of developing the disease or condition of interest. They can also determine if there is an associational relationship between the condition and risk factor.
  d) Example: colon cancer and diet.
  e) Less reliable than RCTs and cohort studies.
  f) Cannot directly obtain the absolute risk (incidence) of a bad outcome.
  g) Useful for rare conditions or diseases.
5. Case series or case reports (Figure 29.6)
  a) One or more reports on the treatment of individual patients with a specific disease or condition
  b) Used to illustrate an aspect of a condition, its treatment, or adverse reaction to treatment
  c) Easy to develop and useful for educational purposes
  d) No statistical validity

III. Evaluating research
A. Statistical significance
B. P value: the probability of obtaining the sample data if the null hypothesis is true
C. P value <0.05 = statistical significance
D. 95% confidence interval (CI)
E. Clinical significance

IV. Barriers to evidence-based practice (EBP) and research utilization
A. Lack of understanding about EBP/research process
B. Lack of time
C. Difficulty with access to evidence-based guidelines
D. Lack of administrative support/mentorship
E. Research/research utilization is not a priority
F. Not part of my role as a provider

RESOURCES

1. Sackett DL, Rosenberg WMC, Gray JAM, et al. Evidence-based medicine: what is and what isn't. *BMJ.* 1996; 312(7023):71-2.
2. Armstrong EC. The well-built clinical question: the key to finding the best evidence efficiently. *WMJ.* 1999 Mar-Apr; 98(2):25-8.
3. Ryan S, Perrier L, Sibbald RG. Searching for evidence-based medicine in wound care: an introduction. *Ostomy Wound Manage.* 2003; 49(11):67-75.
4. Warriner RA III. Evidence-based wound care. In: Sheffield PJ, Fife CE, editors. *Wound Care Practice.* 2nd ed. North Palm Beach: Best Publishing Company; 2007: 175-94.
5. Roe E, Williams DL. Using evidence-based practice to prevent hospital-acquired pressure ulcers and promote wound healing. *Am J Nurs.* 2014 Aug; 114(8):61-5.
6. Edwards H, Finlayson K, Courtney M, Graves N, Gibbs M, Parker C. Health service pathways for patients with chronic leg ulcers: identifying effective pathways for facilitation of evidence based wound care. *BMC Health Serv Res.* 2013 Mar 8; 13:86. doi: 10.1186/1472-6963-13-86.
7. Munn Z, Kavanagh S, Lockwood C, Pearson A, Wood F. The development of an evidence based resource for burns care. *Burns.* 2013 Jun; 39(4):577-82. doi: 10.1016/j.burns.2012.11.005. Epub 2012 Dec 3. Accessed at: http://fionawoodfoundation.com/files/106/files/2013%20JBI%20burn%20node%20development.pdf.
8. van Rijswijk L, Gray M. Evidence, research, and clinical practice: a patient-centered framework for progress in wound care. *J Wound Ostomy Continence Nurs.* 2012 Jan-Feb; 39(1):35-44.

SAMPLE QUESTIONS

1. Evidence-based medicine is the conscientious, explicit, and judicious use of current best evidence in making decisions about the care of:
   a) Individual patients
   b) Selected categories of patients
   c) Selected classes of wounds
   d) None of the above

2. The hierarchy of strength of evidence for treatment decisions includes which of the following:
   a) Systematic reviews of randomized clinical trials
   b) Single randomized controlled trial
   c) Physiologic studies
   d) All of the above
   e) Both a and b

3. Which of the following statements regarding the strength of evidence hierarchy is false?
   a) The highest level of evidence is meta-analysis, or the systematic review of multiple randomized controlled trials (RCT).
   b) RCTs are considered to have a higher level of evidence than cohort studies.
   c) Case controlled studies are less reliable than RCTs and cohort studies.
   d) The hierarchy must be considered to be absolute.

See answers on page 262.

NOTES

ANSWER KEY

1. a) Evidence-based medicine is the conscientious, explicit, and judicious use of current best evidence in making decisions about the care of individual patients.

2. d) The hierarchy of strength of evidence for treatment decisions includes systematic reviews of randomized controlled trials, single randomized controlled trial, and physiologic studies.

3. d) As far as strength of evidence is considered, the highest level of evidence is meta-analysis or the systematic review of multiple RCTs. RCTs are considered to be a higher level of evidence than cohort studies, and case controlled studies are less reliable than RCTs and cohort studies; however, this hierarchy should not be considered absolute.

FISTULAE MANAGEMENT 30

Dianne Rudolph, RN, GNP-BC, DNP, CWOCN

INTRODUCTION

A fistula is a pathologic sinus or abnormal passage leading from an abscess cavity or a hollow organ to the surface, or from one abscess cavity or organ to another. This chapter will discuss common fistula locations, the goals of care, management options, and the fitting of fistula pouches.

OBJECTIVES

Participants should be able to define a fistula, describe skin integrity issues associated with fistulae, select appropriate products to manage fistulae, discuss the principles of fitting fistulae with management systems, and describe the use of negative pressure wound therapy (NPWT) for fistulae management.

I. Fistulae

A. Definition and types of fistulae
1. External cutaneous fistula (ECF): an abnormal opening between one hollow organ and the skin (e.g., an abnormal communication between the small or large bowel and the skin) (Figure 30.1). The ECF is the focus of this chapter.
   a) Enterocutaneous fistula—an opening between the small intestine and the skin
      i) Usually high volume liquid drainage
      ii) Usually contains digestive enzymes that are damaging to the skin

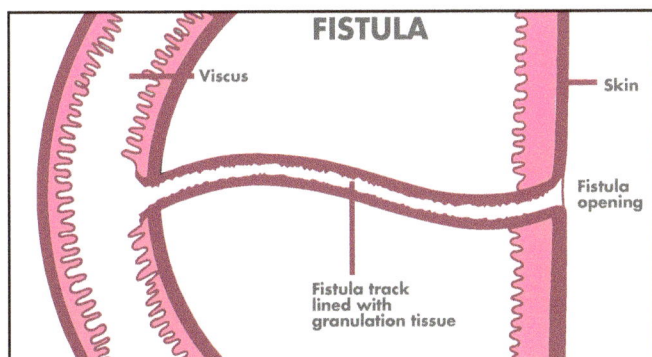

Figure 30.1: External cutaneous fistula.

b) Colocutaneous fistula—an opening between the colon and the skin
   i) The output consistency is usually semi-formed, but there can be liquid drainage.
   ii) Drainage is usually malodorous and may contain gas.
c) Vesicocutaneous fistula—an opening between the bladder and the skin
   i) Drains urine
d) Spit fistula or esophagostomy—an opening between esophagus and skin
   i) Drains mucus
   ii) Oral fluids come out of fistula
2. Internal fistula (IF)—an abnormal opening between two hollow organs. Three main types: enteroenteric, enterovaginal, and enterovesical fistulas.
3. Unexplored fistula—extends in an unknown direction and has an unknown endpoint.

B. Identified by the organs involved
1. Example: an enterocutaneous fistula connects the intestine to the surface of the skin

C. Incidence and etiology
1. High-risk patients
2. Associated with a high risk of morbidity and mortality ranging from 5-20% due to associated sepsis, nutritional abnormalities, and electrolyte imbalances
3. 80% occur following GI surgery (post-operative contributing factors leading to fistula after bowel surgery) (Figure 30.2)
   a) Tension on the suture line
   b) Improper suturing technique
   c) Distal obstruction
   d) Hematoma or abscess formation at anastomotic site
   e) Presence of tumor or inflammatory disease at site of anastomosis
   f) Inadequate blood supply to the anastomosis

D. Associated with
1. Cancer, inflammatory bowel disease, trauma, distal bowel obstruction, pancreatitis, and mesenteric vascular disease

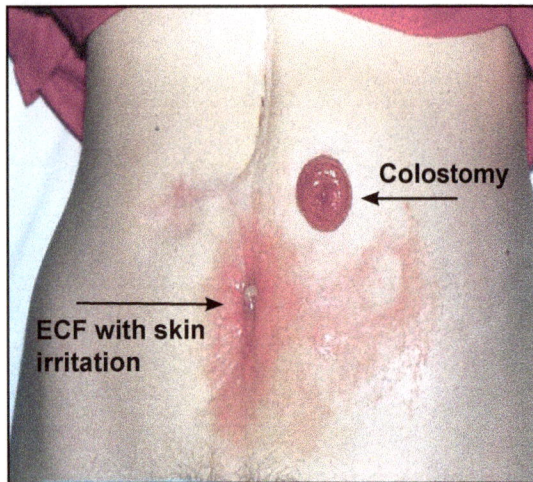

Figure 30.2: ECF after abdominal surgery.

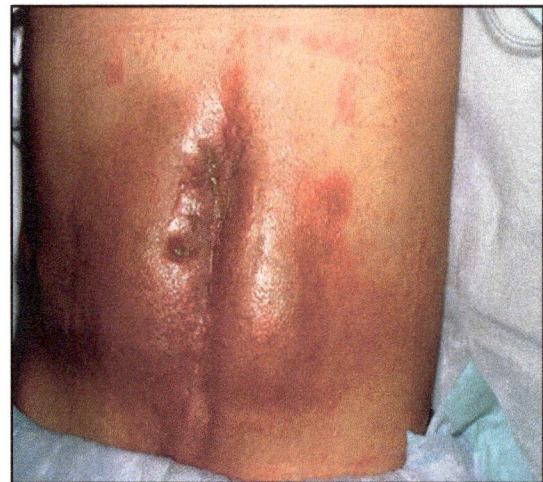

Figure 30.3: Altered skin and tissue integrity around the fistula.

2. Predispositions may include steroid use, radiation therapy, inflammatory bowel disease, enterostomy, malnutrition, hypoxia, diabetes mellitus, cirrhosis of the liver, chemotherapy, anti-inflammatory drugs, sepsis, and GI surgery without bowel prep

E. Common locations
  1. Dehisced wounds
  2. Abscess sites
  3. Incisions
  4. Established drain sites
  5. Site of active disease

F. The type of ECF, as based on the output of the enteric contents, also determines the patient's health status and how the patient may respond to therapy. ECFs are usually classified into three categories:
  1. Low-output fistula (<200 mL/day)
  2. Moderate-output fistula (200-500 mL/day)
  3. High-output fistula (>500 mL/day)
    a) Increases the possibility of fluid and electrolyte imbalance and malnutrition
    b) Typically requires pouching/containment

II. Management of fistulae

A. High resource utilization
  1. Prolonged hospitalization
  2. Nutritional support
  3. Diagnostic tests
  4. Pharmacological interventions
  5. Additional nursing care/time/expertise
  6. Dressings, bandages, and other medical supplies

B. The underlying priority of care
  1. Prevention of altered skin and tissue integrity
    a) The output from a fistula is usually very irritating to the skin, causing pain and discomfort (Figure 30.3).
    b) Skin barriers are used to prevent contact of fistula drainage with skin.

C. Goals of care
  1. Maintain/restore nutrition/hydration
  2. Contain drainage and odor
  3. Maintain/restore skin integrity
  4. Quantify output
  5. Improve quality of life
  6. Contain costs

D. Management options
  1. Medical management
    a) Fluid and electrolytes management
    b) If patient is kept NPO, consideration must be given for total parenteral nutrition until the fistula closes spontaneously.
    c) Complete nutritional assessment and management is needed while the patient is treated for a complex fistula.
    d) Antibiotics and infection control measures also need consideration if a wound becomes infected around the fistula.
  2. Wound care dressings
    a) Dressings to manage exudate
    b) If exudate or fistula output is significant, a pouch is the most efficient and appropriate dressing
  3. Skin care products (protective creams and ointments)
    a) Required to treat skin irritation from fistula drainage or leakage
  4. Skin barriers (wafers, Eakin Cohesive® Seals, pastes, powders)
    a) Prevent fistula drainage from irritating skin by creating a barrier
  5. Wound and fistula pouches (Figure 30.4)
    a) Most efficient way to contain drainage
    b) Protect healthcare providers from exposure to bodily fluids
    c) Easier to measure fistula drainage
    d) More cost effective than frequent dressing changes
    e) Helps to manage odor

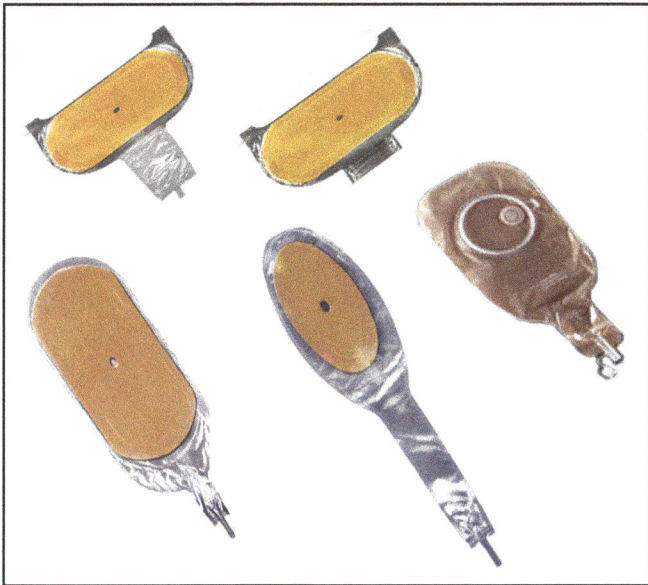

Figure 30.4: Wound and/or fistula pouches.

 f) Patients can usually self-manage pouch changing
 g) Indications for wound and/or fistula pouches
  i) Drainage greater than 100 cc in 24 hours
  ii) Frequent dressing changes
   (1) Are painful
   (2) Damage the skin
   (3) Exhaust the patient
  iii) High-output pouch
   (1) High volume tube or drain
  iv) To facilitate ambulation
 h) Principles of fitting a management system
  i) Wound and/or fistula pouches
   (1) Help control odor
   (2) Decrease change frequency
  ii) Selecting the "right" system
   (1) Size and shape of cutting surface
   (2) Type of skin barrier
   (3) Pouch capacity
   (4) Outlet matches character of drainage
   (5) Access window/transparent film
   (6) Condition of skin (denuded, intact, flat, retracted)
6. Negative pressure wound therapy (NPWT)
 a) Appropriate for complex fistulas (within a wound)
 b) Contraindicated for non-enteric and unexplored fistulas
 c) Used in complex fistulae within a wound with the specific goal of promoting wound healing
7. Change management option to meet the changing needs of the patient, the wound, and the skin
 a) Hospital to home
 b) Increase or decrease in output
 c) Improvement or deterioration of skin integrity

8. Contemporary issues associated with fistula management
 a) Care setting
 b) Cost of care versus cost effectiveness
 c) Product formulary
 d) Reimbursement
 e) Quality of life
 f) Interdisciplinary approach
9. Patient education
 a) Purpose of pouch or NPWT
 b) Etiology of fistula
 c) Routine care and hygiene

III. Case studies

A. Case study 1—Dehisced surgical wound with fistula: 65-year-old patient after multiple surgeries (Figures 30.5a and 30.5b)
 1. Issues
  a) Denuded skin
  b) High volume output
  c) Uneven skin
  d) Need access to wound
  e) Access to site required
 2. Goals
  a) Skin protection
  b) Local management of denuded skin
  c) Containment of output
  d) Less frequent dressing changes
 3. Options for treatment
  a) Large fistula pouch cut to fit fistula

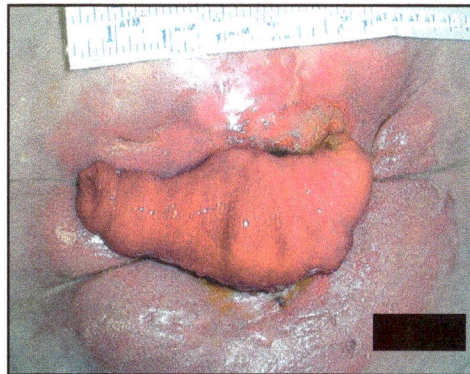

Figure 30.5a: Dehisced surgical wound with fistula.

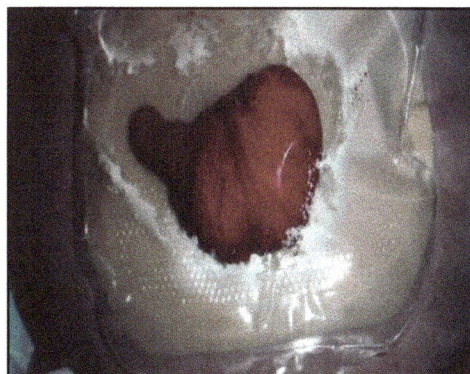

Figure 30.5b: Same patent now covered with fistula pouch.

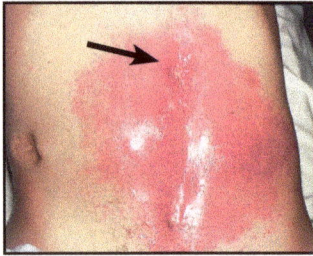

Figure 30.6a: High-output ECF.

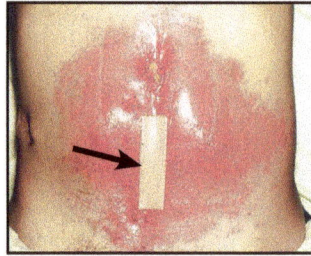

Figure 30.6b: Fill in trough with wound dressings like calcium alginate or collagen.

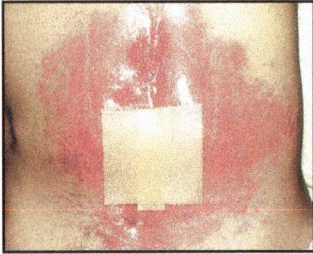

Figure 30.6c: Cover trough.

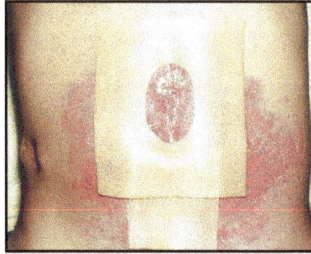

Figure 30.6d: Use skin barriers like wafers, Eakin Cohesive® Seals, pastes, and powders; isolate the fistula with dressing before applying the pouch to protect the surrounding skin.

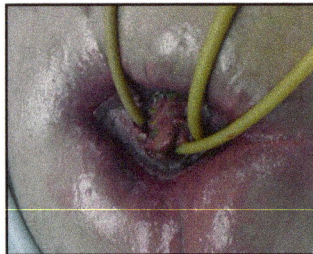

Figure 30.7a: Multiple fistulas isolated by inserting drains.

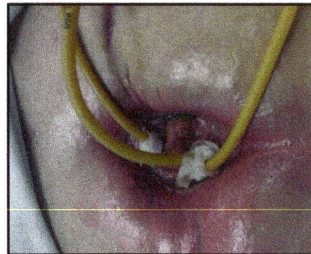

Figure 30.7b Drains covered by Kling to isolate the ECF. Drains are then connected to wall suction.

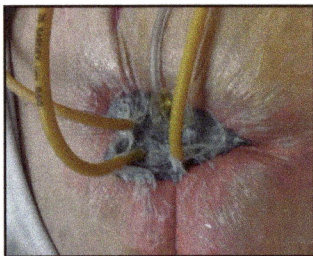

Figure 30.7c: NPWT applied after isolating the fistula to help heal the surrounding wound.

B. Case study 2—High-output enterocutaneous fistulae: 22-year-old patient with a history of Crohn's disease (Figures 30.6a–30.6d)
   1. Issues
      a) Fistula in incision
      b) Extensive damage to skin integrity
   2. Goals
      a) Need to fill in trough
      b) Need to create level skin surface
   3. Options for treatment
      a) Level skin surface achieved
      b) Skin protection provided
   4. Goals achieved
      a) Placement of strips of stoma adhesive wafer and paste to level surface
      b) Placement of two-piece ostomy pouch
      c) Pouch can be applied
C. Case study 3—Fistula management with NPWT: 38-year-old patient with a self-inflicted stab wound (Figures 30.7a–30.7c)
   1. Issues
      a) High-output chronic fistula
      b) Failed surgical intervention
      c) Chronic: 100-125 mmHg continuous
   2. Goals
      a) Goal is to separate the wound from the fistulae to allow for wound healing
   3. Options for treatment
      a) NPWT to treat wound bed, not fistula
      b) Acute: 150-175 mmHg continuous
      c) May be used to encourage wound healing
      d) Not for effluent containment

RESOURCES

1. Bryant R, Rolstad BS. Management of drain sites and fistulas. In: Bryant R, Nix D, editors. *Acute and Chronic Wounds: Current Management Concepts*. St. Louis: Mosby; 2007: 490-516.

2. Brindle CT, Blankenship J. Management of complex abdominal wounds with small bowel fistulae. *J Wound Ostomy Continence Nurs.* 2009; 36(4):396-403.

3. Datta V, Engledow A, Chan S, Forbes A, et al. The management of enterocutaneous fistula in a regional unit in the United Kingdom: a retrospective study. *Dis of the Colon and Rectum.* 2010; 53(2):192-9.

4. KCI Medical. *V.A.C.® Therapy™ Clinical Guidelines. A reference source for clinicians.* KCI Medical; 2010.

5. Deleon JM. Novel techniques using negative pressure wound therapy for the management of wounds with enterocutaneous fistulas in a long-term acute care facility. *J Wound Ostomy Continence Nurs.* 2013; 40(5):481-8.

6. Vikram K, Geibel J. Enterocutaneous fistula [Internet]. 2014 [Updated 2014 Jan 23]. Accessed at: http://emedicine.medscape.com/article/1372132-overview#a1.

7. Hollister Incorporated. Fistula management care tips [Internet]. 2014. Accessed at: http://www.hollister.com/us/files/care_tips/tips_Fistula%20Management.pdf.

8. Cro C, George KJ, Donnelly J, et al. Vacuum assisted closure system in the management of enterocutaneous fistulae. *Postgraduate Med J.* 2002 Jun; 78(920):364-5.

9. Stremitzer S, Dal Borgo A, Wild T, Goetzinger P. Successful bridging treatment and healing of enteric fistulae by vacuum-assisted closure (VAC) therapy and targeted drainage in patients with open abdomen. *Int J Colorectal Dis.* 2011 May; 26(5):661-6. Epub 2011 Jan 7.

10. Goverman J, Yelon JA, Platz JJ, Singson RC, Turcinovic M. The "Fistula VAC," a technique for management of enterocutaneous fistulae arising within the open abdomen: report of 5 cases. *J Trauma.* 2006 Feb; 60(2):428-31; discussion 431.

11. Gunn LA, et al. Management of enterocutaneous fistulas using negative-pressure dressings. *Ann Plast Surg.* 2006 Dec; 57(6):621-5.

12. Bryant RA. Management of drain sites and fistulas. In Bryant, RA, editor. *Acute and Chronic Wounds Nursing Management.* 3rd ed. St. Louis: Mosby; 2000: 490-500.

SAMPLE QUESTIONS

1. Which of the following factors contribute to fistula for-
    mation?
    a) Steroid use
    b) Inflammatory bowel disease
    c) Infection and sepsis
    d) All of the above

2. A high-output fistula has an output of at least:
    a) 250 cc per day
    b) 500 cc per shift
    c) 500 cc per day
    d) None of the above

3. A low-output fistula has an output of less than:
    a) 200 cc per day
    b) 500 cc per shift
    c) 500 cc per day
    d) None of the above

4. A NPWT system is used for fistula management with the
    specific goal of:
    a) Evacuating the effluent
    b) Promoting wound healing
    c) Delaying surgical intervention
    d) Treating wound infection

5. A fistula pouch is indicated when there is:
    a) Denuded skin
    b) High-volume output
    c) Need to access the site
    d) All of the above

See answers on page 270.

NOTES

ANSWER KEY

1. d) Many factors can contribute to fistula formation, including steroid use, radiation therapy, inflammatory bowel disease, enterostomy, malnutrition, hypoxia, diabetes mellitus, cirrhosis of the liver, chemotherapy, anti-inflammatory drugs, infection, sepsis, and GI surgery without bowel prep.

2. c) A high-output fistula has output of at least 500 cc/day.

3. a) A low-output fistula has output of at least 200 cc/day.

4. b) A NPWT system used in a complex fistula within a wound is with the specific goal of promoting wound healing.

5. d) A fistula pouch is indicated when there is denuded skin, high-volume output, and a need to access the site.

HIGHLIGHTS OF NATIONAL TREATMENT GUIDELINES & QUALITY REPORTING IN WOUND CARE

31

Caroline E. Fife, MD, CWSP, FAAFP, FUHM

INTRODUCTION

The AHRQ (Agency for Healthcare Research and Quality—formerly the AHCPR, Agency for Health Care Policy and Research) National Guideline Clearinghouse lists the national treatment guidelines for arterial ulcers, venous ulcers, pressure ulcers, and diabetic foot ulcers. The Wound Healing Society (WHS) and Wound, Ostomy, and Continence Nurses Society (WOCN) are the sources of the national guidelines.

The US outpatient payment system is transitioning from a "volume-driven" model of healthcare to one that is determined by "value" and links cost to improved patient outcomes. Currently, patients who stay in service the longest and receive the most procedures and therapeutic interventions generate the greatest revenue for wound care and hyperbaric medicine clinicians, regardless of whether their outcomes are good. Many Medicare quality programs began with bonus payments to clinicians but are now transitioning to a penalty phase. Clinicians will experience a reduction in Medicare payments if they do not successfully participate in Medicare quality programs.

OBJECTIVES

Participants should be able to explain the guidelines for venous ulcers, diabetic foot ulcers, arterial ulcers, and pressure ulcers. Participants should also be able to identify the quality programs relevant to wound care practitioners and how to report them.

I. National treatment guidelines
A. The following guidelines will be discussed:
   1. WHS guidelines for the treatment of venous ulcers
   2. WOCN guideline for the management of wounds in patients with lower-extremity venous disease
   3. WHS guidelines for the treatment of diabetic foot ulcers
   4. WOCN guideline for management of wounds in patients with lower-extremity neuropathic disease

   5. WHS guidelines for the treatment of arterial insufficiency ulcers
   6. WHS guidelines for the treatment of pressure ulcers
   7. WOCN guideline for prevention and management of pressure ulcers

II. Evidence-based healthcare (different methods)
A. Levels of evidence (refer also to Chapter 29)
   1. Level I: meta-analysis of multiple randomized controlled trials (RCTs) or at least two RCTs that support the intervention of the guideline. Another route would be multiple laboratory or animal experiments with at least two clinical series that support the laboratory results.
   2. Level II: less than level I, but at least one RCT and at least two significant clinical series or expert opinion papers with literature reviews support the intervention. Experimental evidence that is quite convincing but not yet supported by adequate human experience is included.
   3. Level III: suggestive data of proof of principle but lacking sufficient data, such as meta-analysis, RCT, or multiple clinical series.
B. Rating of evidence (per WOCN)
   1. Level A: two or more supporting RCTs in humans (at levels I or II), meta-analysis of RCTs, or Cochrane Systematic Review of RCTs
   2. Level B: one or more supporting controlled trials in humans or two or more trials in an animal model (at level III)
   3. Level C: one supporting controlled trial, at least two supporting case series that were descriptive studies in humans, or expert opinion

III. Guidelines for venous ulcers
A. WHS guidelines for the treatment of venous ulcers (2)
   1. Guideline 1.1: Gross arterial disease should be ruled out by establishing that pedal pulses are present on physical examination and/or that the ankle-brachial index (ABI) is >0.8.

a) In elderly patients, patients with diabetes mellitus, or patients with an ABI >1.2, a toe-brachial index of >0.6 or a transcutaneous oxygen partial pressure of >30 mmHg in the region of the ulcer may help to suggest an adequate arterial flow (level I).

2. Guideline 1.2: Color duplex ultrasound scanning performed with proximal compression or a Valsalva maneuver is useful in providing anatomic and physiologic data helping to confirm a venous etiology for the leg ulcer (level I).

3. Guideline 1.5: Apparent venous ulcers that are excessively painful and that progressively increase in size after debridement and/or despite treatment should be considered for other diagnoses.

   a) This suspicion should be especially high if the ulcer is darker in color, has blue/purple borders, or if the patient has a systemic disease such as Crohn's disease, ulcerative colitis, rheumatoid arthritis, collagen vascular diseases, leukemia, or immunosuppression (level II).

4. Guideline 2.1: The use of a class 3 (most supportive) high-compression system (three layer, four layer, short stretch, paste-containing bandages, e.g., Unna's boot, Duke boot) is indicated in the treatment of venous ulcers.

   a) The degree of compression must be modified when mixed venous/arterial disease is confirmed during the diagnostic workup (level I).

B. WOCN guideline for the management of wounds in patients with lower-extremity venous disease (7)

1. Cleanse the wound at each dressing change, minimizing trauma to the wound. No specific studies demonstrate the benefit of using one cleanser over another for lower-extremity venous disease (LEVD) ulcers.

2. Hydrocolloid or foam dressings may be beneficial in reducing pain associated with LEVD ulcers. (6) Level of evidence = B

3. There is no clear evidence indicating the duration, safety, and efficacy of topical antibiotics. A short course of treatment (approximately two weeks) with a topical antimicrobial such as silver sulfadiazine may be considered if the ulcer has a high level of bacteria (greater than 10^5). Level of evidence = B

4. Cadexomer iodine (Iodoflex™) may be useful in removing slough and thus reducing bacterial bioburden. It has been shown to be more effective than "standard treatments" such as wet-to-dry dressings and thin hydrocolloids and results in faster healing times. Level of evidence = A

5. Two randomized controlled trials (RCTs) found that flavonoids (rutoside) in doses ranging from 250 to 300 mg twice daily improved ulcer healing rates when compared with placebo. Level of evidence = A

6. Treatment with short-stretch compression bandaging may reduce pain. Level of evidence = B

7. Compression therapy heals more venous leg ulcers than no compression therapy and decreases the healing time. Level of evidence = A

8. High compression is more effective than low compression, but there are no differences in the effectiveness of the different types of products available for high compression. Level of evidence = A

9. For individuals with mixed arterial/venous disease and moderate arterial insufficiency (ABI >0.5 to <0.8) who present with ulcers and edema, a trial of modified reduced compression bandaging to a level of 23 to 30 mmHg at the ankle may promote healing. Level of evidence = C

IV. Guidelines for diabetic foot ulcers

A. WHS guidelines for the treatment of diabetic foot ulcers (1)

1. Guideline 1.1: Clinically significant arterial disease should be ruled out by establishing that pedal pulses are clearly palpable or that the ankle-brachial index (ABI) is >0.9.

   a) An ABI >1.3 suggests non-compressible arteries. In elderly patients or patients with an ABI >1.2, a normal Doppler-derived waveform, a toe brachial index of >0.7, or a transcutaneous oxygen pressure of >40 mmHg may help to suggest an adequate arterial flow (level I).

2. Guideline 1.2: The presence of significant neuropathy can be determined by testing with a 10 gram (5.07) Semmes-Weinstein monofilament (level II).

3. Guideline 2.1: Protective footwear should be prescribed in any patient at risk for amputation (e.g., significant arterial insufficiency, significant neuropathy, previous amputation, previous ulcer formation, pre-ulcerative callus, foot deformity, evidence of callus formation) (level II).

4. Guideline 2.2: Acceptable methods of off-loading include crutches, walkers, wheelchairs, custom shoes, depth shoes, shoe modifications, custom inserts, custom relief orthotic walkers, diabetic boots, forefoot and heel relief shoes, and total contact casts (level I).

5. Guideline 3.6: If osteomyelitis is suspected, appropriate diagnostic measures include probing the wound with a sterile cotton-tipped applicator, serial x-rays, MRI, CT, and radionuclide scan (level II).

6. Guideline 4.2: Initial debridement is required to remove the obvious necrotic tissue, excessive bacterial burden, and cellular burden of dead and senescent cells. Maintenance debridement is needed to maintain the appearance and readiness of the wound bed for healing. The healthcare provider can choose from a number of debridement methods, including surgical, enzymatic, mechanical, biological, or autolytic. More than one debridement method may be appropriate; however, sharp surgical debridement is preferred (level I).

B. WOCN guideline for management of wounds in patients with lower-extremity neuropathic disease (LEND) (4)

1. Treatment
   a) Recommend that patients with wounds and LEND seek care guided by a clinical wound expert.
   b) Utilize a multidisciplinary team for persons with foot ulcers. Level of evidence = B
   c) Relate wound treatments to adequacy of perfusion status.

2. Off-loading
   a) Ensure adequate off-loading of pressure through wound closure
   b) Utilize assistive devices (e.g., walking splints, wedge sole shoes, healing shoes with large toe box) to provide support, balance, and off-loading of the affected site

3. Wound management
   a) Maintain dry stable eschar on non-infected, ischemic, neuropathic wounds. Level of evidence = C
   b) Cleanse wound with non-cytotoxic cleansers

4. Debridement
   a) Recommend debridement of neuropathic wounds and calluses, as needed, throughout the healing process. Level of evidence = C
   b) Debride ulcers with extensive cellulitis and/or osteomyelitis and refer for pharmacological (intravenous) intervention. Level of evidence = C

5. Dressings
   a) Choose dressings that promote a moist wound environment. Level of evidence = B
   b) Re-evaluate the wound dressings on a periodic basis throughout the treatment process. Level of evidence = C
   c) Consider the use of growth factors (rh PDGF-BB) for foot ulcers after necrotic tissue has been debrided, infection is cleared, and adequate perfusion has been established. Level of evidence = A
   d) Consider the use of biological wound coverings for the treatment of non-infected diabetic foot ulcers. Level of evidence = B

6. Infection
   a) Observe clinical manifestations of infection, which may be subtle due to reduced blood flow or absence of sensation in the neuropathic foot.
   b) Infected neuropathic wounds may be limb threatening and require immediate referral for assessment of vascular perfusion and for surgical intervention. Level of evidence = C

7. Antimicrobials
   a) Tissue biopsy is considered the gold standard to confirm diagnosis of infection. Quantitative swab cultures have been demonstrated to be a reasonable alternative in clinical practice. Level of evidence = B
   b) Systemic antibiotics are warranted in the management of ulcers when bacteremia, sepsis, advancing cellulitis, or osteomyelitis occurs, and caution must be exercised against multiple antibiotic-resistant organisms. Level of evidence = C

8. Osteomyelitis
   a) As a noninvasive technology, magnetic resonance imaging (MRI) has demonstrated the highest sensitivity and specificity for diagnosing osteomyelitis in patients with diabetes and foot ulcers.
   b) Refer the patient for further evaluation for suspected infection, positive probe to bone, and radiographic changes demonstrating Charcot osteoarthropathy. Level of evidence = C

V. Guidelines for arterial ulcers

A. WHS guidelines for the treatment of arterial insufficiency ulcers (5)

1. All patients with lower extremity ulcers should be assessed for arterial disease.

2. Guideline IV.1.a: Indications for revascularization in patients with ulcers will depend on ambulatory status and the severity of comorbidities along with anatomic factors that determine the likelihood of success.
   a) If the patient is not a candidate for revascularization (e.g., demented, no distal run-off), document that further invasive studies or treatment is inappropriate and, as healing without such intervention is not likely, place the patient in a palliative care mode.

3. Guideline 1.1: All patients with lower extremity ulcers should be assessed for arterial disease. Suspicion of arterial disease in the context of a patient with a lower-extremity ulcer should prompt referral to a vascular specialist (level IA).

4. Guideline 1.2: Patients who have ulcers and present with risk factors for atherosclerosis (smoking, diabetes, hypertension, hypercholesterolemia, advanced age, obesity, hypothyroidism) are more likely to have arterial ulcers and should be carefully and broadly evaluated (level IA).

5. Guideline 1.4: Patients presenting with rest pain or gangrene should be promptly referred to a vascular specialist (level IA).

6. Guideline 2.2: In the presence of an arterial ulceration, the natural history is one of disease progression and eventual limb loss, and the treatment options are revascularization (endovascular or open surgery) or amputation. Adjuvant therapies may improve healing of the ulcer but do not correct the underlying vascular disease and cannot replace revascularization (level IIA).

7. Guideline III.1: Cardiovascular diseases should be identified and managed with a multidisciplinary,

evidence-based approach. Standard treatment guidelines for medical therapy will improve outcomes for not only coronary artery disease, but also ischemic arterial ulcers.

8. Guideline III.1.a: Increases in viscosity and hypercoagulability have been implicated as a factor for poor prognosis in peripheral arterial obstructive disease (PAOD). Use of anti-platelet therapy decreases the incidence of cardiovascular death.

9. Guideline III.1.b: Use of beta blockers in patients without contraindications to its use decreases the incidence of new cardiac events in patients presenting with concomitant coronary artery disease.

10. Guideline III.1.c: Use of lipid-lowering therapies decreases long-term ischemic arterial ulcer development (level I).

11. Guideline III.1.d: Monitoring of blood sugar and management of diabetes mellitus should be continually addressed.

12. Guideline III.2: Interventions to enable patients with PAOD to quit smoking should be consistently pursued.

13. Guideline III.3: Lower extremity protection should be aggressively pursued in patients with known or suspected PAOD whether or not the patient has associated neuropathy from diabetes or other causes. The oxygen requirement for intact skin is significantly lower than for injured skin.

14. Guideline III.4: External pneumatic compression has been shown to improve arterial inflow in ischemic limbs and may be of benefit in treating or preventing arterial ulcers (level II).

15. Guideline III.7: Frequent exercise with increased walking distance improves the distance to claudication pain as well as peripheral circulation and pulmonary function.

VI. Guidelines for pressure ulcers

A. WHS guidelines for the treatment of pressure ulcers (3)
    1. Guideline 1.1: Establish a repositioning schedule and avoid positioning patients on a pressure ulcer (level II).
    2. Guideline 1.3: Assess all patients for risk of developing a pressure ulcer. Use a pressure-reducing surface in those patients at risk (level I).
    3. Guideline 1.6: In patients who have a large stage III or stage IV pressure ulcer or multiple pressure ulcers involving several turning surfaces, a low air loss or air fluidized bed may be indicated (level I).
    4. Guideline 2.3: Ensure adequate dietary intake to prevent undernutrition to the extent that this is compatible with the individual's wishes (level III).
B. WOCN guideline for prevention and management of pressure ulcers (8)
    1. Reduce friction and shear. Level of evidence = C
    2. Turn patient every two hours. Level of evidence = C

3. Utilize positioning devices to avoid placing patient on an ulcer. Level of evidence = C

4. Maintain the head of the bed at 30 degrees elevation for supine positions and 30 degrees or less for side-lying. Level of evidence = C

5. Use pressure relief such as low air loss or air fluidized mattresses/beds for individuals with stage III or IV ulcers or those with multiple ulcers over several turning surfaces. Level of evidence = A

6. Shift weight for chair-bound individuals every 15 minutes; if patient cannot perform shifts, caregivers should reposition every hour. Level of evidence = C

7. Limit time in chair and use pressure-relief chair cushions in the presence of pressure ulcers on sitting surfaces. Level of evidence = C

8. Manage fecal and urinary incontinence. Level of evidence = C

9. Select absorbent underpads, diapers, or briefs to wick effluent away from the skin. Level of evidence = C

10. Ensure adequate nutrient and fluid intake to maximize the potential for wound healing: 35-40 kcalories per kg of body weight/day for total calories and 1.0-1.5 g protein/kg of body weight/day for total protein. Level of evidence = C

11. Cleanse the wound at each dressing change with a non-cytotoxic cleanser, minimizing trauma to the wound. Level of evidence = C

12. Consider the use of high-pressure irrigation to remove slough or necrotic tissue.

13. Debride the ulcer of devitalized tissue. Level of evidence = C

14. Do not debride dry black eschar on heels that is non-tender, nonfluctuant, nonerythematous, and nonsuppurative. Level of evidence = C

15. Perform wound care using topical dressings determined by wound, patient needs, cost, caregiver time, and availability. Level of evidence = C

16. Choose dressings that provide a moist wound environment, keep the periwound skin dry, control exudates, and eliminate dead space. Level of evidence = C

17. Reassess the wound with each dressing change to determine whether modifications are needed as the wound heals or deteriorates. Level of evidence = C

18. Manage wound infections and differentiate between contamination, colonization, and infection. Level of evidence = C

19. Obtain a quantitative culture or tissue biopsy if high levels of bacteria ($>10^5$) are suspected in a wound exhibiting clinical signs of infection, such as absence of healing.

20. Use topical antibiotics in wounds cautiously and selectively. Level of evidence = C

21. Consider use of topical antimicrobials if a high level of bacteria is present ($>10^5$). Level of evidence = C

22. Use systemic antibiotics in the presence of bacteremia, sepsis, advancing cellulitis, or osteomyelitis.

Level of evidence = C

23. Consider adjunctive therapies to enhance the healing of recalcitrant stage III and IV wounds such as:
    a) Growth factors: platelet-derived growth factor BB (rPDGF-BB). Level of evidence = A
    b) Electrical stimulation. Level of evidence = A
    c) Noncontact normothermic radiant heat therapy. Level of evidence = A
    d) Topical negative pressure wound therapy (e.g., vacuum-assisted wound closure). Level of evidence = A

24. Evaluate the need for operative repair for patients with stage III and IV ulcers who do not respond to conservative therapy. Level of evidence = C

25. Implement measures to eliminate or control pain. Level of evidence = C

26. Educate patients, caregivers, and healthcare providers involved in the continuum of care about prevention, treatment, and factors contributing to recurrence of pressure ulcers. Level of evidence = C

27. Monitor vigilantly for recurrence of any pressure ulcers, and emphasize to patients and families that measures to prevent and manage pressure ulcers are lifelong endeavors. Level of evidence = C

VII. Quality reporting in wound care

A. Physician Quality Reporting System (PQRS)
  1. Penalty/bonus
     a) Began in 2008. Bonus payments increased from 2% to a total of 4% of billed Medicare payments in 2011 and then began to decrease.
     b) Clinicians who do not participate in 2014 will experience a 2% reduction in total Medicare payments in 2016.
     c) Penalties increase to 3% in 2016 and beyond for nonreporters.
  2. Which quality measures?
     a) Standard PQRS measures (382 in 2014): The measures CMS has included in PQRS are released each year: http://www.cms.gov/Medicare/Quality-Initiatives-Patient-Assessment-Instruments/PQRS/MeasuresCodes.html
        i) The number of measures that eligible professionals (EPs) are required to report to obtain bonus money or avoid penalties changes each year. In 2014, providers must report at least nine measures across three National Quality Strategy (NQS) domains in order to obtain the 0.5% bonus available (final year of bonus).
        ii) CMS rarely selects measures for PQRS unless they have been endorsed by a major quality organization, such as the National Quality Forum, which is a laborious and expensive process that has not been favorable to small organizations like wound care

or hyperbaric medicine.
        iii) As of 2015 there are no wound care related quality measures within PQRS, although there are measures of diabetic footwear and examination of diabetics for neuropathy. Other measures may be relevant to a wound care practice (e.g., smoking cessation, hemoglobin A1C).
     b) Qualified Clinical Data Registry (QCDR): In 2014, CMS provided another quality reporting option via a QCDR. The provider must report at least nine measures, and one must be an outcomes measure covering at least three NQS domains.
        i) The biggest advantage of QCDRs is that they can develop their own measures rather than be limited to the measures CMS has selected for traditional PQRS.
  3. Reporting mechanism
     a) Initially reported via claims
     b) Registry reporting—began in 2008
     c) QCDRs: the list of CMS-approved QCDRs is available at: https://www.cms.gov/Medicare/Quality-Initiatives-Patient-Assessment-Instruments/PQRS/Downloads/2014QCDRPosting.pdf
        i) A QCDR has to have at least one outcome measure and must be able to stratify patients by severity or risk.
        ii) The US Wound Registry (part of the Chronic Disease Registry) has 12 wound care specific quality measures designed to capture as many wound care clinical practice guidelines as possible.
           (1) Uses the Wound Healing Index to stratify patients for outcomes reporting
           (2) Specifications for measures can be found at: http://www.uswoundregistry.com/Specifications.aspx
        iii) US Wound Registry measures for reporting
           (1) Adequate off-loading of diabetic foot ulcers at each visit
           (2) Diabetic foot ulcer (DFU) healing or closure
           (3) Plan of care creation for DFU patients not achieving 30% closure at four weeks
           (4) Diabetic foot and ankle care: comprehensive diabetic foot examination
           (5) Adequate compression at each visit for patients with venous leg ulcers (VLU)
           (6) VLU: healing or closure
           (7) Plan of care for venous leg ulcer patients not achieving 30% closure at four weeks
           (8) Appropriate use of hyperbaric oxygen therapy for patients with diabetic foot ulcers

(9) Appropriate use of cellular or tissue-based products (CTPs) for patients aged 18 years or older with a DFU or VLU

(10) Vascular assessment of patients with chronic leg ulcers

(11) Wound bed preparation through debridement of necrotic or nonviable tissue

(12) Patient reported experience of care: wound-related quality of life

B. Value-based purchasing (VBP)
   1. Penalty/bonus
      a) Created under the Affordable Care Act (ACA).
      b) Exact percentage of revenue at risk under the ACA is not yet known, but it will cause potentially substantial reductions in payment to both clinicians and hospitals tied to PQRS performance.
      c) Clinicians not participating in PQRS will be automatically issued a 1.0% reduction to all 2015 calendar year Medicare payments.

C. Meaningful use of an electronic health record (EHR)
   1. Bonus/penalty
      a) Health Information Technology for Economic and Clinical Health (HITECH) Act was passed in 2009.
      b) Provided $44,000 per clinician as an incentive for the purchase and "meaningful use" (MU) of a certified EHR.
      c) Incentive money obtained in installments by meeting requirements of the "stages" of MU. In 2014, requirements for stage 2 were released; stage 3 requirements were still being developed.
      d) Incentive phase has ended: Clinicians who have not adopted a certified EHR face a potential reduction of 1.0% of Medicare payments in 2015.
      e) Penalty for not adopting an EHR increases 1% annually to a maximum of 3% in 2017 and beyond.
      f) Electronic prescribing (eRx) is a requirement for QHPs to achieve MU of their EHR.
   2. Stage 2 MU measures (total of 20) http://www.healthit.gov/sites/default/files/meaningfulusetables-series2_110112.pdf
      a) Core: 17 objectives that all providers must meet
      b) Menu: Providers must meet three menu objectives by selecting from a list of six
         i) Implement five clinical decision support interventions related to four or more clinical quality measures at a relevant point in patient care for the entire EHR reporting period.
      c) Under stage 2 of MU beginning in 2015, providers wishing to obtain EHR bonus money must share data with a public health agency or a specialty registry by transmitting the data directly from their EHR

D. Overall implications for clinicians
   1. In 2015, clinicians who do not participate in PQRS, MU, or eRx will risk up to 5.5% of their Medicare payments when the penalties of all these programs are added together.
   2. Penalties will escalate in subsequent years.

RESOURCES

1. Robson MC, et al. Guidelines for the best care of chronic wounds. *Wound Repair Regen.* 2006; 14(6):647-8.

2. Robson MC, et al. Guidelines for the treatment of venous ulcers. *Wound Repair Regen.* 2006; 14(6):649-62.

3. Whitney J, et al. Guidelines for the treatment of pressure ulcers. *Wound Repair Regen.* 2006; 14(6):663-79.

4. Wound, Ostomy, and Continence Nurses Society (WOCN). Guideline for management of wounds in patients with lower-extremity neuropathic disease [Internet]. 2012. Accessed at: http://www.guideline.gov/content.aspx?id=38248.

5. Hopf HW, et al. Guidelines for the treatment of arterial insufficiency ulcers. *Wound Repair Regen.* 2006; 14(6):693-710.

6. Arnold TE, Stanley JC, Fellows EP, Moncada GA, et. al. Prospective, multicenter study of managing lower extremity venous ulcers. *Ann Vasc Surg.* 1994 Jul; 8(4):356-62.

7. Wound, Ostomy, and Continence Nurses Society (WOCN). Guideline for management of wounds in patients with lower-extremity venous disease [Internet]. 2011. Accessed at: http://www.guideline.gov/content.aspx?id=38249.

8. Wound, Ostomy, and Continence Nurses Society (WOCN). Guideline for prevention and management of pressure ulcers [Internet]. 2010. Accessed at: http://www.guideline.gov/content.aspx?id=23868.

9. Assessment and management of foot ulcers for people with diabetes. 2005 Mar (revised 2013 Mar). NGC:01010: Registered Nurses' Association of Ontario - Professional Association.

10. SOLUTIONS® wound care algorithm. 1994 (revised 2013 Sep). NGC:010274 ConvaTec - For Profit Organization.

11. Diabetic foot problems. Inpatient management of diabetic foot problems. 2011 Mar. NGC:008758 National Institute for Health and Care Excellence (NICE) – (Britain)

12. Clinical practice guideline for type 2 diabetes. 2008 Jul 1. (reaffirmed 2013 Jun). NGC:009014 Basque Office for Health Technology Assessment, Osteba - State/Local Government Agency [Non-US]; GuiaSalud - National Government Agency [Non-US]; Ministry of Health (Spain) - National Government Agency [Non-US].

13. ACR Appropriateness Criteria® suspected osteomyelitis of the foot in patients with diabetes mellitus. 1995 (revised 2012). NGC:009220 American College of Radiology - Medical Specialty Society.

14. 2012 Infectious Diseases Society of America clinical practice guideline for the diagnosis and treatment of diabetic foot infections. 2004 Oct 1 (revised 2012 Jun). NGC:009111.

15. Guideline for management of wounds in patients with lower-extremity neuropathic disease. 2004 (revised 2012 Jun 1). NGC:009275 Wound, Ostomy, and Continence Nurses Society - Professional Association.

16. Association for the Advancement of Wound Care guideline of pressure ulcer guidelines. 2010 Oct 1. NGC:008120.

Nonprofit Organization.

17. AHRQ link for venous leg ulcers. http://www.guideline.gov/search/search.aspx?term=venous+leg+ulcers.

18. AHRQ link for pressure ulcers. http://www.guideline.gov/search/search.aspx?term=pressure+ulcers.

19. US Department of Health & Human Services. The Affordable Care Act [Internet]. 2010 [cited 30 April 2013]. Accessed at: http://www.healthcare.gov/law/full/index.html.

20. Centers for Medicare & Medicaid Services. 2013 Physician Quality Reporting System [Internet]. 2013 [cited 30 April 2013]. Accessed at: http://www.cms.gov/Medicare/Quality-Initiatives-Patient-Assessment-Instruments/PQRS/MeasuresCodes.html.

21. American Society of Plastic Surgeons, Physician Consortium for Performance Improvement, and National Committee for Quality Assurance. Chronic Wound Care Physician Performance Measurement Set [Internet]. 2008 [cited 30 April 2013]. Accessed at: http://www.ama-assn.org/resources/doc/pcpi/wound-care-worksheets.pdf.

22. Fife CE, et al. Electronic Health Records, Registries, and Quality Measures: What? Why? How? *Adv Wound Care* (New Rochelle). 2013 Dec; 2(10):598-604.

23. Centers for Medicare & Medicaid Services. Qualified Registries for the 2012 Physician Quality Reporting System (PQRS) and Electronic Prescribing (eRx) Incentive Programs [Internet]. 2012 [cited 30 April 2013]. Accessed at: http://www.cms.gov/Medicare/Quality-Initiatives-Patient-Assessment-Instruments/PQRS/downloads/2012_Qualified_Registries_Posting_Phase1.pdf.

24. Fife CE, Carter MJ, Walker D. Why is it so hard to do the right thing in wound care? *Wound Repair Regen.* 2010; 18(2):154–8.

25. Fife, CE, Carter MJ, Walker D, Thomson, B, Eckert KA. Diabetic foot ulcer off-loading: The gap between evidence and practice. Data from the U.S. Wound Registry. *Adv Skin Wound Care.* 2014 July; 27(7): 310-16.

26. Horn SD, Fife CE, Smout RJ, Barrett RS, Thomson B. Development of a wound healing index for patients with chronic wounds. *Wound Repair Regen.* 2013; 21(6): 823–32.

27. Medicare Program; Revisions to Payment Policies under the Physician Fee Schedule, Clinical Laboratory Fee Schedule & Other Revisions to Part B for CY 2014. A Rule by the Centers for Medicare & Medicaid Services on 12/10/2013 [Internet]. 2013 [cited 29 Dec 2014]. Accessed at: https://www.federalregister.gov/articles/2013/12/10/2013-28696/medicare-program-revisions-to-payment-policies-under-the-physician-fee-schedule-clinical-laboratory.

28. National Qualify Forum. Measure Evaluation Criteria [Internet]. 2012 [cited 30 April 2013]. Accessed at: http://www.qualityforum.org/docs/measure_evaluation_criteria.aspx.

29. Huang ET, Mansouri J, Murad MH, Joseph WS, Strauss MB, Tettelbach W, Worth ER. A clinical practice guideline for the use of hyperbaric oxygen therapy in the treatment of diabetic foot ulcers. *Undersea Hyperb Med.* 2015; 42(3):205-47.

SAMPLE QUESTIONS

1. All national guidelines agree on which of the following:
   a) A vascular screen should be performed before initiating compression.
   b) Diabetic patients need a vascular screen.
   c) Suspected arterial ulcer patients need a vascular assessment.
   d) All of the above

2. All national guidelines agree that the primary treatment for arterial ulceration is revascularization if possible.
   a) True
   b) False

3. With regard to wound care, all guideline recommendations for all wound types include:
   a) Debriding necrotic material
   b) Maintaining a moist wound environment
   c) Controlling infection
   d) All of the above

4. Which of the following statements is true about PQRS for eligible providers (EPs) in 2015?
   a) There will be no measures specifically relating to wound care among the nearly 400 quality measures chosen by CMS for the PQRS program.
   b) EPs who do not participate in PQRS could experience up to a 2% decrease in their Medicare payments.
   c) The USWR QCDR provides several wound care specific quality measures from which EPs can select to satisfy the requirements of PQRS.
   d) Providers can select from both QCDR measures and traditional PQRS measures in order to meet their reporting requirements.
   e) All of the above

5. Which of the following programs have the potential for the largest percent reduction in Medicare payments for providers who are not participating fully in quality initiatives?
   a) PQRS (physician quality reporting system)
   b) ACA (Affordable Care Act)
   c) Meaningful use of an EHR (electronic health record)

6. The reason quality programs have become critically important to wound and hyperbaric clinicians is that outpatient payment is moving away from a system based on "volume" to one based on "value" defined by the performance of quality metrics.
   a) True
   b) False

See answers on page 280.

NOTES

ANSWER KEY

1. d) All national guidelines agree that a vascular screen should be performed before initiating compression, diabetic patients need a vascular screen, and suspected arterial ulcer patients need a vascular assessment.

2. a) All national guidelines agree that the primary treatment for arterial ulceration is revascularization, if possible.

3. d) With regard to wound care, all guideline recommendations for all wound types include debriding necrotic material, maintaining a moist wound environment, and controlling infection.

4. e) As of 2015 there are no wound care related quality measures within PQRS, although there are measures of diabetic footwear and examination of diabetics for neuropathy. The USWR QCDR provides several wound care specific quality measures from which EPs can select to satisfy the requirements of PQRS. Providers can select from both QCDR measures and traditional PQRS measures in order to meet their reporting requirements. EPs who do not participate in PQRS could experience up to a 2% decrease in their Medicare payments.

5. b) There could be potentially substantial reductions in payment to both clinicians and hospitals tied to PQRS performance under the Affordable Care Act (ACA).

6. a) It is true that quality programs have become critically important to wound and hyperbaric clinicians as outpatient payment is moving away from a system based on "volume" to one based on "value" defined by the performance of quality metrics.

CLINICAL PATHWAYS: BEST PRACTICE RECOMMENDATIONS FOR THE PRACTITIONER

32

Jayesh B. Shah, MD, CWSP, FAPWCA, FACCWS

INTRODUCTION

Chronic wounds are challenging to manage. Dr. Shah has combined more than 15 years of experience in wound care with available evidence on wound management to develop these pathways. Also included are some modifications to existing pathways created by previous authors and other wound care experts. This chapter looks to simplify the process of assessment and management of various wounds. It is recommended that wound care providers look at the Clinical Wound Management Master Pathway on page 282 for evaluating all patients and consulting other algorithms based on the patient's diagnosis. Wound care providers will find these pathways useful not only in the preparation for various certification exams but also to manage wounds on a daily basis.

OBJECTIVES

Participants should be able to use these pathways as a guide for managing wound care patients.

Pathway 1
Clinical Wound Management Master Pathway

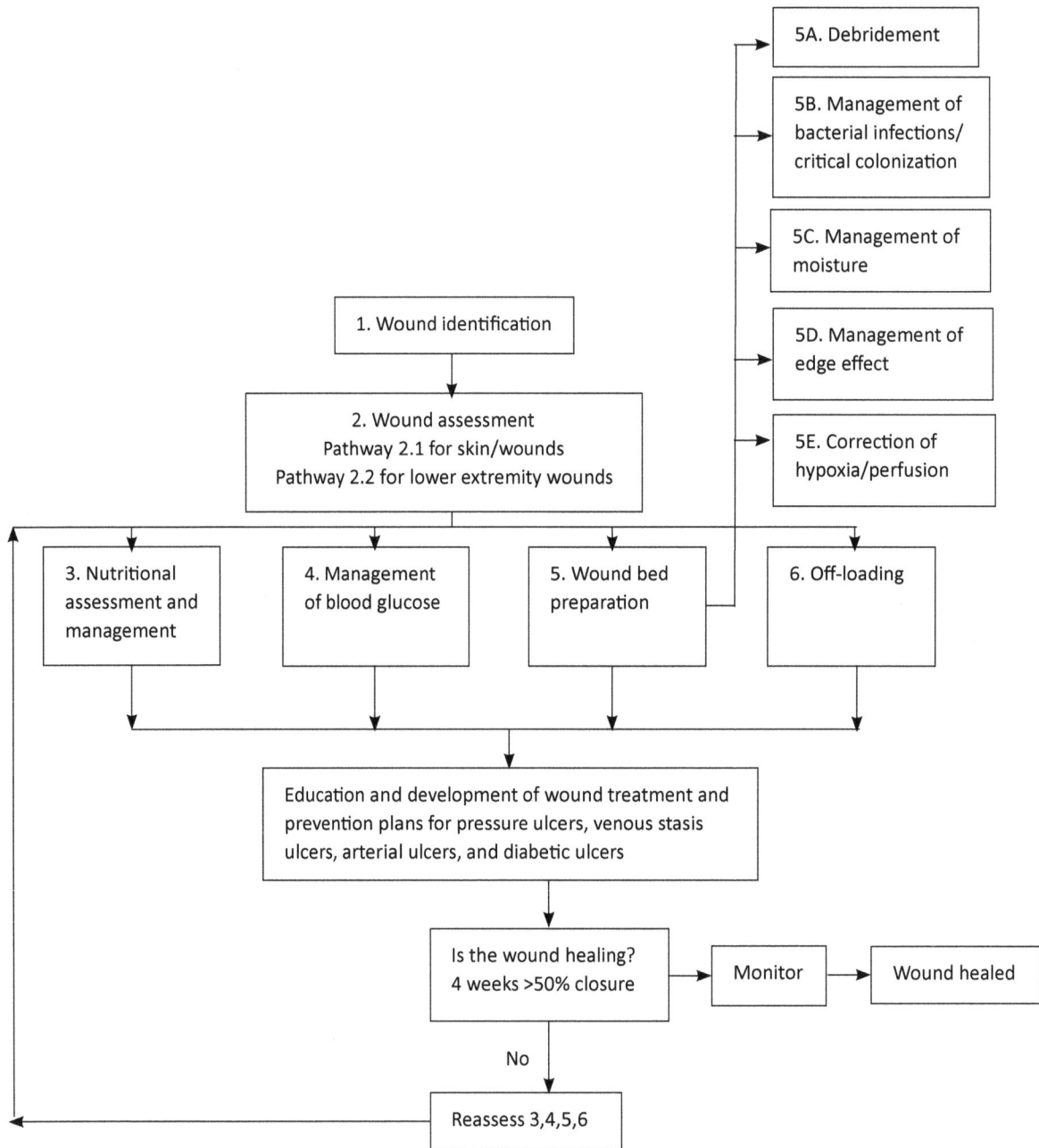

Pathway 2.1
Wound/Skin Assessment

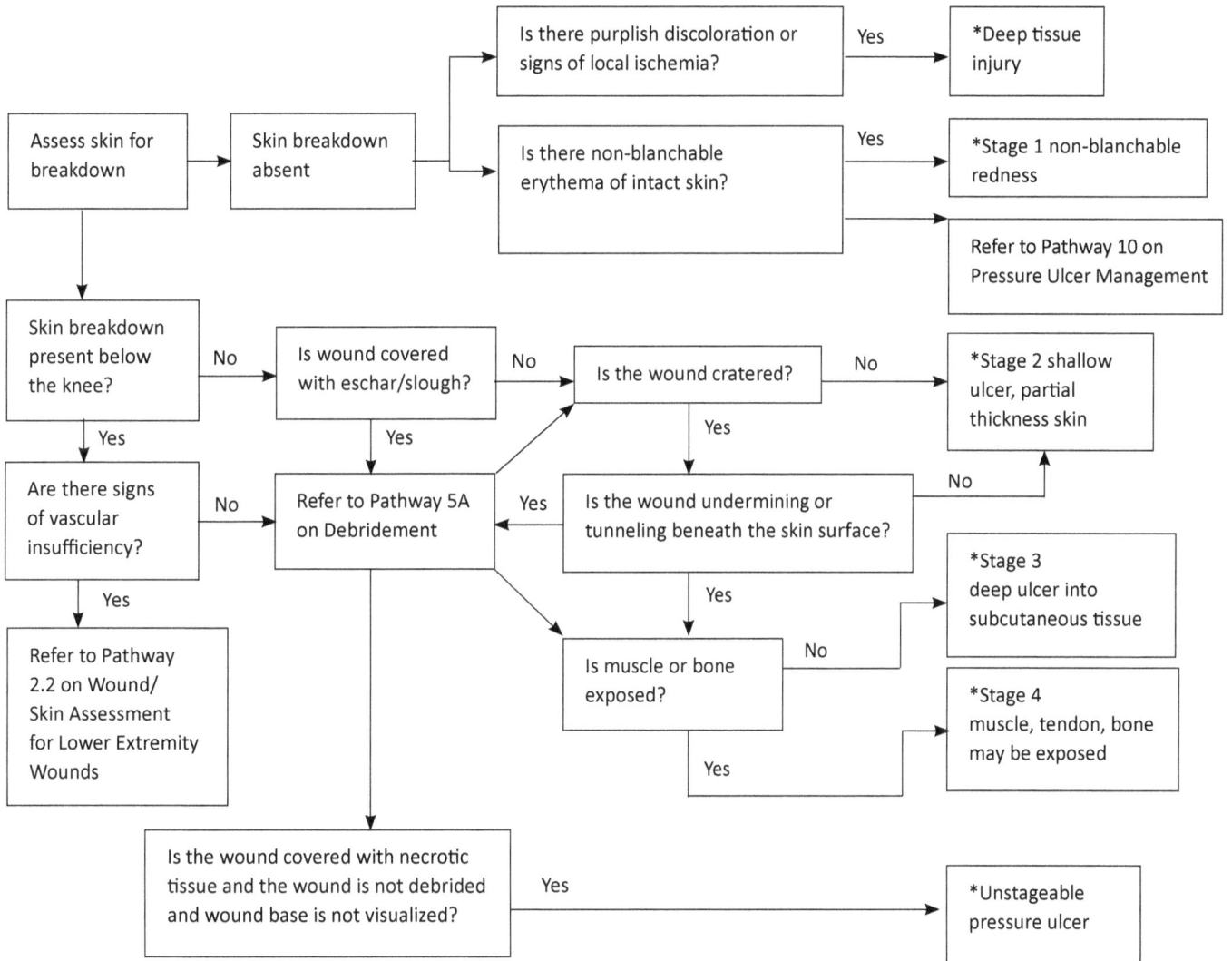

* Refer to Pathway 10 on Pressure Ulcer Management

Pathway 2.2
Wound/Skin Assessment for Lower Extremity Wounds

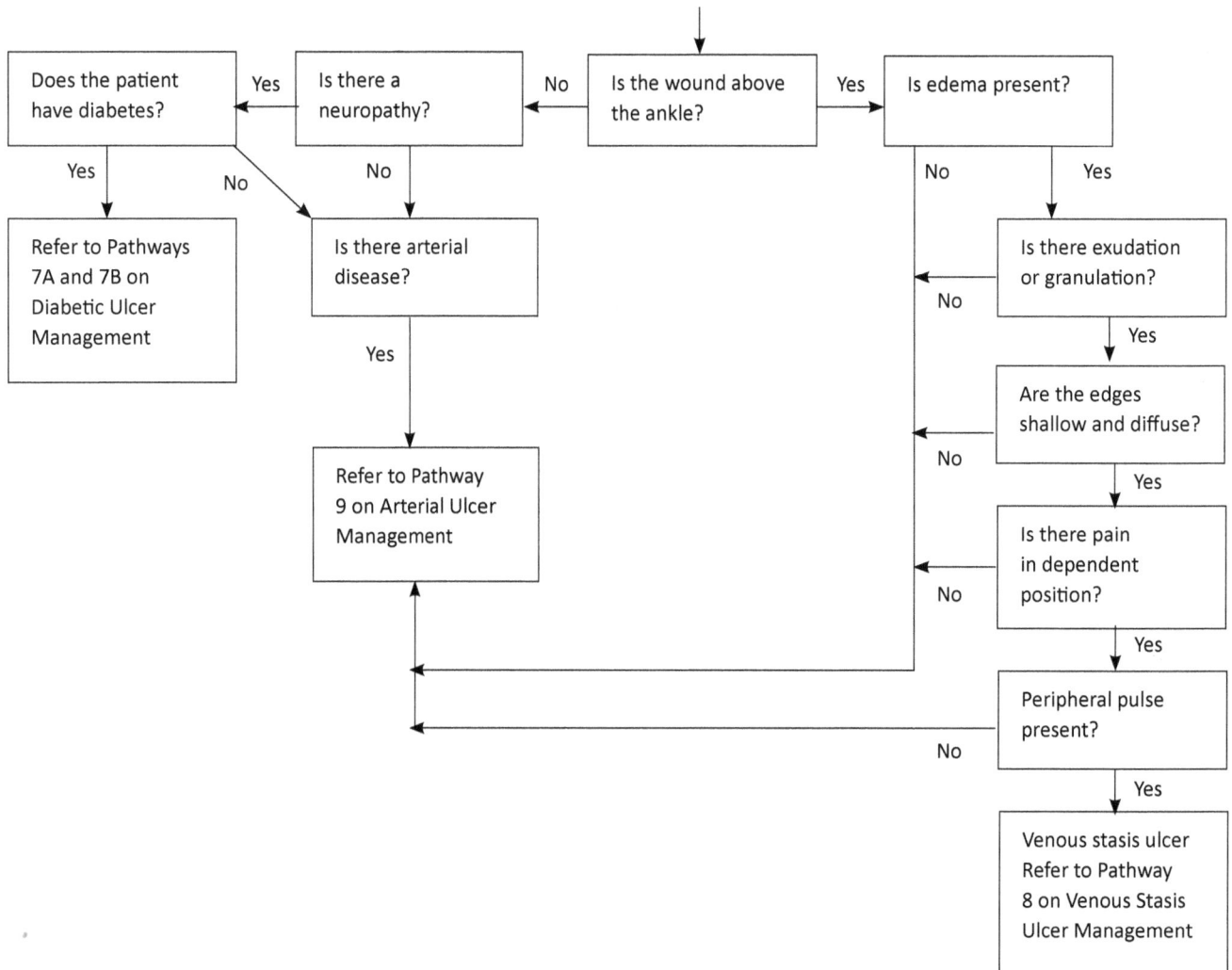

Does the patient have diabetes? → Yes → Is there a neuropathy? → No → Is the wound above the ankle? → Yes → Is edema present?

Does the patient have diabetes? — Yes → Refer to Pathways 7A and 7B on Diabetic Ulcer Management

Does the patient have diabetes? — No →

Is there a neuropathy? — No → Is there arterial disease?

Is there arterial disease? — Yes → Refer to Pathway 9 on Arterial Ulcer Management

Is edema present? — No →

Is edema present? — Yes → Is there exudation or granulation?

Is there exudation or granulation? — No →

Is there exudation or granulation? — Yes → Are the edges shallow and diffuse?

Are the edges shallow and diffuse? — No →

Are the edges shallow and diffuse? — Yes → Is there pain in dependent position?

Is there pain in dependent position? — No →

Is there pain in dependent position? — Yes → Peripheral pulse present?

Peripheral pulse present? — No →

Peripheral pulse present? — Yes → Venous stasis ulcer Refer to Pathway 8 on Venous Stasis Ulcer Management

Pathway 3
Nutritional Assessment and Management
Modified from Bergstrom N, Bennett MA, Carson CE, et al.,1994 (9)

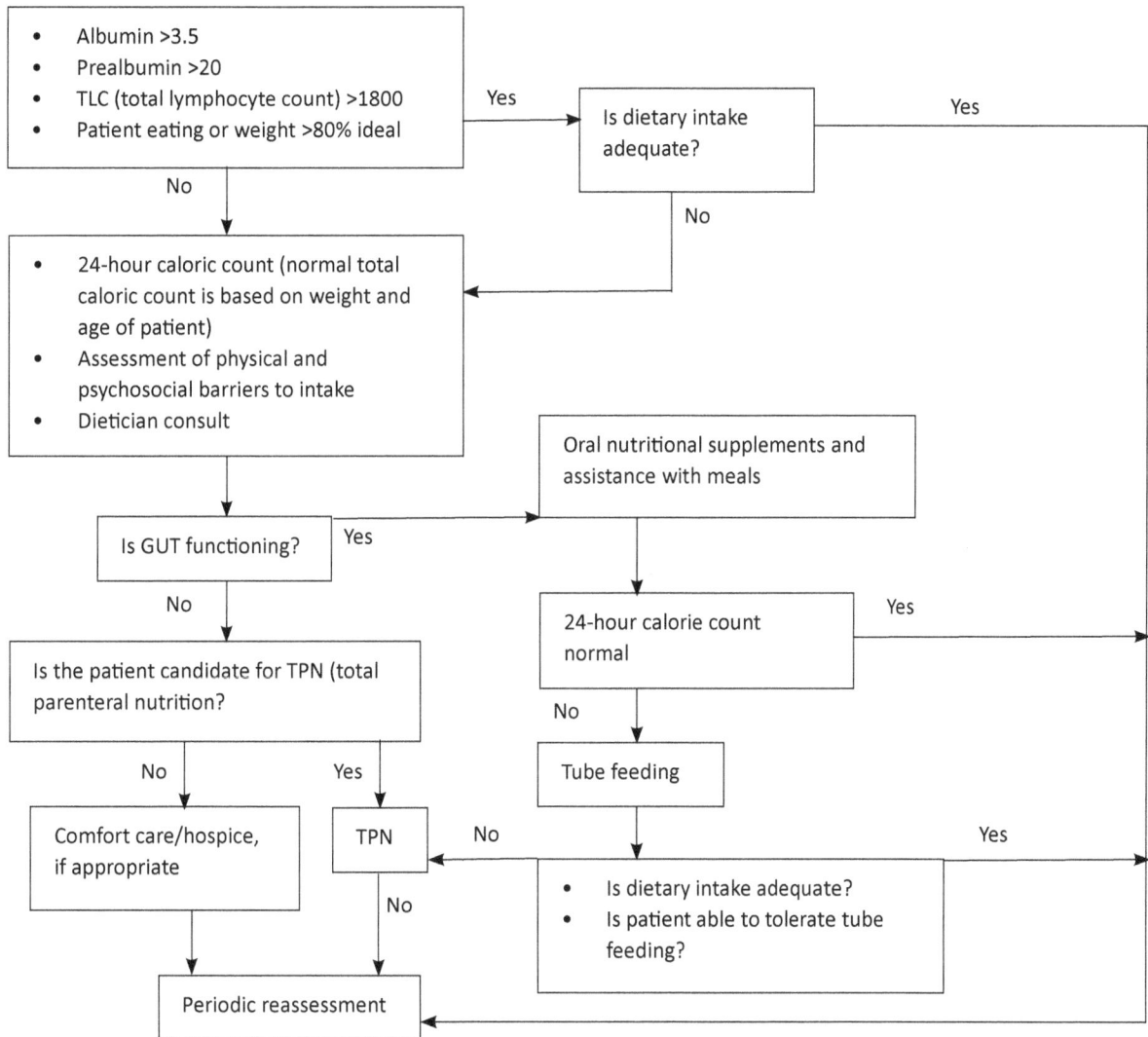

Pathway 4
Management of Blood Glucose

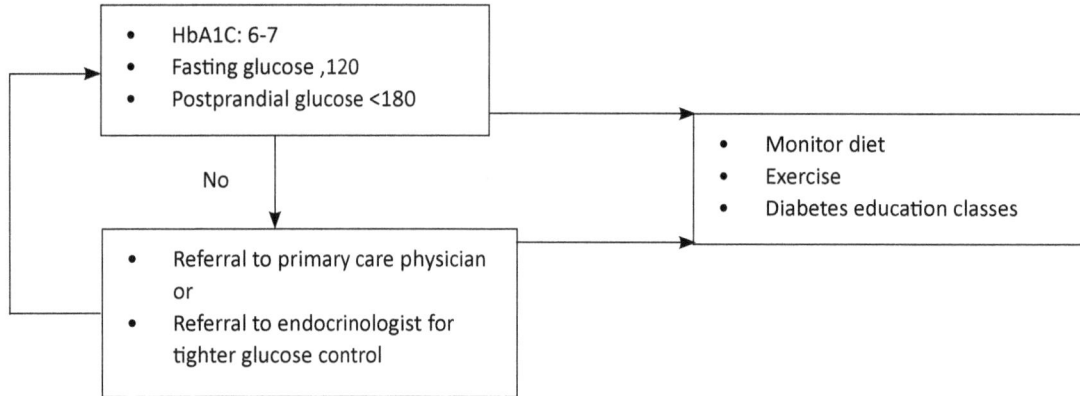

```
┌──────────────────────────────────┐
│  •  HbA1C: 6-7                   │ ─────────────────────┐
│  •  Fasting glucose ,120         │                      │
│  •  Postprandial glucose <180    │                      │
└──────────────────────────────────┘                      │
                 │                                          ▼
                No                         ┌────────────────────────────────────┐
                 ▼                          │  •  Monitor diet                   │
┌──────────────────────────────────┐       │  •  Exercise                       │
│  •  Referral to primary care      │       │  •  Diabetes education classes     │
│     physician                     │ ─────▶└────────────────────────────────────┘
│     or                            │
│  •  Referral to endocrinologist   │
│     for tighter glucose control   │
└──────────────────────────────────┘
```

Pathway 5
Wound Bed Preparation TIME O$_2$ Principles (7)
Modified from TIME Principles (5,6)

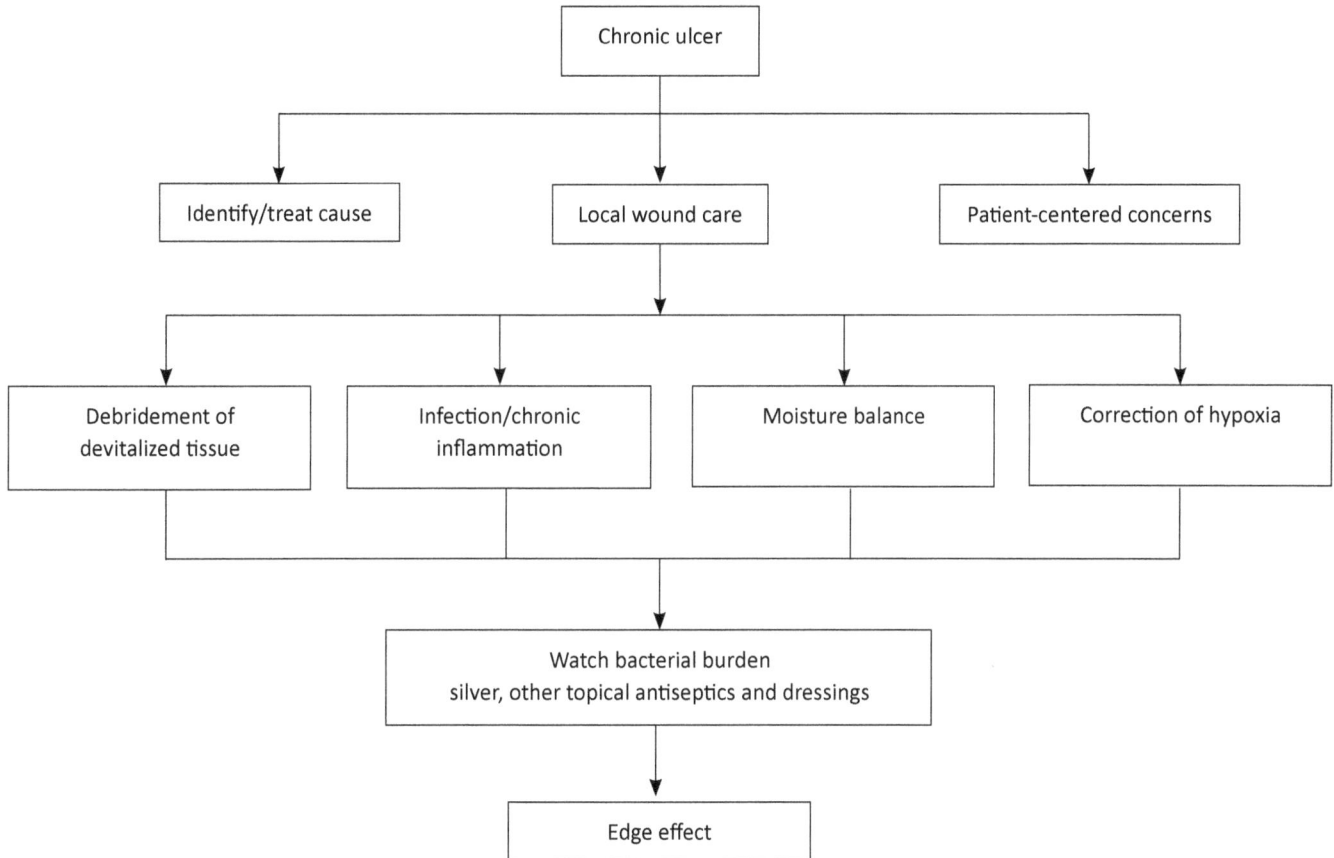

```
                         ┌─────────────────┐
                         │  Chronic ulcer  │
                         └─────────────────┘
         ┌───────────────────────┼───────────────────────┐
         ▼                       ▼                       ▼
┌──────────────────┐   ┌──────────────────┐   ┌──────────────────────────┐
│ Identify/treat   │   │ Local wound care │   │ Patient-centered concerns│
│ cause            │   │                  │   │                          │
└──────────────────┘   └──────────────────┘   └──────────────────────────┘
                                │
      ┌─────────────────┬───────┴───────┬─────────────────┐
      ▼                 ▼               ▼                 ▼
┌─────────────┐ ┌──────────────┐ ┌──────────────┐ ┌──────────────────┐
│ Debridement │ │ Infection/   │ │ Moisture     │ │ Correction of    │
│ of          │ │ chronic      │ │ balance      │ │ hypoxia          │
│ devitalized │ │ inflammation │ │              │ │                  │
│ tissue      │ │              │ │              │ │                  │
└─────────────┘ └──────────────┘ └──────────────┘ └──────────────────┘
      └─────────────────┴───────┬───────┴─────────────────┘
                                ▼
              ┌──────────────────────────────────────────┐
              │ Watch bacterial burden                   │
              │ silver, other topical antiseptics and    │
              │ dressings                                │
              └──────────────────────────────────────────┘
                                │
                                ▼
                    ┌──────────────────────┐
                    │      Edge effect     │
                    └──────────────────────┘
```

Pathway 5A
Debridement (5,6,7)

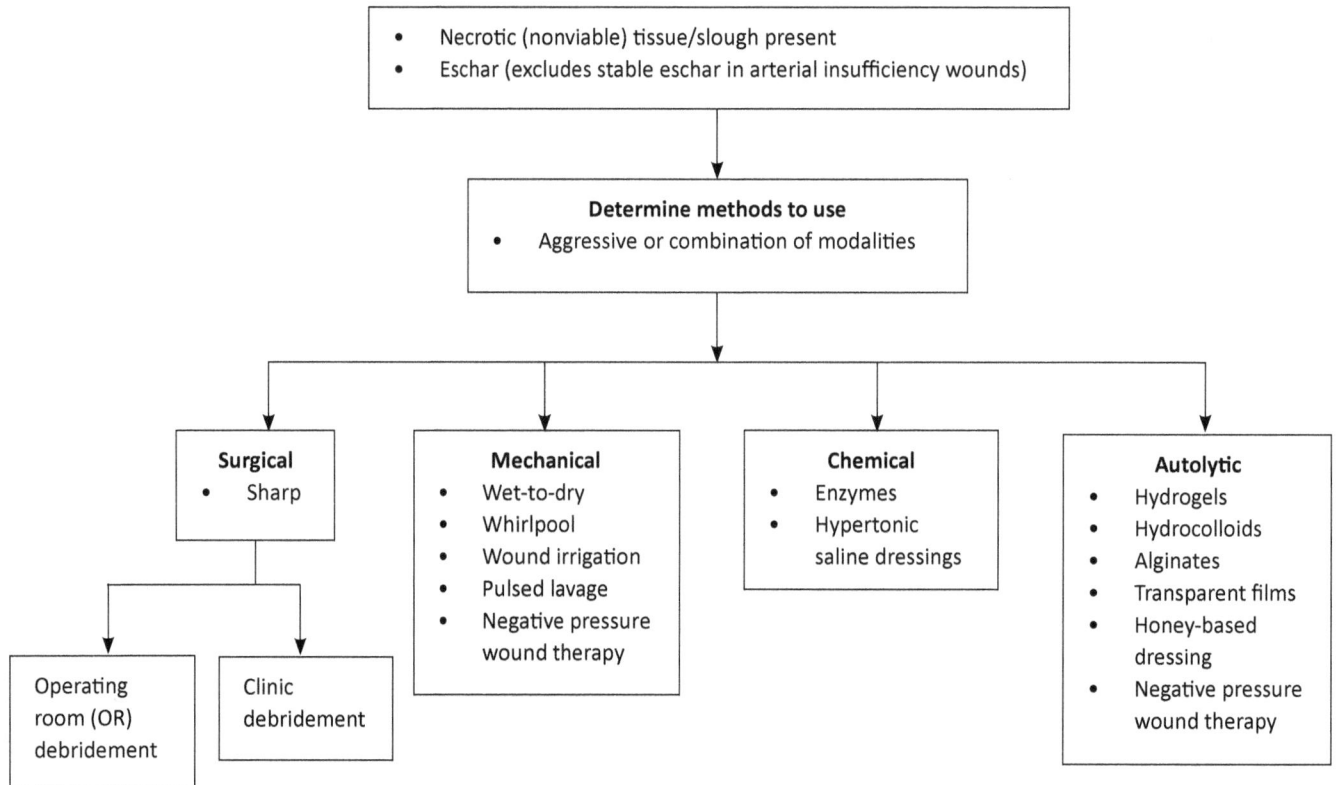

```
┌─────────────────────────────────────────────────────────────┐
│  •  Necrotic (nonviable) tissue/slough present                │
│  •  Eschar (excludes stable eschar in arterial insufficiency  │
│     wounds)                                                    │
└─────────────────────────────────────────────────────────────┘
                              │
                              ▼
          ┌───────────────────────────────────────┐
          │      Determine methods to use          │
          │  •  Aggressive or combination of        │
          │     modalities                          │
          └───────────────────────────────────────┘
                              │
```

Surgical	Mechanical	Chemical	Autolytic
• Sharp	• Wet-to-dry • Whirlpool • Wound irrigation • Pulsed lavage • Negative pressure wound therapy	• Enzymes • Hypertonic saline dressings	• Hydrogels • Hydrocolloids • Alginates • Transparent films • Honey-based dressing • Negative pressure wound therapy

Operating room (OR) debridement	Clinic debridement

Pathway 5B
Wound Infection (5,6,7)

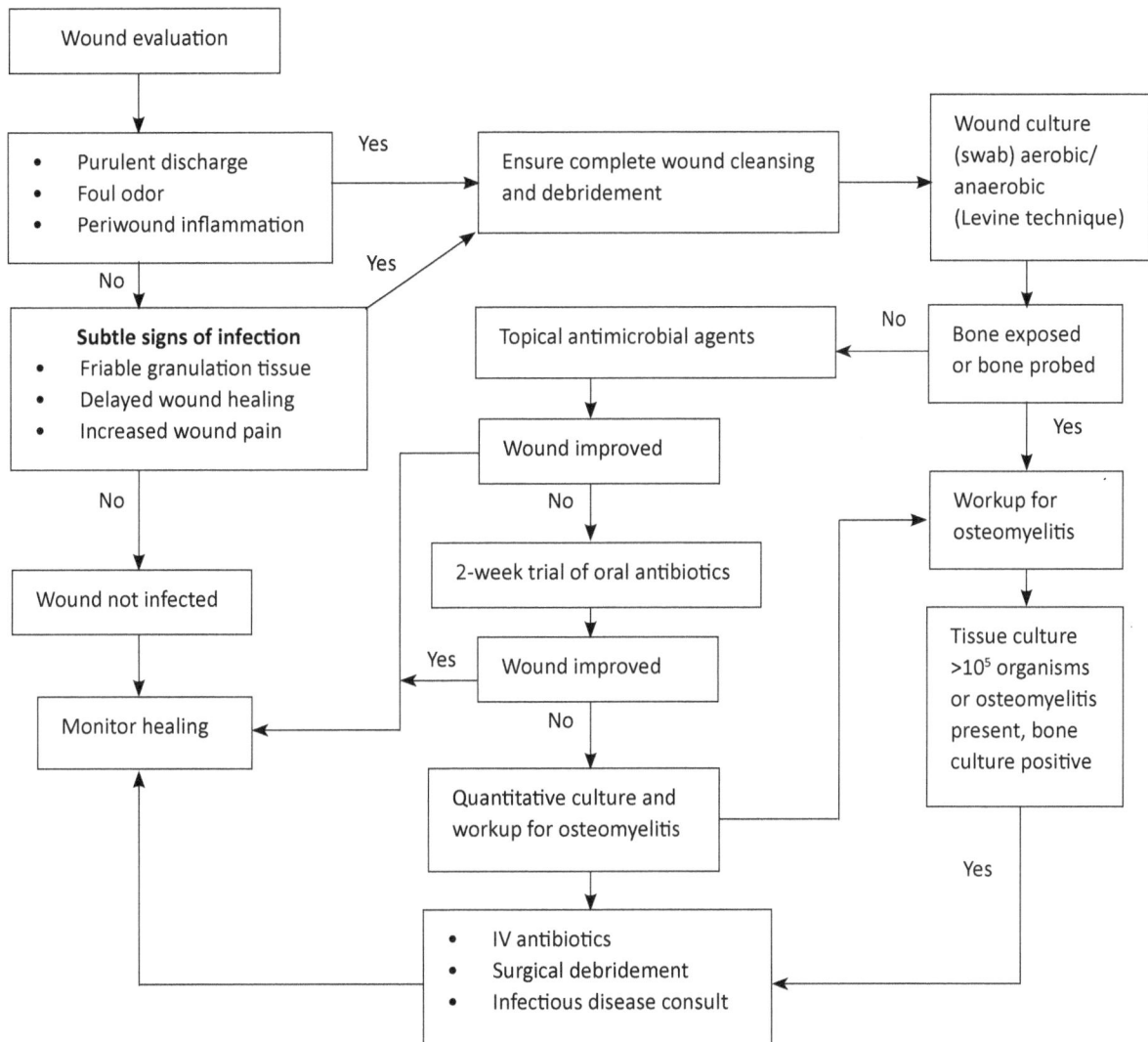

Pathway 5C
Moisture Balance (5,6,7)

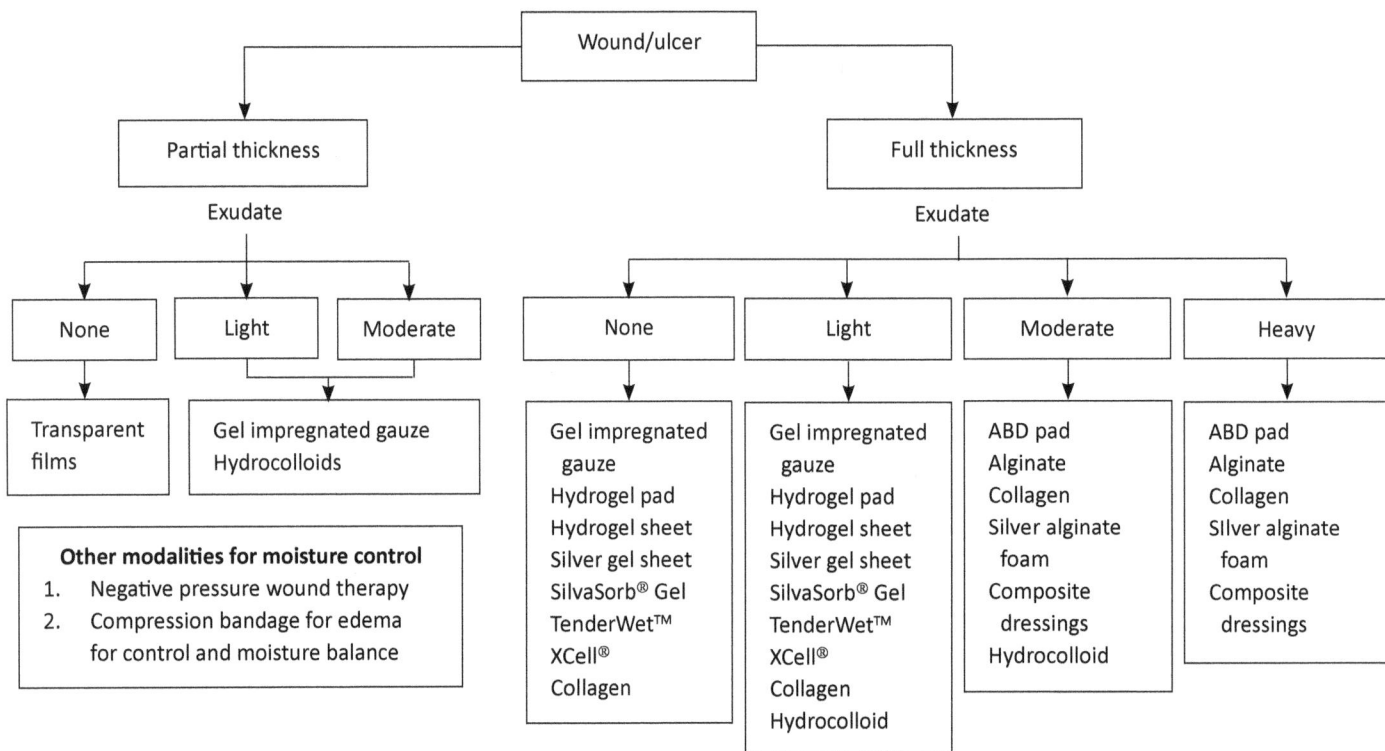

```
                          ┌──────────────┐
                          │ Wound/ulcer  │
                          └──────────────┘
          ┌──────────────────────┴──────────────────────┐
┌────────────────────┐                        ┌────────────────────┐
│ Partial thickness  │                        │  Full thickness     │
└────────────────────┘                        └────────────────────┘
        Exudate                                      Exudate
```

Partial thickness — Exudate			Full thickness — Exudate			
None	**Light**	**Moderate**	**None**	**Light**	**Moderate**	**Heavy**
Transparent films	Gel impregnated gauze Hydrocolloids		Gel impregnated gauze Hydrogel pad Hydrogel sheet Silver gel sheet SilvaSorb® Gel TenderWet™ XCell® Collagen	Gel impregnated gauze Hydrogel pad Hydrogel sheet Silver gel sheet SilvaSorb® Gel TenderWet™ XCell® Collagen Hydrocolloid	ABD pad Alginate Collagen Silver alginate foam Composite dressings Hydrocolloid	ABD pad Alginate Collagen SIlver alginate foam Composite dressings

Other modalities for moisture control
1. Negative pressure wound therapy
2. Compression bandage for edema for control and moisture balance

---

Examples of dressings

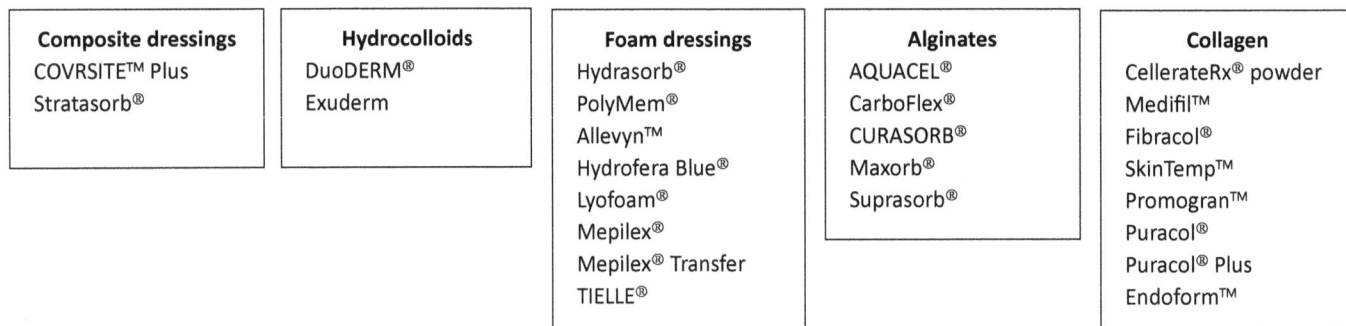

Composite dressings	**Hydrocolloids**	**Foam dressings**	**Alginates**	**Collagen**
COVRSITE™ Plus Stratasorb®	DuoDERM® Exuderm	Hydrasorb® PolyMem® Allevyn™ Hydrofera Blue® Lyofoam® Mepilex® Mepilex® Transfer TIELLE®	AQUACEL® CarboFlex® CURASORB® Maxorb® Suprasorb®	CellerateRx® powder Medifil™ Fibracol® SkinTemp™ Promogran™ Puracol® Puracol® Plus Endoform™

Pathway 5D
Management of Edge Effect (5,6,7)

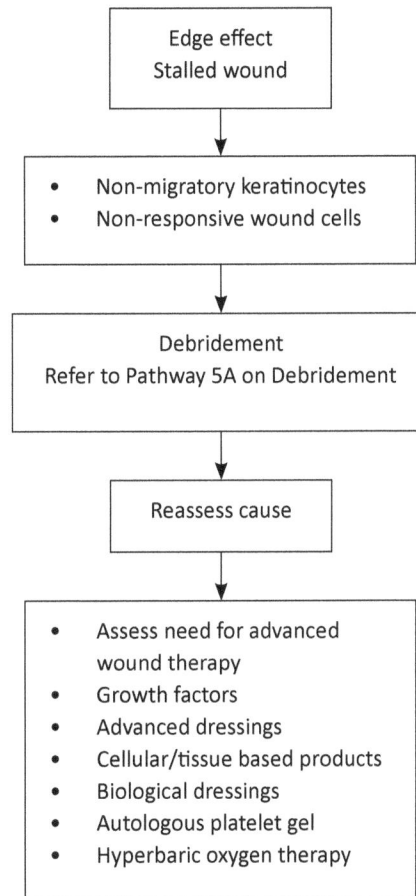

```
                    ┌─────────────────────────┐
                    │      Edge effect        │
                    │     Stalled wound       │
                    └─────────────────────────┘
                                 │
                                 ▼
        ┌─────────────────────────────────────────────┐
        │  •  Non-migratory keratinocytes             │
        │  •  Non-responsive wound cells              │
        └─────────────────────────────────────────────┘
                                 │
                                 ▼
        ┌─────────────────────────────────────────────┐
        │             Debridement                      │
        │   Refer to Pathway 5A on Debridement         │
        └─────────────────────────────────────────────┘
                                 │
                                 ▼
                    ┌─────────────────────────┐
                    │     Reassess cause      │
                    └─────────────────────────┘
                                 │
                                 ▼
        ┌─────────────────────────────────────────────┐
        │  •  Assess need for advanced                 │
        │     wound therapy                            │
        │  •  Growth factors                           │
        │  •  Advanced dressings                       │
        │  •  Cellular/tissue based products           │
        │  •  Biological dressings                     │
        │  •  Autologous platelet gel                  │
        │  •  Hyperbaric oxygen therapy                │
        └─────────────────────────────────────────────┘
```

Pathway 5E
Correction of Hypoxia (1,2,3,7)

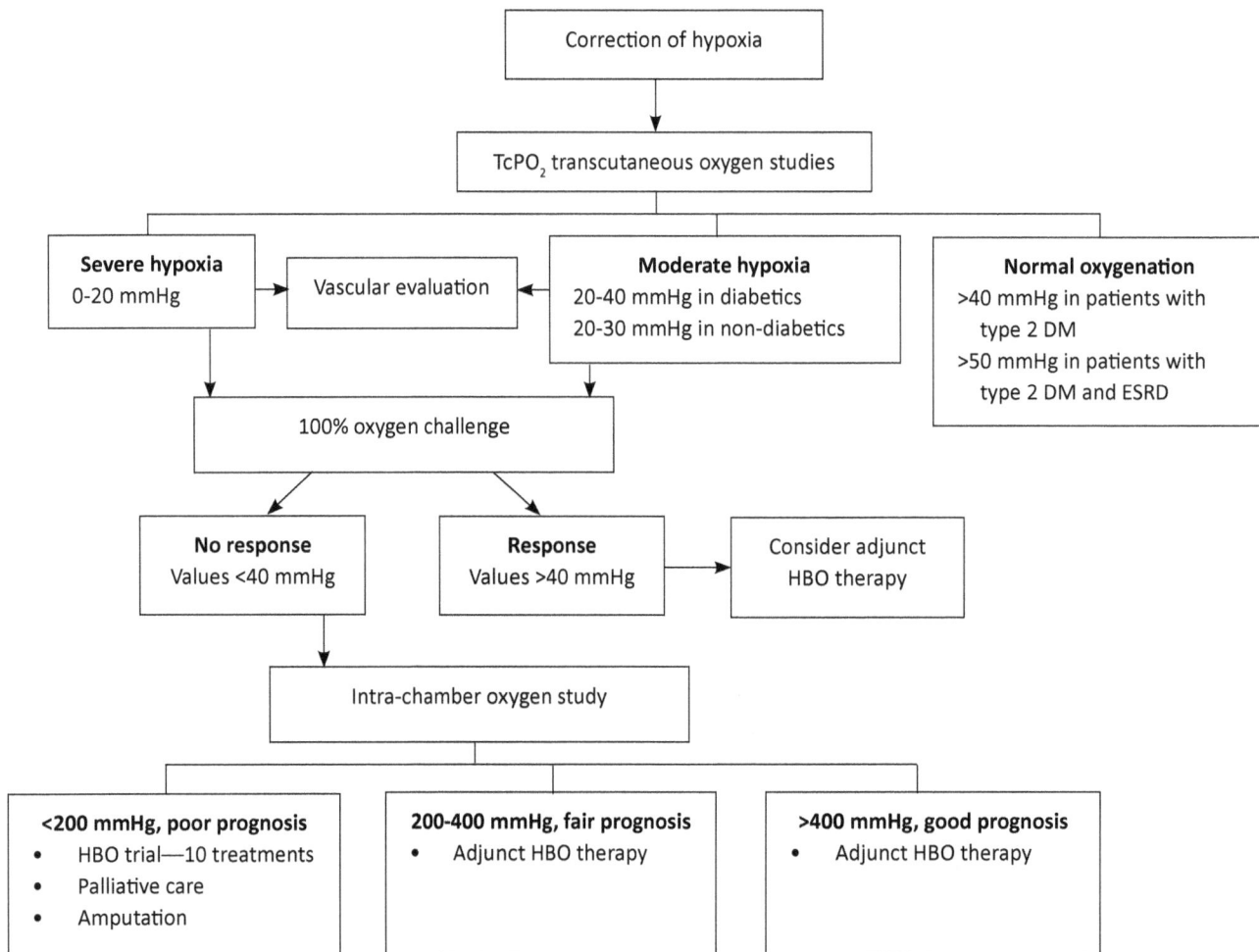

Correction of hypoxia

↓

$TcPO_2$ transcutaneous oxygen studies

Severe hypoxia
0-20 mmHg

→ Vascular evaluation ←

Moderate hypoxia
20-40 mmHg in diabetics
20-30 mmHg in non-diabetics

Normal oxygenation
>40 mmHg in patients with
type 2 DM
>50 mmHg in patients with
type 2 DM and ESRD

100% oxygen challenge

No response
Values <40 mmHg

Response
Values >40 mmHg → Consider adjunct
HBO therapy

Intra-chamber oxygen study

<200 mmHg, poor prognosis
- HBO trial—10 treatments
- Palliative care
- Amputation

200-400 mmHg, fair prognosis
- Adjunct HBO therapy

>400 mmHg, good prognosis
- Adjunct HBO therapy

Pathway 6.1
Off-Loading Foot Orthotics (4)

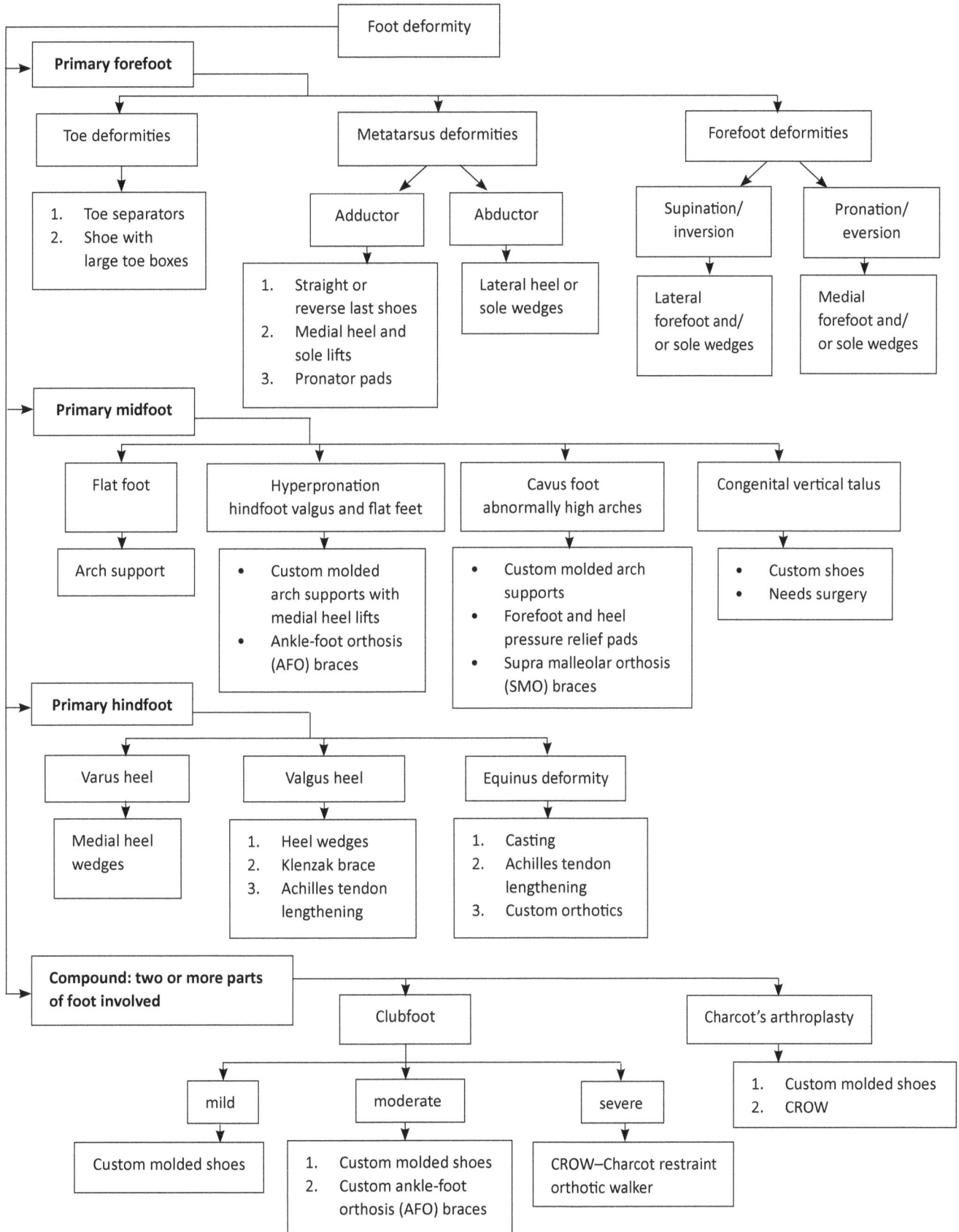

```
                          ┌──────────────────┐
                          │  Foot deformity  │
                          └──────────────────┘

┌─────────────────────┐
│  Primary forefoot   │
└─────────────────────┘
```

Primary forefoot

- **Toe deformities**
  1. Toe separators
  2. Shoe with large toe boxes

- **Metatarsus deformities**
  - **Adductor**
    1. Straight or reverse last shoes
    2. Medial heel and sole lifts
    3. Pronator pads
  - **Abductor**
    - Lateral heel or sole wedges

- **Forefoot deformities**
  - **Supination/inversion**
    - Lateral forefoot and/or sole wedges
  - **Pronation/eversion**
    - Medial forefoot and/or sole wedges

Primary midfoot

- **Flat foot**
  - Arch support

- **Hyperpronation hindfoot valgus and flat feet**
  - Custom molded arch supports with medial heel lifts
  - Ankle-foot orthosis (AFO) braces

- **Cavus foot abnormally high arches**
  - Custom molded arch supports
  - Forefoot and heel pressure relief pads
  - Supra malleolar orthosis (SMO) braces

- **Congenital vertical talus**
  - Custom shoes
  - Needs surgery

Primary hindfoot

- **Varus heel**
  - Medial heel wedges

- **Valgus heel**
  1. Heel wedges
  2. Klenzak brace
  3. Achilles tendon lengthening

- **Equinus deformity**
  1. Casting
  2. Achilles tendon lengthening
  3. Custom orthotics

Compound: two or more parts of foot involved

- **Clubfoot**
  - **mild**
    - Custom molded shoes
  - **moderate**
    1. Custom molded shoes
    2. Custom ankle-foot orthosis (AFO) braces
  - **severe**
    - CROW—Charcot restraint orthotic walker

- **Charcot's arthroplasty**
  1. Custom molded shoes
  2. CROW

Pathway 6.2
Prescription Off-Loading Shoe Adjustments (4)

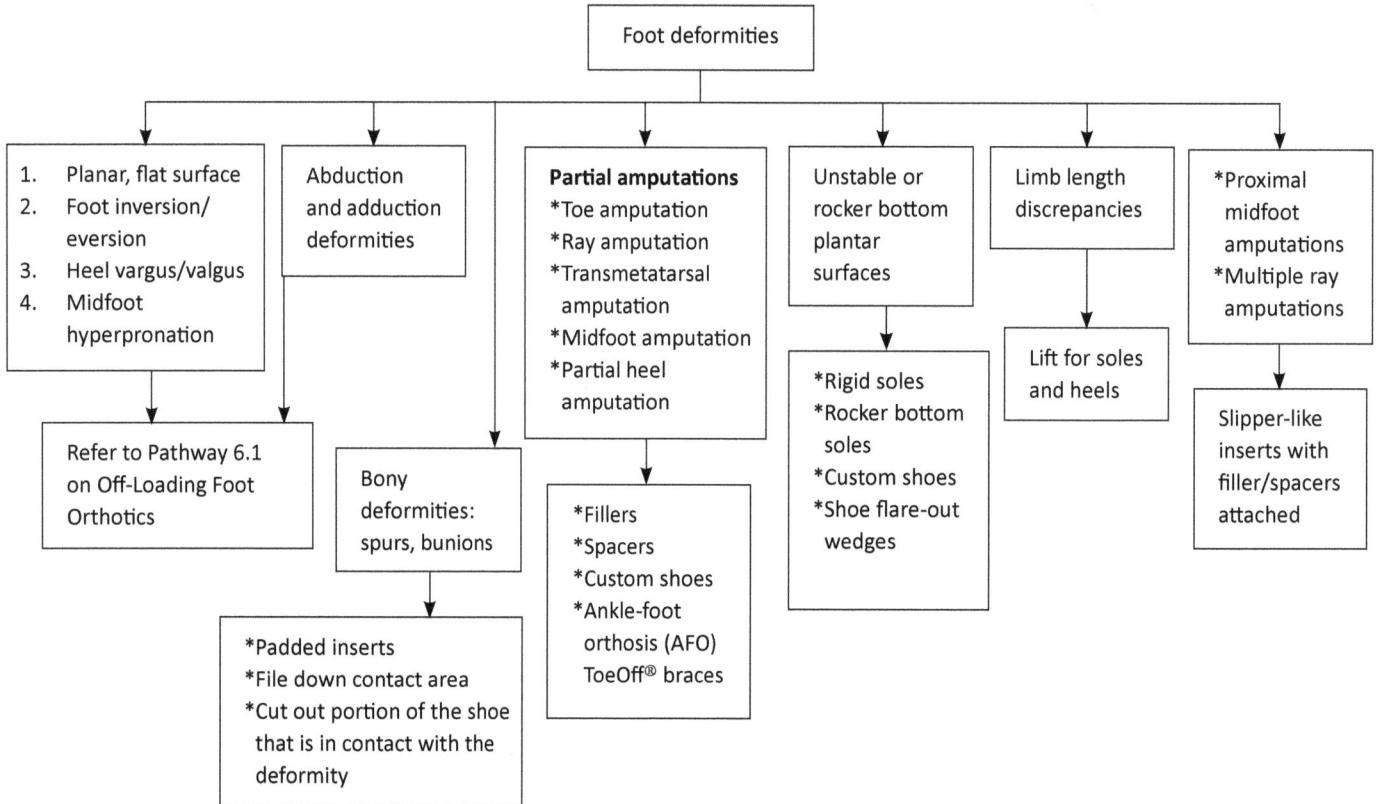

```
                              ┌──────────────────┐
                              │ Foot deformities │
                              └──────────────────┘
```

Foot deformities branches to:

1. Planar, flat surface 2. Foot inversion/eversion 3. Heel vargus/valgus 4. Midfoot hyperpronation	Abduction and adduction deformities

Partial amputations
*Toe amputation
*Ray amputation
*Transmetatarsal amputation
*Midfoot amputation
*Partial heel amputation

Unstable or rocker bottom plantar surfaces

Limb length discrepancies

*Proximal midfoot amputations
*Multiple ray amputations

Refer to Pathway 6.1 on Off-Loading Foot Orthotics

Bony deformities: spurs, bunions

*Fillers
*Spacers
*Custom shoes
*Ankle-foot orthosis (AFO) ToeOff® braces

*Rigid soles
*Rocker bottom soles
*Custom shoes
*Shoe flare-out wedges

Lift for soles and heels

Slipper-like inserts with filler/spacers attached

*Padded inserts
*File down contact area
*Cut out portion of the shoe that is in contact with the deformity

Pathway 7A
Non-Infected Diabetic Foot Ulcers

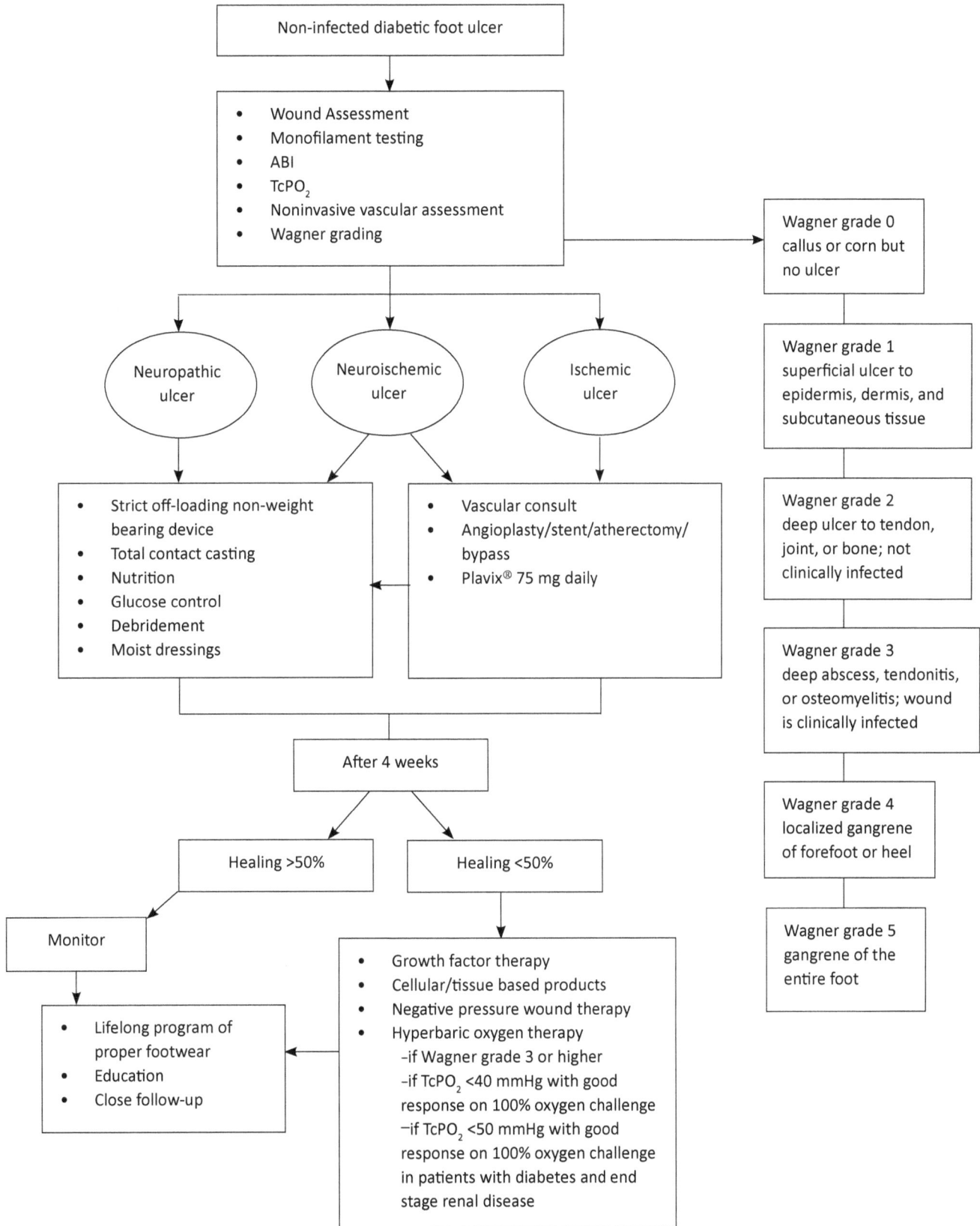

Pathway 7B
Infected Diabetic Foot Ulcers

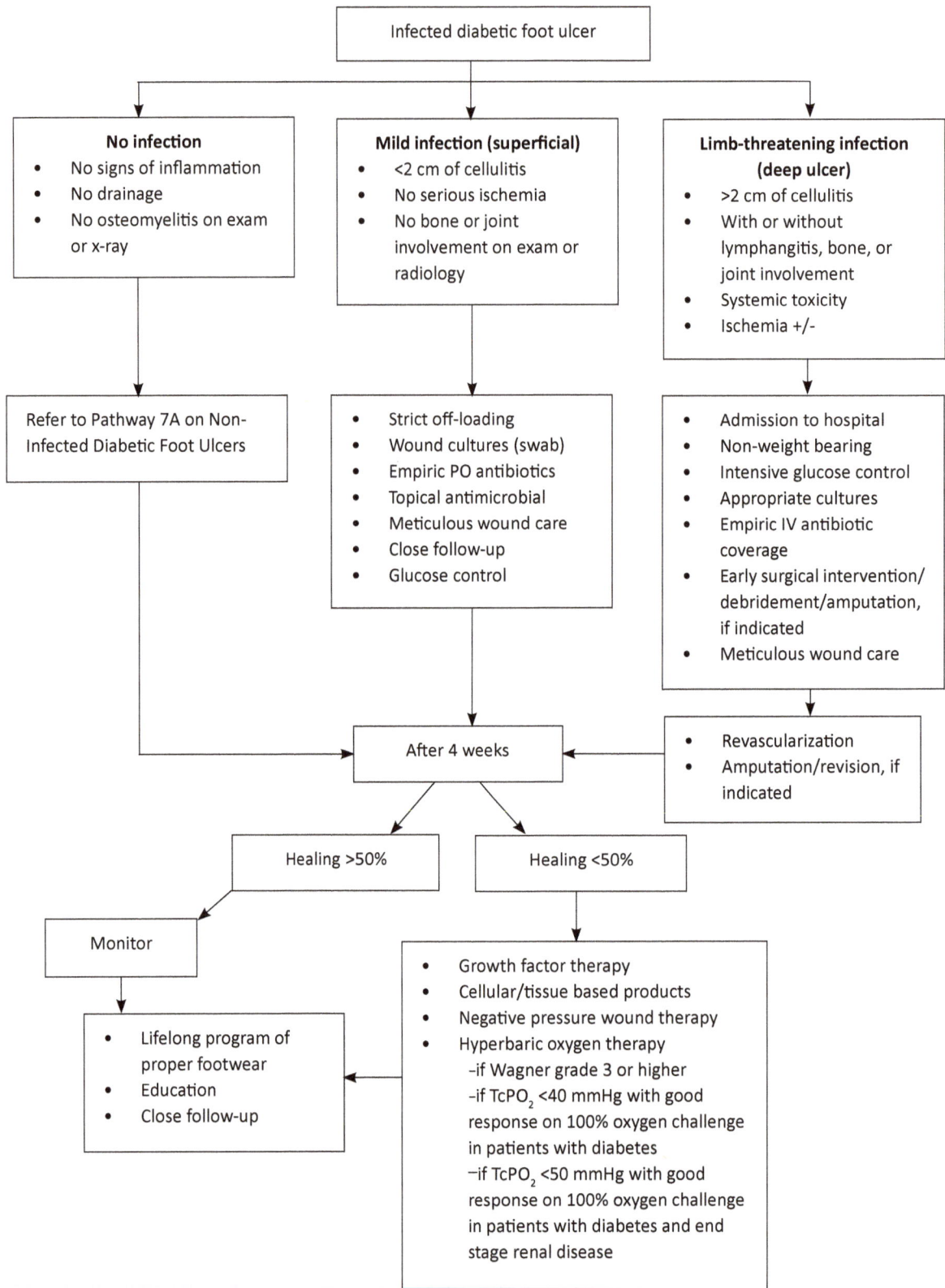

Infected diabetic foot ulcer

No infection
- No signs of inflammation
- No drainage
- No osteomyelitis on exam or x-ray

Mild infection (superficial)
- <2 cm of cellulitis
- No serious ischemia
- No bone or joint involvement on exam or radiology

Limb-threatening infection (deep ulcer)
- >2 cm of cellulitis
- With or without lymphangitis, bone, or joint involvement
- Systemic toxicity
- Ischemia +/-

Refer to Pathway 7A on Non-Infected Diabetic Foot Ulcers

- Strict off-loading
- Wound cultures (swab)
- Empiric PO antibiotics
- Topical antimicrobial
- Meticulous wound care
- Close follow-up
- Glucose control

- Admission to hospital
- Non-weight bearing
- Intensive glucose control
- Appropriate cultures
- Empiric IV antibiotic coverage
- Early surgical intervention/debridement/amputation, if indicated
- Meticulous wound care

- Revascularization
- Amputation/revision, if indicated

After 4 weeks

Healing >50%

Healing <50%

Monitor

- Lifelong program of proper footwear
- Education
- Close follow-up

- Growth factor therapy
- Cellular/tissue based products
- Negative pressure wound therapy
- Hyperbaric oxygen therapy
  –if Wagner grade 3 or higher
  –if $TcPO_2$ <40 mmHg with good response on 100% oxygen challenge in patients with diabetes
  –if $TcPO_2$ <50 mmHg with good response on 100% oxygen challenge in patients with diabetes and end stage renal disease

Pathway 8
Venous Stasis Ulcer Management

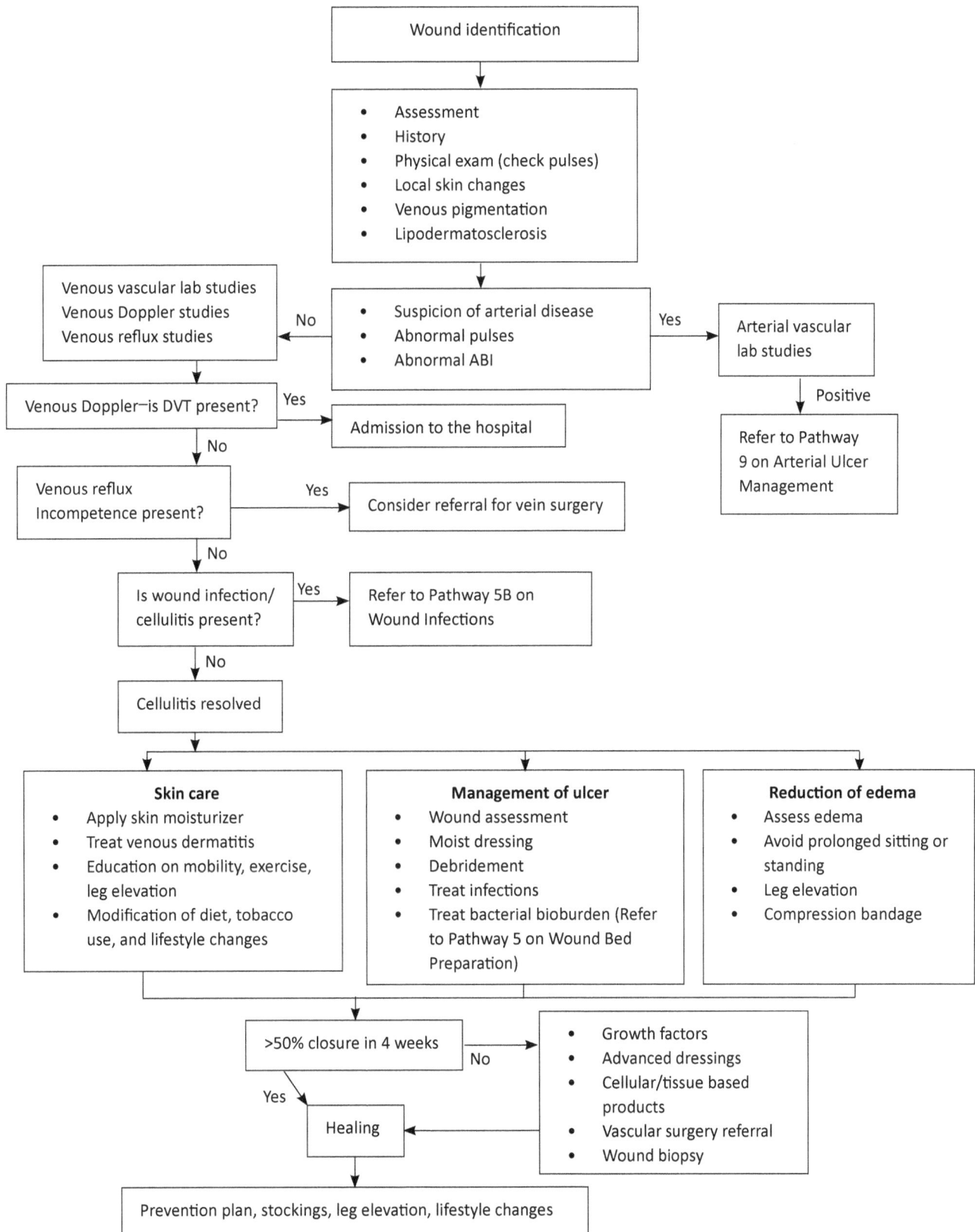

```
                        ┌─────────────────────────────┐
                        │    Wound identification     │
                        └─────────────────────────────┘
                                     │
                        ┌─────────────────────────────┐
                        │  • Assessment               │
                        │  • History                  │
                        │  • Physical exam (check pulses) │
                        │  • Local skin changes       │
                        │  • Venous pigmentation      │
                        │  • Lipodermatosclerosis     │
                        └─────────────────────────────┘
                                     │
┌─────────────────────────┐      ┌─────────────────────────────┐        ┌──────────────────┐
│ Venous vascular lab      │  No  │  • Suspicion of arterial    │  Yes   │ Arterial vascular│
│ studies                  │◄─────│    disease                  │───────►│ lab studies      │
│ Venous Doppler studies   │      │  • Abnormal pulses          │        └──────────────────┘
│ Venous reflux studies    │      │  • Abnormal ABI             │                 │ Positive
└─────────────────────────┘      └─────────────────────────────┘        ┌──────────────────┐
            │                                                            │ Refer to Pathway │
┌─────────────────────────────────┐  Yes  ┌──────────────────────┐      │ 9 on Arterial Ulcer│
│ Venous Doppler—is DVT present?   │──────►│ Admission to the     │      │ Management       │
└─────────────────────────────────┘       │ hospital             │      └──────────────────┘
            │ No                           └──────────────────────┘
┌─────────────────────────┐  Yes  ┌──────────────────────────────────┐
│ Venous reflux           │──────►│ Consider referral for vein surgery│
│ Incompetence present?   │       └──────────────────────────────────┘
└─────────────────────────┘
            │ No
┌─────────────────────────┐  Yes  ┌──────────────────────────┐
│ Is wound infection/     │──────►│ Refer to Pathway 5B on   │
│ cellulitis present?     │       │ Wound Infections         │
└─────────────────────────┘       └──────────────────────────┘
            │ No
┌─────────────────────────┐
│ Cellulitis resolved     │
└─────────────────────────┘
```

Skin care	Management of ulcer	Reduction of edema
• Apply skin moisturizer	• Wound assessment	• Assess edema
• Treat venous dermatitis	• Moist dressing	• Avoid prolonged sitting or standing
• Education on mobility, exercise, leg elevation	• Debridement	• Leg elevation
• Modification of diet, tobacco use, and lifestyle changes	• Treat infections	• Compression bandage
	• Treat bacterial bioburden (Refer to Pathway 5 on Wound Bed Preparation)	

```
        ┌──────────────────────┐   No   ┌────────────────────────────┐
        │ >50% closure in 4 weeks│──────►│ • Growth factors           │
        └──────────────────────┘        │ • Advanced dressings       │
                  │ Yes                  │ • Cellular/tissue based    │
           ┌──────────────┐             │   products                 │
           │   Healing    │◄────────────│ • Vascular surgery referral│
           └──────────────┘             │ • Wound biopsy             │
                  │                      └────────────────────────────┘
  ┌─────────────────────────────────────────────────────────┐
  │ Prevention plan, stockings, leg elevation, lifestyle changes│
  └─────────────────────────────────────────────────────────┘
```

Pathway 9
Arterial Ulcer Management

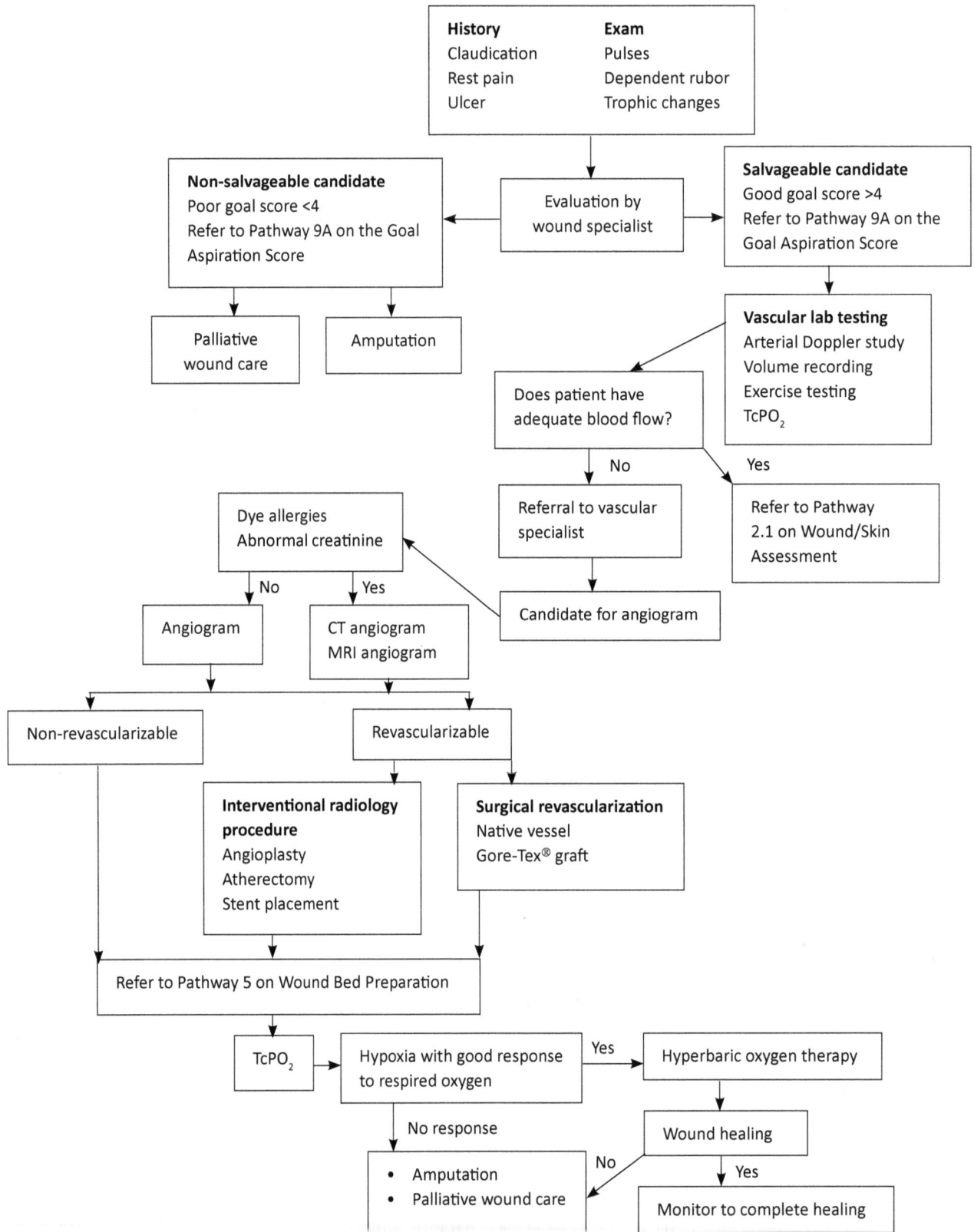

History	Exam
Claudication	Pulses
Rest pain	Dependent rubor
Ulcer	Trophic changes

Evaluation by wound specialist

Non-salvageable candidate
Poor goal score <4
Refer to Pathway 9A on the Goal Aspiration Score

Salvageable candidate
Good goal score >4
Refer to Pathway 9A on the Goal Aspiration Score

Palliative wound care

Amputation

Vascular lab testing
Arterial Doppler study
Volume recording
Exercise testing
TcPO$_2$

Does patient have adequate blood flow?

No → Referral to vascular specialist → Candidate for angiogram

Yes → Refer to Pathway 2.1 on Wound/Skin Assessment

Dye allergies
Abnormal creatinine

No → Angiogram

Yes → CT angiogram
MRI angiogram

Non-revascularizable

Revascularizable

Interventional radiology procedure
Angioplasty
Atherectomy
Stent placement

Surgical revascularization
Native vessel
Gore-Tex® graft

Refer to Pathway 5 on Wound Bed Preparation

TcPO$_2$

Hypoxia with good response to respired oxygen

Yes → Hyperbaric oxygen therapy

No response

Wound healing

- Amputation
- Palliative wound care

No

Yes → Monitor to complete healing

Pathway 9A
The Goal Aspiration Score
Courtesy of Strauss MB, Aksenov IV, Miller SS, 2010 (4)

ASSESSMENTS	COMMENTS, FURTHER ELABORATION	FULL	SOME	NONE
		Use half points if the information is mixed or intermediate between 2 of the grading criteria		
Comprehension	Awareness of the problems and the options for management	2 Point	1 Point	0 Point
Motivation	To heal the wounds and/or avoid lower limb amputations			
Compliance	Attention to diabetes management, weight control, skin and nail care, diet, non-smoking, etc.			
Support	Degree and quality of care provided			
Independence	Ability for patient to perform			

Goal-Aspiration Score: Summate the points for each of the five assessments.

Interpretation: Scores of 4 or greater support the decision for limb salvage and/or surgeries to facilitate wound healing such as contracture releases and major debridements. This score (4 or greater) indicates the patient and/or family are able and willing to take an active part in wound care.

Pathway 10
Pressure Ulcer Management

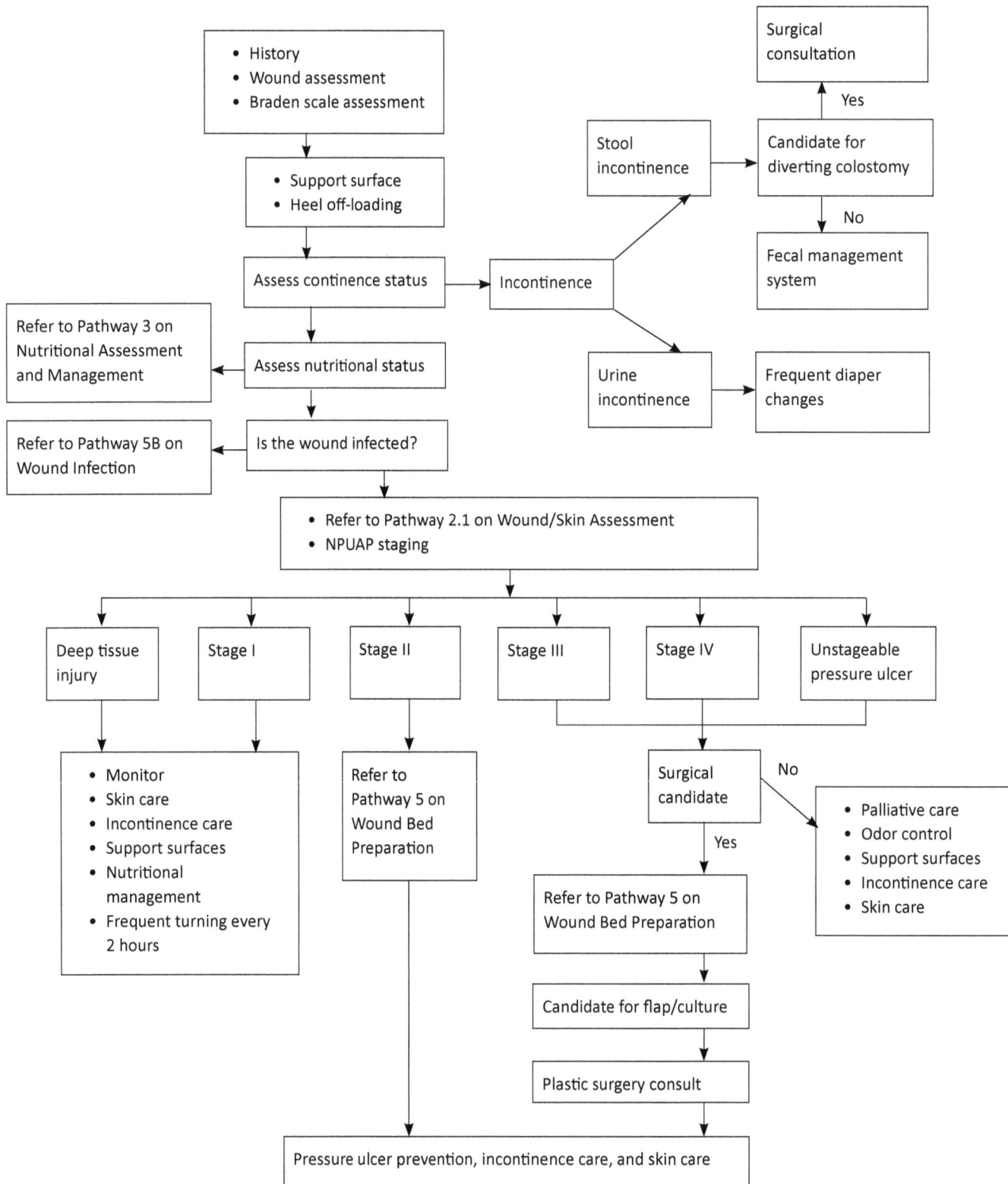

- History
- Wound assessment
- Braden scale assessment

↓

- Support surface
- Heel off-loading

↓

Assess continence status → Incontinence

Incontinence branches to:
- Stool incontinence → Candidate for diverting colostomy
  - Yes → Surgical consultation
  - No → Fecal management system
- Urine incontinence → Frequent diaper changes

Assess continence status ↓

Refer to Pathway 3 on Nutritional Assessment and Management ← Assess nutritional status

↓

Refer to Pathway 5B on Wound Infection ← Is the wound infected?

↓

- Refer to Pathway 2.1 on Wound/Skin Assessment
- NPUAP staging

↓ (branches to)

| Deep tissue injury | Stage I | Stage II | Stage III | Stage IV | Unstageable pressure ulcer |

Deep tissue injury / Stage I →
- Monitor
- Skin care
- Incontinence care
- Support surfaces
- Nutritional management
- Frequent turning every 2 hours

Stage II →
Refer to Pathway 5 on Wound Bed Preparation

Stage III / Stage IV / Unstageable pressure ulcer → Surgical candidate
- No →
  - Palliative care
  - Odor control
  - Support surfaces
  - Incontinence care
  - Skin care
- Yes ↓
  Refer to Pathway 5 on Wound Bed Preparation
  ↓
  Candidate for flap/culture
  ↓
  Plastic surgery consult
  ↓

Pressure ulcer prevention, incontinence care, and skin care

Pathway 11
Unusual Wounds

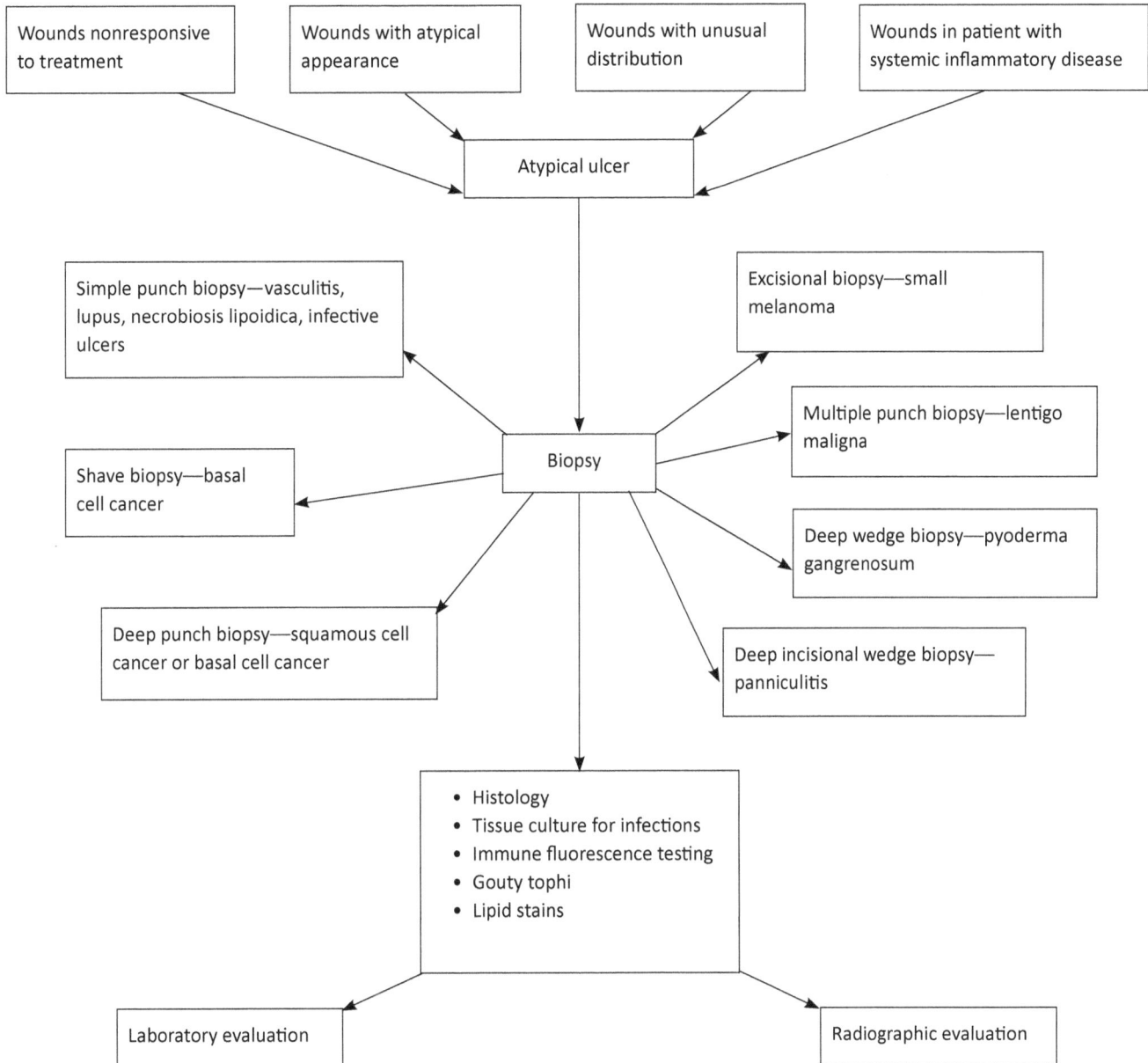

| Wounds nonresponsive to treatment | Wounds with atypical appearance | Wounds with unusual distribution | Wounds in patient with systemic inflammatory disease |

Atypical ulcer

Simple punch biopsy—vasculitis, lupus, necrobiosis lipoidica, infective ulcers

Excisional biopsy—small melanoma

Shave biopsy—basal cell cancer

Biopsy

Multiple punch biopsy—lentigo maligna

Deep wedge biopsy—pyoderma gangrenosum

Deep punch biopsy—squamous cell cancer or basal cell cancer

Deep incisional wedge biopsy—panniculitis

- Histology
- Tissue culture for infections
- Immune fluorescence testing
- Gouty tophi
- Lipid stains

Laboratory evaluation

Radiographic evaluation

Pathway 12
Selection of Support Surfaces
From Bergstrom N, Bennett MA, Carson CE, et al.,1994 (9)

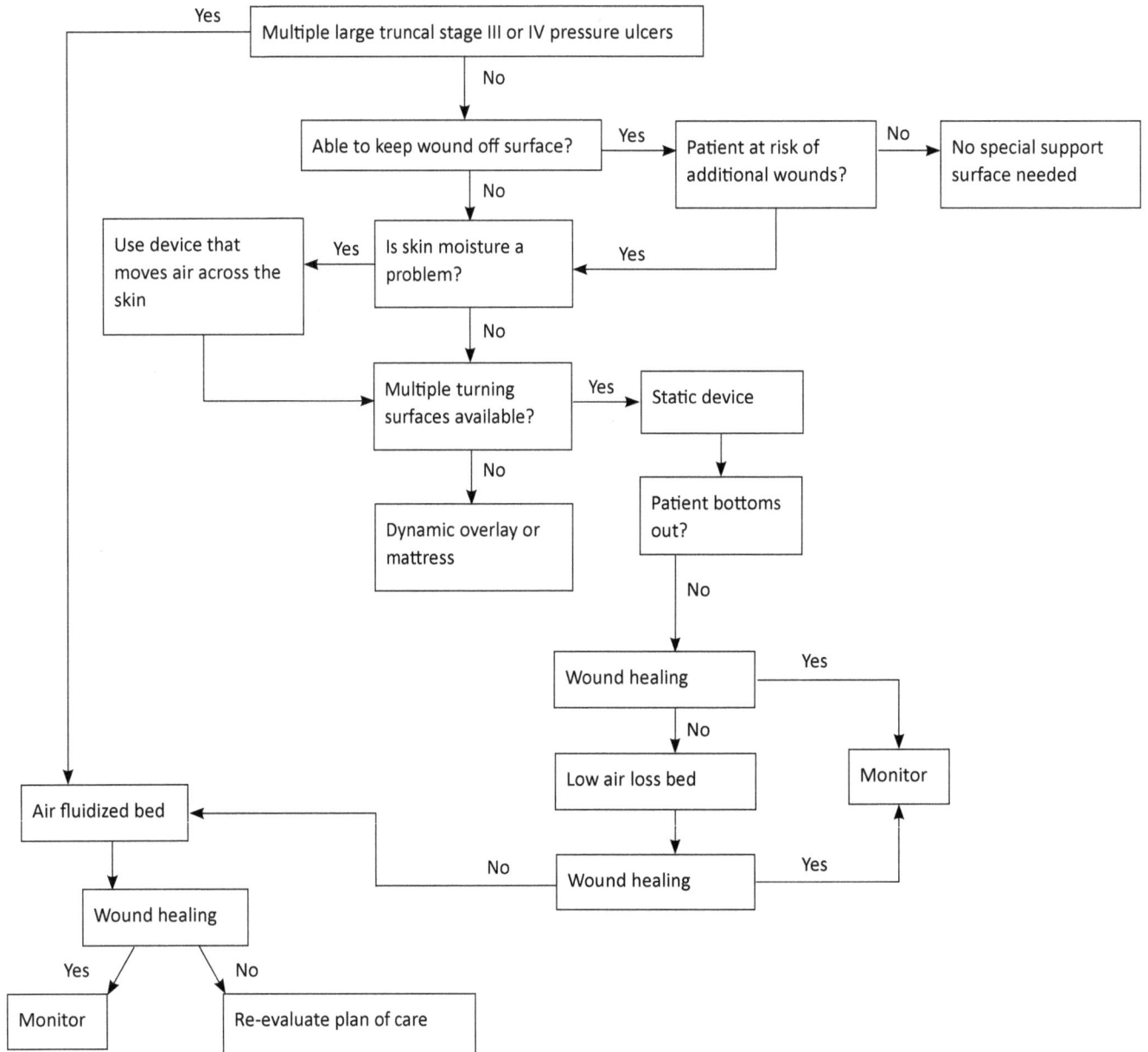

RESOURCES

1. Sheffield PJ. Measuring tissue oxygen tension: a review. *Undersea Hyperb Med.* 1998; 25(3):179-88.

2. Fife CE, et al. The predictive value of transcutaneous oxygen tension measurement in diabetic lower extremity ulcers treated with hyperbaric therapy; a retrospective analysis of 1,144 patients. *Wound Repair Regen.* 2002 Jul-Aug; 10(4):198-207.

3. Fife CE, Smart DR, Sheffield PJ, Hopf HW, Hawkins G, Clarke D. Transcutaneous oximetry in clinical practice: Consensus statements from an expert panel based on evidence. *Undersea Hyperb Med.* 2009 Jan-Feb; 36(1):43-53.

4. Strauss MB, Aksenov IV, Miller SS. *Masterminding Wounds.* North Palm Beach: Best Publishing Company; 2010: 14.

5. Schultz GS, Sibbald RG, Falanga V, et al. Wound bed preparation: a systematic approach to wound management. *Wound Repair Regen.* 2003 Mar; 11 Suppl 1:S1-28.

6. Falanga V. Wound bed preparation and the role of enzymes: A case of multiple actions of therapeutic agents. Wounds 2002; 14(2):47-57. Accessed at: http://www.woundresearch.com/article/209.

7. Shah JB. Correction of hypoxia, a critical element for wound bed preparation Pathways: TIMEO2 principle of wound bed preparation. *J Am Col Certif Wound Spec.* 2011 Oct 9; 3(2):26-32.

8. Bergstrom N, Bennett MA, Carlson CE, et al. Pressure Ulcers in Adults: Prediction and Prevention. Clinical Practice Pathway Number 3. Rockville: Agency for Health Care Policy and Research (AHCPR); 1992.

9. Bergstrom N, Bennett MA, Carlson CE, et al. Treatment of Pressure Ulcers. Clinical Practice Pathway Number 15. Rockville: Agency for Health Care Policy and Research (AHCPR); 1994.

10. National Pressure Ulcer Advisory Panel. National Pressure Ulcer Advisory Panel Support Surface Standards Initiative [Internet]. 2007. Accessed at: http://www.npuap.org/wp-content/uploads/2012/03/NPUAP_S3I_TD.pdf.

NOTES

POST-COURSE PRACTICE EXAM 33

Jayesh B. Shah, MD, CWSP, FAPWCA, FACCWS
Frederick Gale, MD, FACS

INTRODUCTION

This chapter contains questions that are representative of what you may encounter while taking a wound care certification exam. An explanation is provided as to why a specific answer is correct in the answer key. This practice exam supplements the questions provided at the end of each chapter.

OBJECTIVES

Participants should be able to use this post-course exam to identify areas of strength and areas that require additional study before sitting for a certification exam.

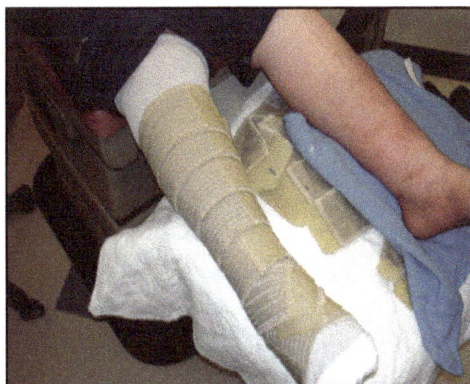

Figure 33.1: A 59-year-old patient with a compression garment for a venous stasis ulcer.

A. A 59-year-old female with a history of congestive heart failure (CHF) and coronary artery disease (CAD) had a recurrent venous stasis ulcer. The patient healed completely with standard wound care and compression; however, she is unable to wear fixed compression stockings and is prescribed the alternate compression garment as seen in Figure 33.1.

1. What is the name of this compression garment?
   a) Burrow wrap
   b) Juzo® zipper Velcro® stocking
   c) FarrowWrap®
   d) Ace bandage with Velcro®

2. Which of the following statements about this type of garment is true?
   a) This type of compression is considered short stretch.
   b) This type of compression has low resting pressure and high working pressure compression.
   c) It has multiple overlapping layers with Velcro® applied to the compression level tolerated by the patient.
   d) It can be applied in the presence of ulcers.
   e) All of the above are true statements.

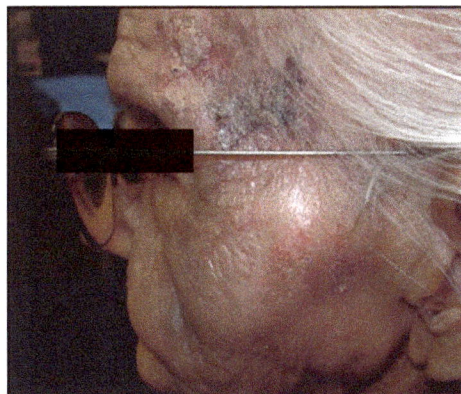

Figure 33.2: A 92-year-old patient with a suspicious facial lesion.

B. A 92-year-old female with a venous stasis ulcer arrives for a follow-up appointment. On general examination, the physician finds a suspicious lesion on her face, as shown in Figure 33. 2. ABCDE (asymmetry, border irregular, color multiple, diameter >5 mm, elevation) is noted.

3. What will be the next step in the management of this patient?
   a) Observe for changes in ABCDE
   b) Send the patient to a plastic surgery consult for an excisional biopsy
   c) This is most likely a benign mole, so just observe
   d) Refer the patient to a dermatologist for an incisional biopsy

4. Biopsy of the lesion is positive for basal cell cancer. All of these statements about basal cell cancer are true except:
   a) Basal cell cancer is also called rodent ulcer.
   b) Basal cell cancer arises from keratinizing epidermal cells.
   c) Basal cell cancer arises from epidermal basal cells.
   d) Basal cell cancer is the most common skin ulcer malignancy.

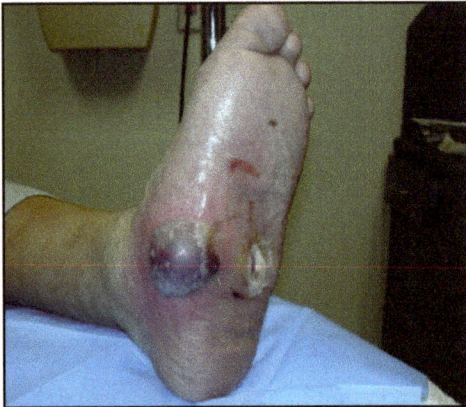

Figure 33.3: A 70-year-old diabetic female with a bullae on the medial aspect of the foot and an ulcer on the plantar aspect of the foot.

C. A 70-year-old female with a history of type 2 diabetes mellitus (DM), critical aortic stenosis, CAD, and an ejection fraction (EF) of 25%, presents to the clinic because of a one-week history of low grade fever, soft tissue swelling on the left leg with bullae on the medial aspect of the foot, and a small 3 × 2 cm ulcer on the plantar aspect of the foot with undermining from the 12 to 5 o'clock position. The wound also has tunneling at the 3 o'clock position for 4 cm, which continues all the way up to the bullae. The base of the wound has bone exposed, and there is moderate seropurulent drainage. The patient has 2+ edema, DP/PT is faintly palpable, and ankle-brachial index (ABI) is non-compressible. TcPO$_2$ at foot level shows baseline numbers of 20 mmHg while breathing air (Figure 33.3).

5. What is the diagnosis?
   a) Acute Charcot's arthropathy
   b) Venous stasis ulcer with blister formation
   c) Cellulitis with possible osteomyelitis
   d) Gas gangrene

6. What is the first step in the management of this patient?
   a) Hyperbaric oxygen therapy
   b) Urgent surgical consult for debridement
   c) MRI with and without contrast
   d) Wound culture and start antibiotics

7. If a diabetic foot infection is suspected, all factors listed below should be considered before starting an empiric regimen except:
   a) Patient allergies
   b) Renal dysfunction
   c) Previous antibiotic therapy
   d) Known local antibiotic sensitivity pattern
   e) Patient's HbA1c level

8. What is the most common organism cultured in patients with diabetic foot infections?
   a) *Staphylococcus aureus*
   b) *Enterococcus*
   c) *Pseudomonas*
   d) *Klebsiella*

9. All of the antibiotic regimens from the following choices will be appropriate in moderate to severe diabetic foot infections except:
   a) Ampicillin/sulbactam 3.0 gm IV q6h + vancomycin 15-20 mg/kg IV q8-12h
   b) Piperacillin-tazobactam 4.5 gm IV q8h + linezolid 600 mg IV q12h
   c) Ertapenem 1 gm IV q24h + vancomycin 15-20 mg/kg IV q8-12h
   d) Aztreonam 2 gm IV q8h + metronidazole 1 gm IV q12h + linezolid 600 mg IV q12h
   e) Levofloxacin 500 mg PO q24h +/- clindamycin 300 mg PO q8h

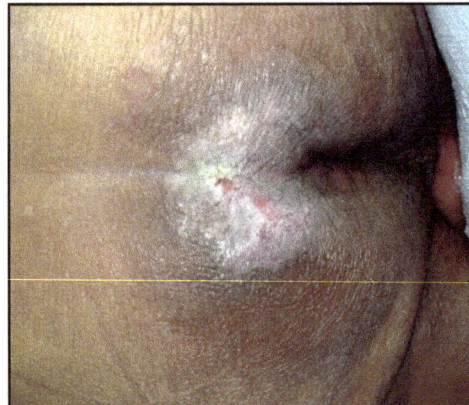

Figure 33.4: A 72-year-old nursing home patient with pressure-induced skin changes.

D. A 72-year-old nursing home patient with cerebrovascular accident (CVA), dementia, CAD, and generalized weakness is admitted to the hospital for pneumonia. On regular skin assessment you notice an ulcer with exposed subcutaneous tissue, as seen in Figure 33.4.

10. What stage pressure ulcer does this patient have?
    a) Stage I
    b) Suspected deep tissue injury
    c) Stage II
    d) Stage III
    e) Stage IV
    f) Unstageable ulcer

11. Static support surfaces, such as water or air overlay mattresses, may be appropriate for patients who are at what level of risk for pressure ulcer development?
    a) Minimal or no risk
    b) Low risk
    c) Moderate risk
    d) High risk

12. All of the following methods of pressure reduction can be used on this patient except:
    a) Turning the patient at least every two hours
    b) Suspending the heels off all surfaces by placing pillows under the calves
    c) Positioning the patient properly
    d) Raising the head of the bed to 45 degrees

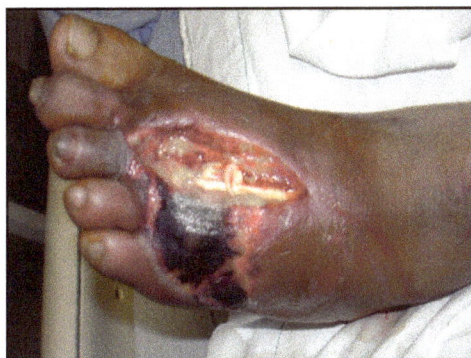

Figure 33.5: A 42-year-old patient with a diabetic foot infection, ulceration, and cellulitis.

E. A 42-year-old male truck driver with type 2 DM is admitted to the hospital because of a diabetic foot infection, ulceration, and cellulitis. The patient was found to have an abscess on the dorsal aspect of his foot for which immediate incision and drainage is performed. The patient is started on broad spectrum antibiotics. Post-operatively the patient is found to have increasing necrosis on the dorsal aspect of his foot. The patient has 2+ edema, arterial Doppler shows monophasic flow of the dorsalis pedis, with an ABI less than 0.4 (Figure 33.5).

13. This patient has:
    a) Normal circulation
    b) Mild peripheral vascular disease
    c) Severe lower extremity ischemia
    d) Venous stasis disease

14. Transcutaneous oxygen study values may be elevated above normal because of:
    a) Active infection
    b) Leak under fixation ring
    c) Acute edema
    d) Thick or sclerotic skin

15. Transcutaneous oxygen sensors can be used to determine the oxygen tension in:
    a) Skin
    b) Bone marrow
    c) Muscle
    d) Tendon

16. A flap must be used in lieu of a split thickness skin graft when:
    a) The recipient bed has poor blood supply
    b) A tendon crosses the recipient bed
    c) The wound is in a weight bearing area
    d) All of the above
    e) None of the above

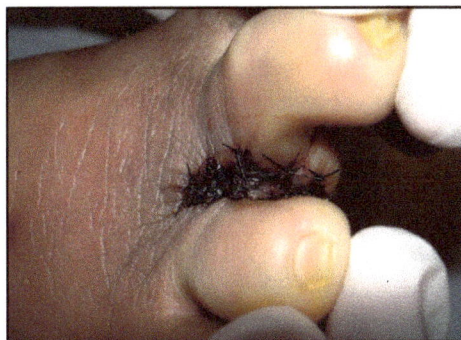

Figure 33.6 A 50-year-old patient with type 2 DM with necrosis of the incision line of a third toe amputation.

F. A 50-year-old male smoker with type 2 DM, end stage renal disease (ESRD), and peripheral vascular disease (PVD) undergoes bypass surgery and a third toe amputation due to gangrene. Subsequent to surgery the patient develops necrosis of the incision line. You are asked to assess this patient and take the ABI as a part of your evaluation (Figure 33.6).

17. The right ABI can best be accurately calculated by:
    a) Dividing the higher right ankle pressure (whether DP or PT) by the systolic pressure from whichever arm gives the higher reading
    b) Dividing the highest brachial diastolic pressure by ankle pressure
    c) Dividing the higher of the two systolic pressures on both arms by ankle pressure
    d) Subtracting two systolic pressures of both arms and divide by ankle pressure

18. All of the following are risk factors for developing arterial ulcers in this patient except:
    a) Smoking
    b) Diabetes mellitus
    c) Hypercholesterolemia
    d) Hypertension
    e) Alcohol use

19. A patient asks you about anodyne therapy to improve circulation. You review the evidence for anodyne therapy for PVD and you find multiple studies. The hierarchy of strength of evidence for treatment decisions includes which of the following?
    a) Systematic reviews of randomized clinical trials
    b) Physiologic studies
    c) Cohort studies
    d) Single randomized clinical trial
    e) All of the above

20. Implementing a palliative wound care plan would be most appropriate for which of the following patients?
    a) A diabetic, ESRD patient with multiple calciphylactic wounds undergoing hyperbaric oxygen therapy
    b) A patient with 10 years of recurrent ulceration secondary to lymphedema and venous stasis
    c) A cachectic nursing home resident with protein calorie malnutrition despite tube feeding, with a stage IV sacral pressure ulcer
    d) A morbidly obese patient whose post-operative bariatric surgery has been complicated by a large, non-healing surgical wound and an enterocutaneous fistula

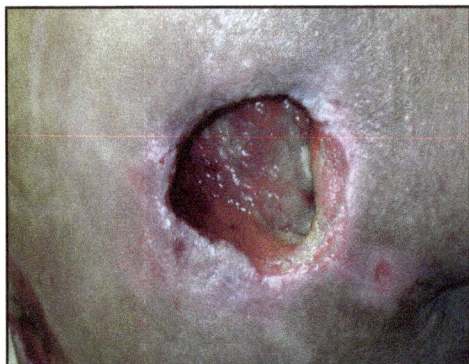

Figure 33.7: A 58-year-old diabetic patient with a pressure ulcer.

G. A 58-year-old female with a history of type 2 DM, ESRD, and paraparesis subsequent to a gunshot wound has developed a pressure ulcer. The wound is 6 × 6 cm with undermining of 3 cm from the 12 to 4 o'clock position. There is 90% granulation tissue and moderate serosanguinous drainage (Figure 33.7).

21. Based on the description and picture, what is the NPUAP stage of this patient's wound?
    a) Stage I pressure ulcer
    b) Stage II pressure ulcer
    c) Stage III pressure ulcer
    d) Stage IV pressure ulcer

22. Which of the following dressing choices would be most appropriate for this patient?
    a) Impregnated gauze
    b) Hydrocolloid dressings
    c) Alginate dressings
    d) Growth factor therapy

23. The preferred biochemical indicator of protein status in this patient is:
    a) Albumin level
    b) Transferrin level
    c) Prealbumin level
    d) Vitamin K level

24. This patient weighs 125 pounds, has poor appetite, and has a prealbumin level of 20 mg/dL. This patient's recommended daily protein requirement is:
    a) 55-115 gm
    b) 68-107 gm
    c) 68-85 gm
    d) 85-113 gm

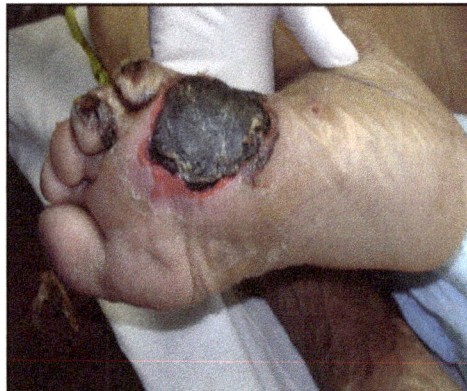

Figure 33.8: An 82-year-old nursing home patient with multiple pressure ulcers and gangrene of the foot.

H. An 82-year-old nursing home patient with right hemiparesis secondary to a stroke and a history of type 2 DM, hypertension (HTN), PVD, and CAD presents with multiple pressure ulcers and gangrene of the foot. On examination she has severe contractures and no palpable peripheral pulse (Figure 33.8).

25. Which of the following management strategies would constitute palliative care in this patient?
    a) Wet-to-dry dressing changes every four hours around the clock
    b) Calcium alginate dressings used on a necrotic appearing wound with minimal exudate
    c) Silver impregnated dressing
    d) Betadine dressing to keep the wound dry

26. You are assessing the pain level in this patient. Which of the findings below most accurately reflects the level of pain that the patient has been experiencing between visits?
    a) It is an objective finding based on the patient's vital signs, including pulse, heart rate, and blood pressure.
    b) It is whatever the patient describes as his or her level of pain.
    c) It is whether or not the patient is able to sleep.
    d) It is the degree of pain the patient experiences during wound care.

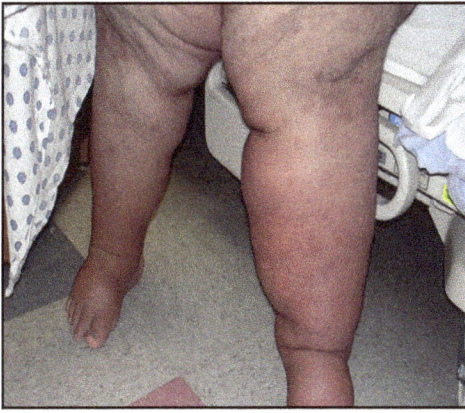

Figure 33.9: A 36-year-old patient with swelling of both legs.

I. A 36-year-old female presents with a history of morbid obesity, cleft palate, and bilateral leg swelling, with the left leg greater than the right leg (Figure 33.9).

27. What clinical sign will differentiate between lymphedema and lipedema?
    a) Stemmer's sign
    b) Homan's sign
    c) Patch testing sign
    d) Koebner phenomenon

28. If this patient is diagnosed with lymphedema what will be the standard of care?
    a) Unna's boots
    b) Lymphedema pump
    c) Complete decongestive therapy
    d) Bandaging

29. The number of neutrophils in the wound is decreased by:
    a) 2-3 days
    b) 3-7 days
    c) 7-10 days
    d) 10-14 days

30. A 60-year-old diabetic male develops a small wound (2 × 3 cm) on the dorsal aspect of the foot. There is moderate greenish drainage that has a fruity odor. The wound is cultured for aerobes/anaerobes. After the cultures, which of the following antibiotics would be the most appropriate empiric choice?
    a) Tetracycline
    b) Doxycycline
    c) Clindamycin
    d) Ciprofloxacin
    e) Augmentin

31. Which of the following patients is at the highest risk for developing a pressure ulcer?
    a) A 70-year-old type 2 DM male whose left hip replacement surgery took more than five hours, and is now on an orthopedic bed that limits movement
    b) A 40-year-old female with morbid obesity subsequent to gastric bypass surgery
    c) A 60-year-old male with type 2 DM, HTN, and prior CHF now admitted with another episode of decompensated heart failure.
    d) An 80-year-old male with a history of dementia admitted to hospital with a change in mental status

32. A 60-year-old diabetic male has wound (2 × 4 cm) on the planter aspect of his foot. In this patient, removing or debriding periwound callus will help with wound healing by:
    a) Decreasing periwound pressure
    b) Increasing wound margins
    c) Decreasing the bacterial bioburden
    d) Increasing growth factors

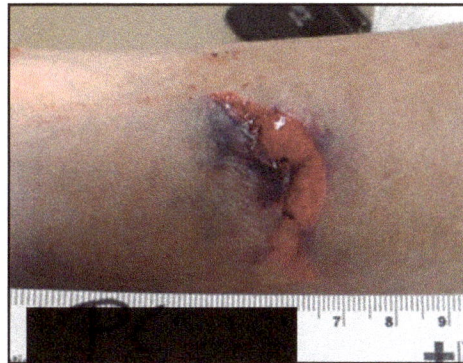

Figure 33.10: An 87-year-old nursing home patient with a wound on her left forearm.

J. An 87-year-old female nursing home patient with a history of multiple falls is referred for consult on the left forearm wound as shown in Figure 33.10.

33. What is the etiology of this wound?
    a) Trauma
    b) Diabetes
    c) Infection
    d) Pressure

34. What is the Payne-Martin category of skin tear?
    a) Category I
    b) Category II
    c) Category III

35. What would be the most appropriate treatment?
    a) Topical film
    b) Calcium alginate
    c) Foam
    d) Any of the above

K. General questions

36. A 37-year-old female with a history of Crohn's disease has a 5 × 7 cm ulcer with a necrotic center and undermined edges on her right leg. The most likely diagnosis would be:
    a) Vasculitis
    b) Pyoderma gangrenosum
    c) Necrobiosis lipoidica
    d) Arterial ulcer

37. When testing for neuropathy on a patient who cannot feel anything, what amount of pressure would be considered the limit for protective sensation?
    a) 5 gm
    b) 10 gm
    c) 15 gm
    d) 20 gm

38. A 40-year-old female with a history of lupus has severe pain from an ulcer on her left lower extremity. There is no sign of infection, but her pain is increasing. What is the best initial management of the wound?
    a) Topical steroids
    b) Systemic steroids
    c) Topical antibacterial cream
    d) Systemic antibiotics

39. Types of collagen seen in dermis and during wound healing are:
    a) I and III
    b) I, II, and III
    c) II and III
    d) I and II

40. A 12-year-old male is seen in the wound center for full thickness burns of his left forearm and hand. What is the most appropriate course of action?
    a) Apply cellular and/or tissue based products (CTPs)
    b) Apply foam
    c) Apply silver sulfadiazine
    d) Refer the patient to a burn center

41. What is the recurrence rate of a diabetic neuropathic foot ulcer that healed within six weeks of total contact casting?
    a) 0-10 %
    b) 10-20%
    c) 20-30%
    d) >30%

42. Which of the following statements about venous stasis ulcers is true?
    a) The amputation rate is <2%.
    b) Compression therapy is a mainstay in the treatment of venous stasis ulcer.
    c) As compared to compression bandaging alone, corrective venous surgery plus compression bandaging does not quicken the healing of a currently existing ulcer.
    d) As compared to compression bandaging alone, corrective venous surgery plus compression bandaging reduces the recurrence of ulcers at four years and results in a greater proportion of ulcer-free time.
    e) All of the above

43. In a study of two groups of patients, one group receives hyperbaric oxygen therapy and one group does not. What is this type of study called?
    a) A cohort study
    b) A case study
    c) A randomized controlled trial
    d) A prospective study

44. Which of the following statements about biofilms is true?
    a) Biofilms are multicellular bacterial communities that arise on mucosal or exposed surfaces.
    b) Biofilm associated bacteria have different phenotypic characteristic and genetic expression studies.
    c) Biofilm associated bacteria have longer doubling times.
    d) All of the above statements are true.

45. Fetal healing occurs without scarring because of:
    a) Regeneration
    b) Proliferation
    c) Migration
    d) Epithelialization

46. Growth factors work on non-healing chronic wounds by:
    a) Decreasing MMPs
    b) Decreasing enzymes
    c) Attaching to the target cell receptors of viable cells
    d) Decreasing bacterial bioburden

47. The most important cells in the proliferative phase are:
    a) Keratinocytes
    b) Epithelial cells
    c) Fibroblasts
    d) Endothelial cells

48. A 60-year-old male with a diabetic wound on the right leg is advised to get his fasting blood glucose level <200 mg/dL, which would help with healing by:
    a) Improving neutrophil function for phagocytosis
    b) Decreasing necrosis
    c) Decreasing infection
    d) Decreasing MMPs
    e) Increasing function of growth factors

49. Which of the following is a function of keratinocytes?
    a) They release MMPs and growth factors.
    b) They help in thermoregulation.
    c) They provide protection against infection.
    d) They migrate into new tissue to form capillary structures.

50. Which is a function of the endothelial cells?
    a) They secrete growth factors and stimulate production of fibronectin and collagen.
    b) They help in deposition of extracellular matrix.
    c) They convert immature type III collagen into type I dermal collagen.
    d) They secrete MMPs.

51. Which of following wounds will heal mainly by contraction?
    a) A facial wound subsequent to dermal abrasion
    b) An abdominal wound left open to heal
    c) A left great toe amputation subsequent to primary closure
    d) A superficial 2 × 2 cm wound on the right pre-tibial region

52. In the list below, the most appropriate antibiotic for a patient with a MRSA wound infection and cellulitis is:
    a) Vancomycin
    b) Cefepime
    c) Imipenem
    d) Ceftriaxone

53. A 70-year-old female has a 3 × 4 cm wound on her right leg. A Gram stain of the seropurulent discharge shows gram-positive cocci in chains. What is the most likely organism?
    a) *Streptococcus*
    b) *Staphylococcus*
    c) *Actinomyces israelii*
    d) *Pseudomonas*

54. Which nerve will be involved while debriding a deep wound of the posterolateral ankle?
    a) Peroneal nerve
    b) Tibial nerve
    c) Sural nerve
    d) Fibular nerve

55. What is an example of semi-occlusive dressing?
    a) Derma GeL®
    b) AQUACEL® Ag
    c) DuoDERM®
    d) SilvaSorb® Gel

56. An acute long term facility patient has a stage IV ischial wound covered with necrotic slough. Before you do bedside debridement on this patient, what is the most appropriate first step for pain management?
    a) Apply a mixture of 4% lidocaine gel and protamine gel on the wound bed.
    b) Apply a 1% lidocaine gel to the wound bed.
    c) Administer two tablets of ibuprofen one hour before the procedure.
    d) Apply lidocaine spray just before debridement.

57. All of the following are common side effects of radiation therapy on skin except:
    a) Decrease in sebaceous glands, causing dryness of the skin
    b) Alteration of skin pigmentation
    c) Flaking or peeling (dry desquamation)
    d) Decrease in erythema

58. Colonization is defined as:
    a) A microorganism on the surface of a wound and not multiplying
    b) A microorganism on the surface of a wound multiplying with invasion of tissues
    c) A microorganism on the surface of a wound multiplying with no host immune response
    d) A microorganism on the surface of a wound multiplying with host immune response

59. Epibole is:
    a) Rolled-in edges
    b) Often seen in chronic wounds with poor healing dynamics
    c) When the migrating form of epithelial cells is unable to cover the wound cavity, they descend and curl under the edges
    d) All of the above

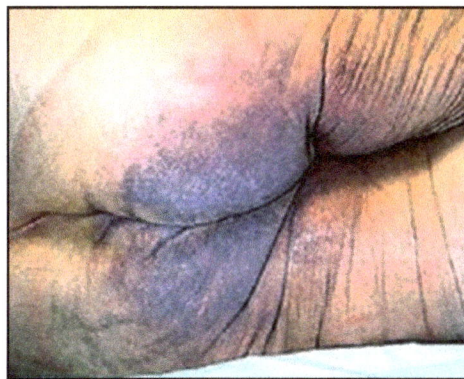

Figure 33.11: Pressure ulcer in need of staging.

60. What would be the NPUAP pressure ulcer stage illustrated in Figure 33.11?
    a) Stage I
    b) Unstageable
    c) Suspected deep tissue injury
    d) Stage III

61. Which method of swab culture has the best chance of identifying the organism causing a wound infection?
    a) Levine technique
    b) Z-technique
    c) Pathergy
    d) Wound biopsy

62. Which water soluble vitamin is helpful for collagen synthesis?
    a) Vitamin A
    b) Vitamin B complex
    c) Vitamin C
    d) Vitamin E

63. Which of the following statements is true regarding pressure ulcer prevention scales?
    a) A Braden scale score of 10 is considered high risk for ulceration.
    b) The Braden scale includes an evaluation of the nursing home staff needed to treat high risk patients prone to ulceration.
    c) The Waterlow scale is mentioned in the AHCPR guidelines.
    d) The Gosnell scale is the most commonly used pressure ulcer assessment scale.

64. What is the most important factor for preventing ulceration in patients with sickle cell disease?
    a) Using moisturizer
    b) Edema control
    c) Off-loading
    d) Restricting dietary iron intake

65. Which of the following causes the greatest risk for developing lymphedema?
    a) Malignancy
    b) Venous stasis ulcer
    c) Diabetes
    d) Pyoderma gangrenosum

66. A patient with long-standing diabetes has had the same leg ulcer for 10 years. What is your primary concern?
    a) This patient may have Marjolin's ulcer.
    b) This patient may have basal cell cancer.
    c) This patient may have vasculitis.
    d) There may be an underlying infection.

67. All of the following are options for lymphedema treatment except:
    a) Exercise
    b) Compression wrapping
    c) Venous valve surgery
    d) Manual lymph drainage

68. All of the following statements about pneumatic compression devices are true except:
    a) They are usually recommended at pressures of 40-60 mmHg for one to four hours daily.
    b) They are contraindicated in patients with anasarca.
    c) They can be used in patients with ulcers if sterile dressing is placed on the ulcer.
    d) They can be safely used in patients with compensated congestive heart failure.

69. A 50-year-old diabetic male complains of calf pain after walking two blocks. The pain gets better with rest. This patient probably has:
    a) Partial occlusion of superficial femoral artery
    b) Complete occlusion of superficial femoral artery
    c) Spinal stenosis at the L4-L5 level
    d) Diabetic neuropathic pain

70. All of the following statements about vascular assessment in diabetic patients are true except:
    a) ABI can be falsely elevated in diabetic patients.
    b) Toe-brachial index is more accurate than ABI in diabetics.
    c) An ABI of >1.2 is considered non-compressible.
    d) A toe pressure of 20 mmHg indicates adequate circulation.

71. A transcutaneous oxygen study is most appropriate in which of these patients?
    a) A 78-year-old female with a non-healing venous stasis ulcer of the right leg
    b) A 60-year-old diabetic male with PVD and a dorsal foot wound that has not healed in more than four weeks
    c) A 38-year-old male with deep full thickness burns on the left forearm
    d) A 50-year-old male with lymphedema on the left leg and a refractory non-healing ulcer on that calf

72. A magnetic resonance angiogram (MRA) has an advantage over a traditional angiogram because of all of the following except:
    a) In MRA there is no arterial puncture.
    b) There is less likelihood of renal complications with dye.
    c) It is safe in patients with dye allergies.
    d) It provides a better diagnostic study than a traditional angiogram.

73. Bone biopsy is considered the gold standard in diagnosing osteomyelitis, but what is the most common disadvantage with this procedure?
    a) It could cause a fracture.
    b) It could introduce an infection (organism) into normal bone.
    c) It may cause sudden ischemia.
    d) It can lead to profuse bleeding and death.

74. A 25-year-old male develops a thermal injury on the left forearm. On exam, the patient's skin is dry, insensate, waxy, and leathery in consistency. What is the depth of the burn?
   a) First degree
   b) Second degree
   c) Third degree
   d) Fourth degree

75. A patient with a terminal illness suddenly develops a pear-shaped ulcer on the sacrum. This patient probably has:
   a) Homan's sign
   b) A Kennedy ulcer
   c) Deep tissue injury
   d) An intensive care unit ulcer

76. Which one of the following procedures is mechanical debridement?
   a) Application of collagenase
   b) Application of DuoDERM®
   c) Application of negative pressure wound therapy
   d) Wet-to-dry dressing

77. When taking the left ABI, at which arteries is the pulse checked?
   a) Left femoral artery or left popliteal artery
   b) Left popliteal artery or left dorsalis pedis artery
   c) Both brachial arteries and the left posterior tibial artery or left dorsalis pedis artery
   d) Left dorsalis pedis artery or left posterior tibial artery

78. An 85-year-old female with a history of DM, non-bypassable PVD, severe dementia, and end stage colon cancer has developed gangrene of the great toe. The patient has selected to receive palliative care. What would be the best treatment option?
   a) Application of collagenase to gangrenous area
   b) Podiatry consult for debridement or amputation
   c) Vascular consult to improve blood flow
   d) Application of betadine to gangrenous area

79. In which of the following patients would primary closure not be recommended?
   a) A 60-year-old patient with type 2 DM who presents with an abscess on the dorsal aspect of her foot
   b) A 30-year-old male intravenous drug abuser (IVDA) with a history of hepatitis C who presents with a progressive necrotizing infection of his left thigh
   c) A 50-year-old female with a history of diabetes now presenting with a carbuncle on her back
   d) All of the above

80. Which is the best tool for the irrigation, debridement, and cleaning of a wound?
   a) Whirlpool
   b) Pulsed lavage
   c) Ultrasound
   d) Infrared therapy

81. What is the recommended pressure for irrigation while doing pulsed lavage?
   a) 0-4 psi
   b) 4-15 psi
   c) 15-21 psi
   d) >21 psi

82. A 50-year-old diabetic patient has a 2 × 2 cm non-healing wound on the left great toe. The patient has a right ABI of 1.2 and a left ABI of 1.4. What do the ABI results suggest?
   a) The patient has normal circulation.
   b) The patient has microvascular disease.
   c) The patient has macrovascular disease.
   d) The ABI results do not give enough information.

83. When applying a multilayer long stretch dressing, the pressure developed beneath any bandage is the sub-bandage pressure. Which of the following statements about sub-bandage pressure is true?
   a) Sub-bandage pressure is directly proportional to the bandage tension and radius of curvature of the limb.
   b) Sub-bandage pressure is inversely proportional to the bandage tension and radius of curvature of the limb.
   c) Sub-bandage pressure is directly proportional to the bandage tension and inversely proportional to the radius of curvature of the limb.
   d) Sub-bandage pressure is inversely proportional to the bandage tension and directly proportional to the radius of curvature of the limb.

84. Pain that occurs to the patient repeatedly because of dressing changes is classified as:
   a) Non-cyclic pain
   b) Cyclic pain
   c) Background pain
   d) Chronic pain

85. All of the following are features of venous stasis ulcers except:
   a) Hemosiderin pigmentation
   b) Irregular wound edges
   c) Shallowness of ulcer
   d) Capillary refill >5 seconds

86. All of the following features are typical of arterial ulcers except:
   a) Painful wounds on toes
   b) Pale wound bed
   c) ABI <0.5
   d) History of deep vein thrombosis (DVT)

87. Fournier's gangrene:
    a) Involves the foot
    b) Is a form of necrotizing soft tissue infection
    c) Involves the perineum
    d) Involves the presacral skin
    e) Both b and c

88. Calcium alginate:
    a) Is manufactured from seaweed
    b) Causes trauma to wounds during removal
    c) Is an occlusive dressing
    d) Never causes desiccation

89. Hydrofiber is:
    a) Indicated for dry eschar
    b) A non-absorptive dressing
    c) Made from sodium carboxymethyl cellulose
    d) Made from seaweed

90. Patch testing is the gold standard for diagnosing
    a) Erythema multiforme
    b) Contact dermatitis
    c) Psoriasis
    d) Lichen planus

91. All of the following are true about negative pressure wound therapy except:
    a) It decreases edema.
    b) It decreases local blood supply.
    c) It increases granulation tissue.
    d) It may decrease bacterial colonization.

92. Weight loss is considered significant or severe if the patient experiences:
    a) >10% weight loss in six months
    b) 5% weight loss in three months
    c) 3% weight loss in one month
    d) 1% weight loss in one week

93. All of the following are risk factors for ulceration and amputation in diabetic patients except:
    a) Hypertension
    b) Hyperglycemia
    c) Age >65 years
    d) Alcohol

94. Which one of the following wounds usually gets worse with debridement?
    a) Diabetic foot ulcer
    b) Venous stasis ulcer
    c) Infected surgical wound
    d) Pyoderma gangrenosum

95. Advanced wound therapies should be considered if the wound fails standard therapy for:
    a) >4 weeks
    b) >8 weeks
    c) >12 weeks
    d) >16 weeks

96. A patient with an ABI of 0.4 states that a total contact cast (TCC) for off-loading was recommended to him. The healthcare provider explains that:
    a) Total contact cast is a good choice for treatment of his diabetic foot.
    b) He cannot receive total contact cast as it is contraindicated with his ABI.
    c) He will not be able to use any off-loading technique due to his ABI.
    d) He can be started on another off-loading device and gradually change to a total contact cast.

97. After starting total contact casting for diabetic neuropathic wounds, what are the chances of healing?
    a) 40%
    b) 50%
    c) 75%
    d) 90%

98. Which of the patients below is most likely to have an inflammatory wound?
    a) A 35-year-old female with a history of chronic lymphedema
    b) A 40-year-old female with a history of scleroderma
    c) A 78-year-old male with a history of pressure ulcers
    d) A 50-year-old-male with history of Kaposi sarcoma

99. A punch or deep wedge biopsy is taken from the central part of the ulcer and sent for culture. By performing this biopsy, we are evaluating for a possibility of:
    a) Pyoderma gangrenosum
    b) Autoimmune blistering
    c) Small vessel vasculitis
    d) Squamous cell cancer

100. What spectral band of ultraviolet light has been demonstrated to be bactericidal?
    a) UVA
    b) UVB
    c) UVC
    d) UVD

101. Optimal wound healing requires:
    a) A phase of acute inflammation
    b) A phase of chronic inflammation
    c) The right amount of moisture
    d) Leaving the wound open so that it can be kept dry
    e) Both a and c

102. In the Wagner scale for diabetic foot ulcers, the hierarchy of severity is broken down into:
    a) Grades
    b) Stages
    c) Levels
    d) Degrees

103. All of the following are from the AHRQ guidelines for pressure ulcer prevention except:
    a) Maintaining elevation of the head of the bed at 45 degrees or less if medical status permits.
    b) Using pillows or wedges to separate bony prominences.
    c) Turning or repositioning the patient's body at least every two hours.
    d) Keeping the patient's heel protected and elevated off the surface of the bed.

104. In the NPUAP scale for pressure ulcers, the hierarchy of severity is broken down into:
    a) Grades
    b) Stages
    c) Levels
    d) Degrees

105. In terms of depth of tissue affected, a Wagner grade 2 foot ulcer is defined as a:
    a) Deep ulcer in which bone, tendon, or ligament may be exposed
    b) Deep ulcer with abscess, tendon infection and/or osteomyelitis
    c) Deep ulcer with gangrene
    d) Superficial ulcer that does not penetrate into the subcutaneous tissue layer

106. A 68-year-old female has a 1 cm ulcer of the anterior lower left extremity a few centimeters above the level of the malleoli. It is just lateral to the tibia, and the wound bed is covered with fibrinous exudate. Debridement is performed with a curette, revealing viable tendon at the base of the wound. What is the proper designation of this procedure?
    a) Surgical debridement
    b) Autolytic debridement
    c) Mechanical debridement
    d) Biologic debridement

107. A 2-year-old male presents with a scald burn in a glove pattern involving the right hand and forearm halfway to the elbow. His work up and care should include which of the following?
    a) Treatment at a burn center
    b) Immediate skin grafting
    c) Temporary dialysis
    d) Notifying social services of potential child abuse

108. Which of the following injuries should be treated at a burn center?
    a) Burns of >10% TBSA in patients under 10 years old
    b) Burns of >10% TBSA in patients over 50 years old
    c) Any second or third degree burns involving the hands or feet
    d) Any second or third degree burns involving the perineum
    e) All of the above

109. A 72-year-old female has type 2 DM, which has long been complicated by peripheral neuropathy. For years she has had no feeling in her feet, and whenever she needs debridement of a foot ulcer she declines analgesia, including topical lidocaine. Yet today, she presents with left foot pain, which has gradually gotten worse over the past three days. She has a low-grade fever, her pulse is regular with a normal rate, and her lungs are clear. On the left heel, she has a 2 × 3 cm plantar ulcer with slough at the base, moderate exudate, and surrounding erythema and warmth. The left ABI is 0.8. Given this presentation, what diagnosis is most likely?
    a) Arthritis of the ankle
    b) Acute Charcot arthropathy
    c) Diabetic foot infection
    d) Arterial embolism

110. What is an abnormal toe-brachial index (TBI)?
    a) >0.9
    b) >0.8
    c) <0.7
    d) >0.7

111. An obese 52-year-old male has had long-standing venous disease of the lower extremities. Over the years, he has had a few ulcerations that healed within a month. However, he now reports that his wound has been open for four months, and does not seem to be healing. There is no exposed bone. What diagnostic technique should you now consider?
    a) Split thickness skin graft
    b) Biopsy of the wound margin
    c) Full thickness skin graft
    d) MRI to look for osteomyelitis

112. The Parkland formula for burn resuscitation stipulates which of the following?
    a) Ringer's lactate 4 ml/kg of body weight/percent of total TBSA for second and third degree burns; half to be given in the first eight hours after arrival at the hospital and the remaining half to be distributed over the next 16 hours.
    b) Normal saline 4 ml/kg of body weight/percent of total TBSA for second and third degree burns; half to be given in the first eight hours after arrival at the hospital and the remaining half to be distributed over the next 16 hours.
    c) Ringer's lactate 4 ml/kg of body weight/percent of total TBSA for second and third degree burns; half to be given in the first eight hours after injury and the remaining half to be distributed over the next 16 hours.
    d) Normal saline 4 ml/kg of body weight/percent of total TBSA for second and third degree burns; half to be given in the first eight hours after injury, and the remaining half to be distributed over the next 16 hours.

113. In the PQRST mnemonic for eliciting a careful pain history, what does the "P" stand for?
　　a) Provocative factors
　　b) Palliative factors
　　c) Pressure factors
　　d) Both a and b

114. Which of the following statements about pain is true?
　　a) Observable changes in vital signs are not required to verify a patient's report of severe pain.
　　b) A patient who can sleep may nonetheless be experiencing moderate to severe pain.
　　c) Analgesics for chronic pain are more effective when administered around-the-clock rather than only as needed.
　　d) The fact that a patient can be distracted from the pain does not indicate that he has less pain than he reports.
　　e) All of the above statements are true.

115. What is the role of ACE™ bandages and T.E.D.™ hose in the compression-wrap treatment of most venous ulcers?
　　a) They are best for patients with lipodermatosclerosis.
　　b) They are best for patients with hyperpigmentation.
　　c) They are best for patients without ulceration.
　　d) None of the above

116. A 76-year-old nursing home resident has been treated for a stage IV sacral pressure ulcer during the past four months. After a multidisciplinary approach coordinated by wound care specialists, all that remains is a 1 cm granulating wound that is 1 mm deep. Now that this patient's ulcer is nearly healed, what is the correct designation of its NPUAP Staging?
　　a) Stage I
　　b) Stage II
　　c) Stage III
　　d) Stage IV
　　e) None of the above

117. During hospitalization, if a patient develops a stage III or IV pressure ulcer that wasn't present on admission, CMS regards this as:
　　a) A hospital-acquired condition (HAC) for which the hospital may receive a payment supplemental to the DRG payment
　　b) A hospital-acquired condition (HAC) for which the hospital cannot receive supplemental payment
　　c) A serious, preventable event
　　d) Both b and c

118. The imaging technology most sensitive and specific for diagnosing osteomyelitis in patients with diabetes and foot ulcers is:
　　a) CT scan
　　b) 4-D CT scan
　　c) MRI
　　d) Color Doppler ultrasound
　　e) X-ray with at least two views

119. What is the definition of full thickness skin loss?
　　a) Loss of both epidermis and dermis only
　　b) Loss of all tissue normally overlying muscle, bone, or tendon
　　c) The part of skin sacrificed as the tumor margin in an excisional skin biopsy
　　d) A sacral ulcer deep enough to reveal presacral fascia in its base

120. Normal skin-surface pH is:
　　a) Acidic: 4.5 to 5.5
　　b) Alkaline: 7.8 to 8.8
　　c) Neutral: 7.2 to 7.6
　　d) It largely depends on ambient temperature

121. Faced with a patient's worsening stage III or IV pressure ulcer, despite optimum body positioning and turning frequency, the clinician should next consider:
　　a) The off-loading adequacy of the patient's bed and mattress
　　b) The patient's continence status and its management
　　c) Surgical consultation for potential repair by a graft or flap operation
　　d) Initiating hyperbaric oxygen therapy
　　e) Answers a, b, and c

L. A 62-year-old female with type 2 DM, CAD, and stage 3 chronic kidney disease (CKD) presents with a 1.5 cm plantar ulcer under the metatarsal head of her left great toe. The ulcer rim has considerable callus.

122. What is the most likely etiology of this ulcer?
　　a) Venous insufficiency
　　b) Arterial insufficiency
　　c) Diabetic neuropathy
　　d) Pyoderma gangrenosum

123. Which of the physical findings below is more likely to be seen in foot ulcer patients who have diabetes versus foot ulcer patients who do not have diabetes?
　　a) Hyperpigmentation in the gaiter area of the leg
　　b) Decreased femoral pulse
　　c) Loss of dermal appendages in the foot
　　d) A positive Semmes-Weinstein test

124. As part of this patient's complete physical exam you check her femoral, popliteal, dorsalis pedis, and posterior tibial artery pulses. Which of the following noninvasive vascular studies should be done next?
    a) Ultrasound of the arteries
    b) Ultrasound of the veins
    c) CT angiogram
    d) ABI

125. What wound care principle underlies the approach to healing this woman's ulcer?
    a) Compression with a four layer wrap
    b) Off-loading
    c) Whirlpool therapy
    d) Callus debridement
    e) Both b and d

M. A 63-year-old diabetic male's brachial BP is 150 mmHg in both arms. In his left foot, only the posterior tibial artery pulse is detectable by Doppler. While collecting data to calculate the left ABI, you find that the posterior tibial artery pulse on that side remains audible even when the ankle blood pressure cuff is inflated to 250 mmHg. In other words, his only audible left pedal artery is non-compressible.

126. What number should you report as this patient's left ABI?
    a) 0
    b) 1
    c) Unable to be determined
    d) Whatever you calculate for his right ABI

127. Other noninvasive tests that might be helpful to get a better idea of this patient's lower left extremity perfusion include which of the following?
    a) Homans' Sign
    b) Stemmer's Sign
    c) Toe-brachial index
    d) TcPO$_2$
    e) Both c and d

N. A 72-year-old male with CAD and a long smoking history has an apparently mixed arterial-venous ulcer of the right lower extremity. However, while completing your physical examination, you discover an exaggerated popliteal pulse on the left side.

128. What potential diagnosis must you be concerned about on the left side?
    a) Venous hypertension
    b) Popliteal aneurysm
    c) Secondary lymphedema
    d) Venous incompetence with varicose veins

129. What are the most important potential complications to know about this condition?
    a) Arterial embolism, resulting in acute ischemia in distal parts of the limb
    b) Arterial thrombosis, threatening the entire distal limb
    c) Fatigue when ambulating beyond a certain distance
    d) Chronic pain
    e) Both a and b

130. Now that you have found a popliteal pulse that you think is abnormally prominent, what should you do next?
    a) Follow up with the patient every six months.
    b) Have the patient call you if he develops symptoms.
    c) Request a diagnostic ultrasound.
    d) Refer the patient to a vascular surgeon for evaluation.
    e) Either c or d

See answers on page 318.

ANSWER KEY

1. c) For patients who are unable to tolerate fixed compression stockings, such as class 3 or 4 stockings, or for patients with chronic lymphedema, alternative compression wraps shown in the picture (Farrow wrap) or CircAid® wrap could be used as a maintenance therapy for control of edema.

2. e) The FarrowWrap® or CircAid® Wrap have multiple overlapping layers of short stretch bandaging with Velcro® such that the compression can be applied to the length of the limb according to patient tolerance. These devices have a low resting pressure and a high working pressure, as do all low stretch options. In addition, they can be applied in patients with ulcers. Stockings and high stretch bandages can cause ischemia because they have a high resting pressure and a low working pressure.

3. d) Once cancer is suspected, the next step is a dermatology referral and incisional biopsy. Observing for changes in ABCDE is mainly for melanoma. A dermatology referral is most appropriate as this patient should most likely receive local therapy.

4. b) This patient has nodular basal cell cancer, which is the most common skin ulcer malignancy. Basal cell cancer, also called rodent ulcer, arises from epidermal basal cells while squamous cell cancer arises from keratinizing epidermal cells.

5. c) This patient has chronic Charcot arthropathy but is presenting with clinical signs of infection: low-grade fever, seropurulent drainage, and exposed bone. This patient most likely has cellulitis, and possibly osteomyelitis as well.

6. d) Although any closed space, undrained infection requires adequate and early drainage, this patient's wound is at least partially draining already, which is consistent with her history of subacute, rather than urgent, presentation. Among the choices given, the most reasonable first step is to culture the wound and start antibiotics. However, note that there are a few fine points for best accomplishing wound cultures. The drainage from tunneled wounds is notorious for giving rise to cultures not representative of the actual deep tissue infection. A classic mistake is to take a swab culture of such drainage, and then start empiric antibiotics, making later identification of the true pathogens more difficult. Instead, take the following steps: prep and drape the area as you would for a sterile procedure. Then determine if there is an abscess from which you can sample pus. If so, aspirate some of the abscess's pus into a syringe, thoroughly expel the air, safety-cap the syringe, and send it off for Gram stain and culture. This technique allows for the responsible culturing of anaerobes as well as aerobes, and its clinical yield is superior to any type of Q-tip or swab culture. In the setting with no abscess pus to sample, a qualified colleague should explore the wound, unroofing superficial detritus as appropriate. Then take samples of the deeper infected tissue, and place them in a sterile jar with saline. Request Gram stain and culture. Note that even a 3mm piece of tissue collected this way can be processed for anaerobes as well as aerobes. Having thus secured the best sample possible for the clinical context, you have now cleared the way for starting an empiric antibiotic regimen.

7. e) An empiric regimen for starting antibiotics depends on the patient's allergies, the extent of renal dysfunction, previous antibiotic therapy, and known local antibiotic sensitivity pattern. It does not depend on HbA1c, a test that evaluates long term control of a patient's diabetes, which is not a factor when choosing antibiotics.

8. a) The most common organism isolated in diabetic foot infections is *Staphylococcus aureus*.

9. e) When confronted with a moderate to severe diabetic foot infection, empiric antibiotics should be administered by IV (not orally), because such patients are at high risk of either limb loss or death. In terms of coverage, an empiric regimen for a moderate to severe diabetic foot infection should cover at least MRSA and strep. If inflammation extends to the fascia, adding coliform coverage is appropriate; if there is systemic toxicity, further adding anaerobic coverage is appropriate. Choice (e) would be appropriate for moderate or mild diabetic foot infection, but not appropriate for severe diabetic foot infection, for two reasons: this regimen is PO, and clindamycin is not sufficiently useful against non-community-acquired MRSA. All of the other regimens listed cover strep, hospital- and community-acquired MRSA, as well as a reasonable number of gram-negative and anaerobic organisms.

10. d) Based on the image showing full thickness tissue loss and visible subcutaneous tissue, but no exposed bone, tendon, or muscle, the patient has a NPUAP stage III pressure ulcer. In stage III pressure ulcers slough may be present, but it is not enough to obscure the depth of tissue loss. Undermining and tunneling may also be present.

11. b) Static support surfaces are recommended for patients with a low risk of developing pressure ulcer (refer to Chapter 32, Selection of Support Surfaces Pathway).

12. d) Pressure reduction can be accomplished in this patient by all of the choices except raising the head of the bed to 45 degrees. In order to minimize shear forces over the ischial tuberosities and presacral area, when the patient is not eating, head elevation should

be limited to 30 degrees or less. In addition, pressure reduction is optimized by turning the patient at least every two hours, placing pillows under the calves to suspend the heels off of all surfaces, and by positioning the patient properly.

13. c) This patient has monophasic flow in dorsalis pedis with an ABI of <0.4, both of which suggest the patient has severe lower extremity ischemia.

14. b) A transcutaneous oxygen study may show elevated oxygen (above normal) if there is leak under the fixation ring. Usually in patients with active infection, acute edema, and thick or sclerotic skin, the tissue will be hypoxic and the oxygen values will be below normal.

15. a) Transcutaneous oxygen sensors help to determine oxygen tension of skin and effectively evaluate the adequacy of skin perfusion.

16. d) A flap is indicated in all three scenarios: when the recipient bed has poor blood supply, when a tendon crosses the wound bed, and when the wound is in a weight-bearing area.

17. a) The left ankle-brachial index (ABI) is calculated by dividing the higher systolic ankle pressure (whether left dorsalis pedis or left posterior tibial pressure) by the higher of the two systolic arm pressures. The right ABI is calculated by dividing the higher systolic ankle pressure on that side (whether right dorsalis pedis or right posterior tibial pressure) by the same systolic arm pressure used as the denominator for the left ABI. Note that at least for the feet, systolic pressures are measured with the aid of a Doppler.

18. e) Smoking, diabetes mellitus, hypercholesterolemia, and hypertension are all known risk factors for the development of atherosclerosis and arterial ulcers. Alcohol (one to two drinks a day) has been considered protective for atherosclerosis and is not a risk factor in the development of arterial ulcers.

19. e) The hierarchy of evidence of treatment decisions will include a systematic review of randomized clinical trials, a single randomized clinical trial, physiologic studies, and cohort studies.

20. c) Depending on further case details, a palliative wound care plan could be indicated for all of the patients listed. However, palliative care would be most appropriate for the patient in a nursing home with a stage IV sacral ulcer, cachexia, and severe protein calorie malnutrition while on tube feeding. This patient has a high risk for non-healing and of failure with flap closure.

21. c) In this patient, the pressure ulcer has undermining, and the wound goes all the way to the subcutaneous tissue, but bone and muscle is not exposed. This is categorized as a stage III pressure ulcer.

22. c) As this patient has moderate drainage, alginate dressing is the most appropriate dressing choice because it will help contain the exudate. Impregnated gauze would be a good dressing to keep a dry wound moist. Hydrocolloid dressings are used for patients who need autolytic debridement and have minimal exudate. Growth factor therapy is premature for this wound: at this point, the goal is exudate control.

23. c) Among all of the choices listed, prealbumin level is the best biochemical indicator of protein status. Prealbumin is the most sensitive and cost-effective method of assessing the severity of illness resulting from malnutrition in patients who are critically ill or have a chronic disease. Prealbumin levels have been shown to correlate with patient outcomes and are an accurate predictor of patient recovery. In high-risk patients, prealbumin levels, determined twice weekly during hospitalization, can alert the physician to declining nutritional status and improve patient outcome. Prealbumin's short half-life (2 days versus 20 days for albumin) gives it a more "current event" value. Albumin levels have been used as a determinant of nutritional status, but albumin is relatively insensitive to recent changes in nutrition, both because of its long half-life and large body pool. The level typically takes 14 days to return to normal when the pool has been depleted. Serum albumin concentrations are also affected by the patient's state of hydration and renal function. It is customary to test for transferrin level (instead of TIBC or UIBC) when evaluating a patient's nutritional status or liver function; however, because it is produced in the liver, transferrin will be low in patients with liver disease. Transferrin levels also drop when there is not enough protein in the diet and is used more to detect iron deficiency anemia. Vitamin K levels play a role in evaluating clotting abnormalities.

24. c) The recommended daily protein requirement is 1.2-1.5 gm/kg body weight/day. First convert pounds into kilograms. This patient weighs 125 pounds, that is, 56.8 kg (125 pounds divided by 2.2 pounds per kg = 56.8 kg). Second, multiply the kg body weight by protein requirement to obtain protein needs. For protein requirement per day at 1.2 gm/kg: 56.8 kg × 1.2 gm = 68.2 gm protein and for 1.5 gm/ kg: 56.8 kg × 1.5 gm = 85.2 gm protein, so the correct answer is (c) 68-85 gm.

25. d) This patient has multiple significant comorbidities in addition to the dry gangrene of her foot. If palliative care is considered, applying betadine to both keep the gangrenous area dry and minimize the nearby bioburden is the most appropriate management.

26. b) Pain assessment should be based on whatever patient describes as his or her level of pain. Pain level has not been correlated with patient's vital signs, ability to

sleep, or as a consequence of wound care.

27. a) The clinical sign that differentiates between lymph-edema and lipedema is the Stemmer's sign. Stemmer's sign is positive when the examiner is unable to pick up a fold of skin between his/her thumb and forefinger at the base of the second toe. If the skin can be lifted, then the Stemmer's sign is negative. Homan's sign is used to rule out deep vein thrombosis. Patch test sign is for contact dermatitis, and the Koebner phenomenon, also called the Koebner response or the isomorphic response, refers to skin lesions appearing on lines of trauma.

28. c) Complete decongestive therapy is the most acceptable and effective standard of care in the treatment of lymphedema. Unna's boots and bandaging are also useful in decreasing edema in patients with lymphedema. Lymphedema pumps may also be used for maintenance therapy in patients with chronic lymphedema.

29. a) Neutrophils are usually depleted in wounds after 2-3 days by the process of apoptosis, and they are replaced by tissue monocytes.

30. d) This patient's greenish, fruity smelling drainage is suggestive of *Pseudomonas aeruginosa* infection. Of the antibiotics listed, the only appropriate choice is ciprofloxacin, a synthetic chemotherapeutic of the fluoroquinolone drug class. The fluoroquinolones are very effective against aerobic gram-negative rods and can be useful in the treatment of *Pseudomonas* infections. In some hospital catchment areas, *Pseudomonas* clinical isolates have more often been sensitive to ciprofloxacin than to the other fluoroquinolones, but this is not always the case. What matters most is the antibiograms for the area where you practice. Clindamycin, which does not cover *Pseudomonas*, is highly effective for the treatment of gram-positive and gram-negative anaerobes. It has some effect on gram-positive aerobic activity, including some forms of streptococci, MSSA, and community-acquired MRSA; however, it is not effective against hospital-acquired MRSA or gram-negative aerobes. Tetracycline and doxycycline have a very broad spectrum of activity and are drugs of choice for chlamydia, mycoplasma, or borrelia infections, but do not cover *Pseudomonas*. Augmentin has good coverage for *E. coli*, *Proteus*, *Salmonella*, *Shigella*, gram-positive, and spirochete infections, but does not cover *Pseudomonas*.

31. a) All of the patients listed will have an increased risk of developing pressure ulcers, but the patient in choice (a) has the highest risk. This patient was immobilized during a long surgery and placed in an orthopedic bed, which further limits movement and greatly increases the risk of pressure ulcer development.

32. a) In this patient, debriding periwound callus will help with healing by decreasing periwound pressure. Any debridement may increase wound size, but the increase per se is not what assists wound healing. While debridement of a wound bed can decrease bacterial bioburden, debriding periwound callus does not. Nor will callus debridement increase growth factors, so (a) is the correct choice.

33. a) This patient developed a wound because of a fall so the primary etiology is trauma.

34. b) This patient has a Payne-Martin category II skin tear as there is 25-50% skin loss. Category I is skin tear without tissue loss, category II includes a tear with partial skin loss, and category III is skin tear with complete tissue loss.

35. d) The goals of care in the treatment of skin tear are to control bleeding, prevent infection, control pain, restore skin integrity, and promote patient comfort. There are multiple choices when treatment of skin tear is considered, including petrolatum ointment, hydrogel, collagen dressing, foam, transparent film, hydrocolloids, Telfa™, and adhesive strips. There is little published on preferred treatment, so correct answer is (d).

36. b) This 37-year-old female with history of Crohn's disease has pyoderma gangrenosum. Patients with pyoderma gangrenosum have undermined edge and central necrosis. Also, pyoderma gangrenosum is associated with Crohn's disease. Necrobiosis lipoidica is associated with diabetes. The patient does not have any risk factors for arterial disease, so arterial ulcer is very unlikely. Vasculitis usually has punched-out edges and is often associated with systemic symptoms as part of a systemic disease like lupus, rheumatoid arthritis, or other connective tissue disorder.

37. b) When testing for neuropathy, 5.07 (10 gm) monofilament gives the amount of pressure that is considered the limit for protective sensation.

38. b) This patient is experiencing increasing pain due to vasculitis and would benefit from oral steroids to decrease pain. Topical steroids will inhibit healing and will not help decrease pain. The patient has no signs of infection, so choices (c) and (d) would not be correct.

39. a) There are 19 different kinds of collagen, but during wound healing types I and III collagen are seen in the dermis. In normal skin, types I and IV are the most common collagens found in skin.

40. d) The patient has full thickness burns on the left forearm and hand. Any second or third degree burn of the hand meets criteria for referral to a burn center. Criteria for burn center referral include: burns >10% TBSA in patients under 10 years old or over 50 years

old; burns >20% in all other ages (burns of this magnitude also mandate IV fluid resuscitation); special nursing needs such as those required for burns of the face/neck/hands/feet/perineum; the need for surgery or specialized hospital care; full thickness burns needing grafting; associated injuries needing hospital care; concurrent medical conditions that either caused the burn injury (e.g., stroke while smoking) or that complicate burn care (e.g., diabetes, asthma, immune compromise); inhalation injury or other respiratory compromise; electrical burns (which can cause cardiac and/or neurological injury as well as extensive muscular injury and necrosis, compartment syndrome, or visceral injury even without visible skin injury); chemical burns with systemic toxicity; and possible child or elder abuse.

41. d) Total contact casting is an excellent tool for healing neuropathic diabetic foot ulcers, but after the wound is healed the patient has a recurrence rate of >30% due to the underlying problems of neuropathy and foot deformity.

42. e) Pure venous stasis ulcers usually have <2% chance of amputation. Compression therapy is the standard of care for venous stasis ulcer patients. The ESCHAR study showed that vein surgery does not improve venous ulcer healing rates. It also showed that as compared to compression alone, vein surgery added to compression bandaging *does* reduce the rate of ulcer recurrence at four years from 56% (compression alone) to 31% (compression plus surgical correction of superficial venous reflux; p<0.01).

43. a) A cohort study is a longitudinal study that observes two groups over time: one which gets an exposure or treatment, and another group that does not. For example, a study that looked at wound healing in smokers versus nonsmokers would be a cohort study. A cohort study could be prospective or retrospective, but in either circumstance, researchers do not decide which patients smoke. They merely compare what happens to smokers versus nonsmokers. In a case study, only one patient is reported. In a randomized controlled study, one or more groups are each exposed to a given treatment, and the research process (via randomization) assigns which similar patients get sorted into which group. Randomized controlled studies are always prospective.

44. d) All of the statements are true. Biofilms are multicellular bacterial communities that arise on mucosal or exposed surfaces. Biofilm-associated bacteria have different phenotypic characteristic (including longer doubling times) and genetic expression studies.

45. a) Fetal healing occurs without scarring because of regeneration.

46. c) Growth factors work on non-healing chronic wounds

by attaching to the target cell receptors of viable cells. Growth factors do not increase MMPs and enzymes. Increased enzymes and MMPs will delay rather than facilitate wound healing. Growth factors do not decrease bacterial bioburden.

47. c) The most important cell in the proliferative phase is the fibroblast. Endothelial cells help with neovascularization. Epithelial cells and keratinocytes are useful for epithelialization.

48. a) Better glucose control in diabetic wound patients helps with wound healing by improving neutrophil function for phagocytosis. It does not decrease necrosis or MMPs, and it does not increase the function of growth factors.

49. a) Keratinocytes release MMPs and growth factors. Skin helps in thermoregulation and provides protection against infection. Endothelial cells migrate into new tissue to form capillary structures.

50. d) Endothelial cells secrete MMPs. Fibroblasts secrete growth factors, stimulate production of fibronectin and collagen, and help in the deposition of extracellular matrix. During the maturation phase, immature type III collagen is converted into type I dermal collagen.

51. b) Wound contraction will be largest contributor primarily in option (b), the abdominal wound left open to heal.

52. a) Among all the choices provided, vancomycin is the drug of choice for MRSA wound infection. As compared to third generation cephalosporins, cefepime (a fourth generation) has increased activity against gram-positive cocci (especially *Streptococcus viridans* and penicillin-resistant pneumococci); however, it is not useful for MRSA. Ceftriaxone is generally effective for *Streptococcus* and has some activity against MSSA, *E. coli*, and *Klebsiella*. Imipenem has a broad spectrum of activity against many gram-positive and gram-negative, aerobic or anaerobic infections, but is not clinically useful against MRSA.

53. a) A Gram stain showing cocci in chains is diagnostic for *Streptococcus*. Staphylococci are seen in clusters. *Actinomyces israelii* is a gram-positive filamentous rod and sulphur granules are diagnostic. *Pseudomonas aeruginosa* is a gram-negative rod.

54. c) The tibial nerve is derived from the anterior portions of roots L4-S3 and travels with the common peroneal nerve as the sciatic nerve. It usually separates from the sciatic nerve high in the popliteal fossa and passes between the heads of the gastrocnemius muscle. The common peroneal (fibular) nerve divides into the sural communicating nerve, superficial fibular (peroneal) nerve, and deep fibular (peroneal, anterior tibial) nerve. The sural nerve is formed by

contributions from the tibial and common peroneal nerves and passes on the posterolateral aspect below the lateral malleolus. So when debriding a deep wound on the posterolateral ankle, the nerve that may be involved is the sural nerve.

55. a) Semi-occlusive dressings are waterproof dressings through which water and gas can pass. Examples of semi-occlusive dressings are DermaGeL® and film dressings like OPSITE™, PolyMem®, etc. Hydrocolloids are waterproof occlusive dressings that aid in the prevention of bacterial contamination. Hydrocolloids absorb exudates and protect the natural wound bed environment, but unlike semi-occlusive dressings, water and gas cannot pass through them. Hydrogels like SilvaSorb® are hydrophilic gels that increase moisture at the wound site. Hydrogels rehydrate the wound bed and soften necrotic tissue. AQUACEL® Ag is an alginate dressing with silver that can be considered an occlusive dressing.

56. c) Before debriding the wound at bed side, it is important to provide oral pain medication. As oral medication needs time to take effect, it is better to administer it before the planned procedure. Answer (c) is the only option where oral medications (ibuprofen, two tablets) are to be given one hour before the procedure. Topical anesthesia is useful, but the first step is to give oral medication and then use local topical anesthesia as needed.

57. d) The most common skin reactions associated with radiation include flaking or peeling of skin, erythema, alteration in pigmentation, hair loss, loss of perspiration, decreased sebaceous glands, changes in superficial blood vessels, edema, ulceration, and scarring. Radiation will cause increased, not decreased, erythema, so (d) is the correct answer.

58. c) Contamination is the presence of bacteria on the wound surface with no multiplication of bacteria. Colonization is characterized by the replication of microorganisms on the wound surface without invasion of the wound tissue and no host immune response. The first sign of critical colonization may be delayed wound healing, as evidenced by no change in wound size (L × W) or increasing exudates. Wound infection means invasion of the wound tissue with resulting host immune response and corresponds to bacterial counts exceeding 10^5 organisms per gram of tissue.

59. d) Epibole is defined as rolled-in epithelial edges. It is often seen in chronic wounds with poor healing dynamics. The epibole is formed because the migrating front of epithelial cells is unable to cover the wound cavity, so they descend and curl under the edges.

60. c) This is classified as suspected deep tissue injury per the NPUAP classification.

61. a) The best method for doing swab culture is by Levine technique: rotating a swab over a 1 square cm area with sufficient pressure to express fluid from within the wound tissue. This technique is more reflective of "tissue bioburden" than swabs of exudates or swabs taken by Z-technique, which samples a large area and may reflect surface contamination. Pathergy is a sign where any trauma can lead to more necrosis. It is found in patients with pyoderma gangrenosum. A wound biopsy would give better results, but it is not a swab culture.

62. c) Vitamins B and C are water soluble. Vitamin C is essential for collagen synthesis, while vitamin B is necessary for the production of energy from glucose, amino acid, and fat. Vitamins A, D, E, and K are fat soluble, and while vitamins A and E are also helpful for collagen formation, they are not water soluble.

63. a) All of the statements about pressure ulcer prevention scales are false except answer (a). Braden scale scores of 15-18 are considered at risk, scores of 13-14 are at moderate risk, scores of 10-12 are at high risk, and scores of 9 or below are considered very high risk. The Braden scale does not include an evaluation of nursing home staff needed to treat high risk patients prone to ulceration. The Waterlow scale is not mentioned in AHCPR guidelines, and the Gosnell scale is most appropriately used in neurologic and orthopedic conditions.

64. b) In sickle cell patients, edema is a critical indicator before ulceration, and the most important ulcer prevention therapy in patients with sickle cell disease is edema control. Skin care (keeping it moist, and avoiding trauma) are important for prevention, but edema control is the most important.

65. a) In patients with malignancy, pathologic lymph node enlargement and blockage causes a high risk of developing lymphedema. Patients with venous stasis ulcer can also develop phlebolymphedema, but the greatest risk for developing lymphedema is in patients with malignancy. In patients with diabetes and pyoderma gangrenosum, there is no increased risk of lymphedema.

66. a) The primary concern in this scenario is that the long-standing ulcer may transform into a malignancy. The most common malignancy associated with chronic wounds is squamous cell cancer, also called Marjolin's ulcer.

67. c) Complete decongestive therapy includes manual lymph drainage, compression bandaging, exercises, and skin care, all of which are considered extremely important in the treatment of lymphedema. Venous valve surgery is not indicated in patients with chronic lymphedema.

68. d) Pneumatic compression devices are contraindicated

in congestive heart failure. Right ventricular failure inevitably results in damage to the myocardium of the left ventricle because generalized venous hypertension causes increased pressures that back up through the heart. Eventually, this increased pressure reaches the left side of the heart, straining the left ventricle as it tries to pump out its blood. Lymphatic drainage is also reduced in this region, i.e., the lymphatic preload and afterloads are simultaneously elevated. If edema fluid is mobilized by massage or bandaging, the volume of circulating blood increases even more and can burden the already damaged left ventricular muscles to such a degree that left ventricular failure develops. Cardiac asthma and pulmonary edema can also develop.

69. a) This patient has exercise-induced claudication, since after walking two blocks, he has calf pain that relieves with rest. The superficial femoral artery is the most commonly occluded artery in legs of patient with peripheral vascular disease. In patients with partial occlusion, this manifests as ischemic pain, cramping, or fatigue when the muscle works beyond its oxygen and blood flow supply. Usually patients with complete occlusion will have rest pain of the foot or gangrene. Patients with spinal stenosis will have calf pain associated with muscle weakness, and the pain is usually present at rest. Diabetic neuropathic pain is usually in the plantar area of both feet.

70. d) All the statements of vascular assessment in diabetic patients are true except (d). ABIs can be falsely elevated in diabetic patients, and toe-brachial index is more accurate in diabetics. An ABI of >1.2 is considered non-compressible. A toe pressure of 40 mmHg or greater indicates adequate circulation, not 20 mmHg.

71. b) A transcutaneous oxygen study is most appropriate in the 60-year-old diabetic male with PVD who has a non-healing dorsal foot wound for more than four weeks. In this patient, $TcPO_2$ is an important test to determine if the patient will benefit from hyperbaric oxygen therapy. Hypoxic tissue ($TcPO_2$ <40 mmHg) that has a significant rise (>50% rise to at least 40 mmHg) on respired oxygen at atmospheric pressure is a positive test for hyperbaric oxygen therapy. Another test would be an in-chamber assessment to achieve $TcPO_2$ >200 mmHg while breathing 100% oxygen. Transcutaneous oximetry can be useful for patients with venous stasis, lymphedema, or deep full thickness burns to check for local hypoxia, and if so, whether it is correctable; however, it is most useful in the 60-year-old diabetic male with PVD.

72. d) MRA is better than angiography because it does not require arterial puncture, its contrast load is much lower, and MRA is safe in patients with dye allergies. However, a traditional angiogram is the gold standard and a better diagnostic study than MRA, so (d) is the correct choice.

73. b) Bone biopsy is the gold standard for diagnosing osteomyelitis, but the most common disadvantage of this procedure is that there can be introduction of infection (organism) in the normal bone. It is very rare to have fracture or sudden ischemia. Patients may experience profuse bleeding if they have coagulopathy or are on blood thinners.

74. c) Description of the left forearm area of skin that is leathery in consistency, dry, insensate, and waxy suggests that the patient has a third degree burn. Usually in first degree burns, the patient has erythematous tissue that blanches with pressure, and these wounds are red, dry, and painful. Second degree burns are red, wet, and painful with blisters. In fourth degree burns, usually tendon and bone are exposed.

75. b) The pear-shaped ulcer on the sacrum is most likely a Kennedy ulcer, which is an unavoidable pressure ulcer that some people get as they are dying. Deep tissue injury is possible in a terminal patient, but it is usually a purple or maroon discoloration without ulceration. Homan's sign is a test to detect deep vein thrombosis in the lower part of the leg. A positive Homan's sign is present when there is increase in pain in the calf or popliteal region with the examiner's abrupt dorsiflexion of the patient's foot at the ankle while the knee is flexed to 90 degrees. An intensive care unit ulcer is not a defined terminology.

76. d) The application of collagenase is an example of enzymatic debridement. The application of DuoDERM® is a type of autolytic debridement. Application of negative pressure wound therapy also causes autolytic debridement. Wet-to-dry dressing is the only choice that falls under the category of mechanical debridement.

77. c) When taking the left ABI, the pulse is checked at both brachial arteries and the left posterior tibial artery or left dorsalis pedis artery.

78. d) The best option for a patient electing for palliative care is to apply betadine and keep the gangrenous area dry. All other options are not considered palliative care.

79. d) In options (a), (b), and (c), primary closure will not be recommended, but debridement will be needed. The wound should be left open to ensure it remains non-infected before closure, so answer (d) is the correct choice.

80. b) Among the choices given, pulsed lavage is best for irrigation, debridement, and cleaning the wound. Whirlpool does help with debridement, but it is labor intensive, time consuming, may macerate surrounding periwound skin, and may increase risk for

water-borne infection such as *Pseudomonas*. It can also cause cross contamination. With pulsed lavage, cleaning and debridement is possible without damaging the wound bed if pressures are kept between 4 to 15 psi. Ultrasound also helps with debridement, but it does not help with irrigation and cleaning.

81. b) The recommended pressure for irrigation with pulsed lavage is 4 to 15 psi.

82. d) In the diabetic patient, an ABI >1.2 is most likely secondary to calcified vessels and is not useful for diagnosis, so answer (d) is the correct choice.

83. c) As it relates to compression bandages, Laplace's law states that sub-bandage pressure (P) is directly proportional to bandage tension (T) and inversely proportional to the radius (r) of the limb to which it is applied, so the correct answer is (c). P=T/r (where P = sub-bandage pressure; T = Bandage tension; r = radius of curvature of limb). As the radius of the limb increases, the pressure decreases. In practice the radius is not easily measured, so the circumference is used instead. This means that the pressure is greater at the smaller circumferences of the limb (wrist/ankle) than it is at the larger circumferences (thigh/upper arm), when even bandage tension is applied throughout. It is also important to consider the number of bandage layers applied (N) and the width of the bandage (W). The pressure is expressed in mm Hg; which gives the final equation: P = T × N × constant 4630/C × W (where P = the interface pressure under the bandage [mmHg], also called the compression force; T = the tension of the bandage [Kgf], which depends on the material and its % of stretch; N = the number of layers [defined by the level of overlap and the number of bandages]; C = the circumference at the measurement point [cm]; W = the bandage width [cm]).

84. b) Pain that occurs to patient repeatedly because of dressing changes is classified as cyclic pain. Pain that occurs because of debridement is classified as non-cyclic pain. Pain based on the etiology of the wound (i.e., vasculitis, infection, or malignancy) is called chronic pain or background pain.

85. d) Venous stasis ulcers are often shallow and have irregular wound edges, with surrounding skin showing hemosiderin pigmentation. If the patient has a capillary refill >5 seconds, it suggests arterial disease. Normal capillary refill is <3 seconds.

86. d) Arterial ulcers are painful, and usually located on the toes, or foot. These wounds usually have a pale bed, with the limb's ABI less than 0.5. Patients with history of deep vein thrombosis usually develop venous hypertension, leading to and venous stasis ulcers, not arterial ulcers.

87. e) Fournier's gangrene is a form of necrotizing soft tissue infection involving the perineum. It is most often

regarded as polymicrobial, including anaerobes as well as aerobes. Because it is a necrotizing infection, early aggressive debridement by a qualified surgeon is indicated. In some cases in males, much or all of the scrotum requires excision. However, because of the redundant blood supply to the testes, they almost always remain viable.

88. a) Calcium alginate is manufactured from seaweed. It does not cause trauma during dressing removal and is not classified as an occlusive dressing. It can cause desiccation around the wound.

89. c) Hydrofiber is not indicated for dry eschar. It is classified as an absorptive dressing and is made from sodium carboxymethyl cellulose, not seaweed.

90. b) Patch testing is the gold standard for diagnosing contact dermatitis.

91. b) Negative pressure wound therapy helps to decrease edema. It helps to increase granulation tissue and local blood supply, and may decrease bacterial colonization.

92. a) Weight loss is considered significant or severe if there is >10% weight loss in six months, >7.5% weight loss in three months, >5% weight loss in one month, or >2% weight loss in one week.

93. d) Risk factors for ulceration and amputation in diabetic patients include hypertension, hyperglycemia, and an age >65 years. Alcohol is not a risk factor for ulceration and amputation in diabetic patients.

94. d) In patients with pyoderma gangrenosum, wounds get worse with debridement and this sign is called pathergy.

95. a) Advanced wound therapies should be considered if a wound fails standard therapy for more than four weeks.

96. b) A patient with an ABI of 0.4 has severe peripheral vascular disease, contraindicating a TCC (total contact cast) approach in this patient. The patient should use other kinds of off-loading devices. In addition, unless his severe arterial insufficiency is surgically remediable, he cannot be "gradually changed" to a TCC strategy. TCC is a good standard of care for diabetic foot neuropathic ulcer, but it is not indicated in this patient because of low ABI.

97. d) Neuropathic diabetic foot wounds treated by total contact casting heal in 90 % of cases.

98. b) Of the choices listed, the 40-year-old female with a history of scleroderma, who may have a mixed connective tissue disease, is the most likely to have an inflammatory wound.

99. a) A punch or deep wedge biopsy is taken from the central part of the ulcer in patients with a diagnosis of pyoderma gangrenosum. In patients with squa-

mous cell cancer, a deep punch biopsy is needed from the edge of the wound. In patients with small vessel vasculitis, a simple punch biopsy is taken from edge of the wound. In autoimmune blistering a biopsy is taken of the skin, not the wound.

100. c) The UVC spectral band of ultraviolet light has been demonstrated to be bactericidal. UVC is capable of killing strains of bacteria in laboratory cultures, animal tissues, and in patients with chronic ulcers infected with methicillin-resistant *Staphylococcus aureus* (MRSA). UVA and UVB cause pigmentation and erythema, and UVB has been shown to induce an inflammatory reaction that stimulates the growth of granulation tissue and debridement of necrotic tissue.

101. e) The acute inflammatory phase is highly important for the initiation of normal wound healing. Coming right after the hemostatic phase, it helps set the stage for the migratory, proliferative, and maturation phases to follow. In contrast, chronic non-progressive inflammation is inhibitory to healing. The cytokine environment of chronic wounds is more pro-inflammatory than that of acute wounds. In addition, proteases are significantly elevated in chronic wound fluid. Modern wound management also stresses the importance of neither letting the healing tissues dry out nor letting them become overwhelmed by exudate/fluids that can cause maceration. The need to preserve the right amount of moisture throughout a wound's healing cycle is why the same wound in the same patient may call for different dressings and products at different times.

102. a) Diabetic foot ulcers are usually graded by the Wagner scale, which refers to its levels of severity as grades. Wagner grade 1 is a superficial ulcer that may penetrate (but not all the way through) the subcutaneous tissue layer. Wagner grade 2 reaches to the subcutaneous tissue, and deep tendon, capsule, or bone may be exposed. Wagner grade 3 is also deep, and further involves abscess, tendon infection, or infected bone (osteomyelitis). Wagner grade 4 is localized gangrene of the foot (e.g., toes, forefoot, or heel). Wagner grade 5 is gangrene of the entire foot.

103. a) The AHRQ Pressure Ulcer Prevention Guidelines include: using pillows or wedges to separate bony prominences, turning or repositioning the patient's body at least every two hours, keeping the patient's heel protected and elevated off the surface of the bed, and keeping the elevation of the head of the bed at 30 degrees or less, not 45 degrees.

104. b) The NPUAP classification of pressure ulcers includes stages I-IV and two additional categories. Stage I is intact skin with non-blanchable erythema. In very dark skin, this stage may present as an area of intact skin that may be painful, firm, soft, and warmer or cooler than adjacent tissue. Stage II involves the epidermis and dermis (i.e., the skin), but not the underlying subcutaneous tissue. Stage III reaches into the subcutaneous tissue. Stage IV reaches to tendon, muscle, or bone. In addition to these four stages, the NPUAP classification of pressure ulcers includes two other categories. Suspected deep tissue injury (sDTI) refers to purplish or maroon discoloration of the skin over one or more bony prominences. Experienced pressure ulcer clinicians recognize this presentation as almost certainly harboring significant tissue loss underneath. In very dark skin, sDTI may present as an area that feels different in either texture or temperature from the surrounding skin. The other recognized NPUAP category of pressure ulcer is called unstageable. When an area of pressure injury is covered with fibrinous exudate or eschar, the clinician cannot see which tissue type lies at the base of the wound; therefore, these wounds are necessarily deemed unstageable. In many cases it will be appropriate to debride the wound, and once the underlying tissues are revealed, it is possible to stage the pressure ulcer. Note that in selected circumstances, such as a dry, black eschar overlying the heel of a patient with poor arterial circulation, it is best to do no debridement, leaving the eschar as a natural biologic dressing until the patient has been evaluated for possible surgical restoration of adequate blood flow. Such heel ulcers are often painted with betadine in order to minimize bioburden and to keep the heel from becoming macerated.

105. a) A Wagner grade 2 diabetic foot ulcer penetrates through the subcutaneous fat layer to tendon or joint capsule, but there is no abscess or osteomyelitis. Wagner grade 1 is a superficial foot ulcer that includes disruption of skin extending into the subcutaneous fat layer. In addition, superficial infection (with or without cellulitis) may be present. Wagner grade 3 is a deep ulcer that may probe to the bone, with abscess, osteomyelitis, or joint sepsis. Wagner grade 4 is localized gangrene of the foot (e.g., toes, forefoot, or heel). Wagner grade 5 is gangrene of the entire foot.

106. a) Surgical debridement refers to using sharp instruments (curette, scalpel, or surgical scissors) to remove fibrinous exudate, bioburden, or devitalized tissue (e.g., skin, subcutaneous tissue, muscle, tendon, bone). Mechanical debridement includes wet-to-dry dressings (currently not used very often because of the importance of optimizing wound moisture), pulsed lavage, and whirlpool. Biologic debridement refers to maggot therapy, in which medical grade maggots selectively liquefy necrotic material without damaging healthy tissue. In addition, their secretions possess broad-spectrum antimicrobial activity and stimulate wound healing. Autolytic debridement refers to the

liquification of necrotic tissue by the body's own natural enzymes, which is a process that only works if the wound stays moist. Chemical debridement, also known as enzymatic debridement, invokes the use of collagenase or papain.

107. d) When a patient who is dependent on family members for his or her daily care becomes a burn victim, the clinician must think about the possibility of abuse. Your hospital is likely to have resource people with special training and expertise in this area. Typically, they can interview family members directly, render an assessment, and take action to protect the patient as necessary. Note that in many geographic areas, including the United States, clinicians are legally obligated to consider the possibility of abuse and to see that it is properly assessed.

108. e) Burn wounds of the types listed should all be referred to a burn center. Second and third degree burns totaling over 10% of body surface area carry particular morbidity and mortality in patients under 10 and over 50 years of age. In addition, burns involving the hands, feet, perineum, face, or neck are technically demanding because of the high stakes involved and the challenges in optimizing long-term outcomes.

109. c) It is important to realize that although patients with insensate feet do not feel the pain of a plantar ulcer, they do feel the pain caused by infection that might complicate that ulcer or the pain of either acute ischemia or acute Charcot arthropathy. All three of these conditions require prompt attention. In this case the gradual onset points away from embolism and acute Charcot arthropathy, and toward infection, which is also the most common of these three conditions. The presence of an ulcer with exudate and surrounding erythema in a febrile patient also points toward infection. Acute Charcot arthropathy can present with an impressively edematous, erythematous, and warm foot with a relatively bounding dorsalis pedis pulse, but the patient is typically afebrile (and the white blood cell count non-elevated). Note that if this patient had been portrayed as having an acutely red, warm, and swollen foot, but had no fever and no break in the skin, the diagnosis of acute Charcot arthropathy would rise in probability. Arthritis of the ankle would likely show local tenderness. Arterial embolism would lead to serious pain of sudden onset, likely forcing the patient to medical attention much earlier than three days. In addition, the physical exam would show at least pulselessness and pallor accompanying the pain. The foot would be cool, not warm, and if treatment were delayed, the patient would go on to experience lower extremity paresthesias and paralysis. The most common source of arterial embolism would be atrial fibrillation, and this patient has a regular rhythm.

110. c) An abnormal TBI is <0.7, and a normal TBI is >0.7 (refer to Chapter 16 on Arterial Insufficiency Ulcers).

111. b) Wounds that do not heal or progress sufficiently (e.g., remain open continuously without signs of healing for three months or do not demonstrate any response to treatment after six weeks) should be biopsied for histological diagnosis. Especially when looking for cancer as the underlying cause, the biopsy should be taken at the wound margin, which may be heaped up. When attempting to make the diagnosis of pyoderma gangrenosum, biopsy should at least include a sample from the wound margin, and for the ulcerative form, some experts recommend taking a biopsy from the central ulcer itself, making sure that it is deep enough to include tissue (and not just exudate) (refer to Chapter 14 on Venous Insufficiency Ulcers).

112. c) The Parkland formula for volume resuscitation after major burns intends that "the first eight hours" refers to the first 8 hours *after injury*. If the clinician misinterprets this to be the first eight hours after presentation to the hospital, volume resuscitation could be seriously delayed.

113. d) The "P" in the PQRST mnemonic stands for provocative and palliative factors. In other words, what seems to make the pain worse or trigger it? Alternatively, what has the patient learned to do to mitigate the pain? Q = quality of pain. Is it stabbing, a dull ache, boring, or lightning-like? R = region and radiation of the pain. Where is the pain? Does it seem to exist in one place, or travel to include another? S = severity. How is the pain affecting the patient's life? T = temporal aspects of the pain. What is the timing of onset? How long has it been going on? Does it come and go? Is it sudden and violent in onset, but then relenting nearly back to normal? Is it gradual in onset? What is the overall trend—is it getting better or worse?

114. e) All of these statements about pain are true, and it is important for clinicians to be well-versed in separating pain facts from pain myths. Fear of addiction causes many patients and clinicians to under-treat pain. Under-treated pain can contribute directly to poor outcomes in patients with wounds. For example, if patients learn that debridement is especially painful they are less likely to keep their appointments, no matter how urgently their wounds need to be debrided.

115. d) ACE™ wraps are difficult for wound patients to keep in place. They often telescope down the leg, and they were not engineered to deliver appropriately sustained pressure for successful compression wrapping. T.E.D.™ hose was also not developed for the management of lower extremity wounds. In contrast, there are many products available for delivering effec-

tive compression wrap treatment.

116. d) This pressure ulcer remains a stage IV. The NPUAP stages are not allowed to be downgraded because in a deep ulcer that heals, the lost subcutaneous, muscle, tendon, and bone tissues never regenerate. Their loss is permanent, and they are replaced only by fibrosis (scar tissue).

117. b) CMS has identified eleven incidents that it deems "reasonably preventable errors," which, if they occur during a patient's hospital admission, are considered "hospital-acquired conditions." Additional hospital payment under DRG is not authorized for these HACs. CMS recognizes only four serious preventable events, Medicare's so-called Never Events (refer to Chapter 28 on Regulatory and Reimbursement Issues in Wound Care).

118. c) An MRI is the most sensitive and specific for diagnosing osteomyelitis in patients with diabetes and foot ulcers.

119. a) Skin is composed of epidermis and dermis, but not the underlying subcutaneous layer. Therefore, full thickness *skin* loss refers to loss of the epidermis and dermis, exposing the subcutaneous tissue. In contrast, full thickness *tissue* loss refers to the loss of epidermis, dermis, and subcutaneous protective tissues, thus exposing the deeper layers of muscle, tendon, joint capsule, and bone. In fact, NPUAP draws on these concepts in the definition of its pressure ulcer staging. Stage III is defined as full thickness *skin* loss: if the subcutaneous tissue is exposed, then the ulcer has definitely gone deeper than both the epidermis and dermis. Similarly, stage IV is defined as full thickness *tissue* loss because if the deeper structural tissues are exposed, then all of the protective layers, including the subcutaneous tissue, have been lost.

120. a) Normal skin is acidic, and some wound care clinicians make use of this fact when they prescribe moisturizers for the flaking, dry skin that is often the backdrop for wound care patients' lower extremity ulcers. Some of the prescription lotions have a pH of 4.5-5.5. Open wounds tend to have a neutral or alkaline pH. A weakly acidic environment, such as that provided by normal skin, may promote healing of open wounds by inhibiting the action of proteases (refer to Chapter 5 on the Physiology of Wound Healing).

121. e) Usually, worsening stage III and IV pressure ulcers may imply inadequate off-loading. Faced with this situation, the clinician should investigate whether the patient's bed and mattress are adequate and evaluate the patient's continence status (both urinary and bowel). The WOCN guidelines for pressure ulcers make the point that clinicians should also consider surgical consultation for debridement and possible

operative repair by grafts or flaps. Hyperbaric oxygen therapy is not indicated in routine pressure ulcer management. It may have a role in salvaging threatened skin grafts or flaps, or when the pressure ulcer occurs in a previously radiated field, or is complicated by refractory osteomyelitis (refer to Chapter 31 on Highlights of National Treatment Guidelines & Quality Reporting in Wound Care).

122. c) Diabetic neuropathy can involve motor, sensory, and autonomic nerves. In the foot, loss of protective sensation sets the diabetic patient up for dangerous wounds that he or she may never be aware of. In addition, motor neuropathy of the intrinsic muscles of the foot can lead to deformities that predispose the foot to areas of increased pressure. Finally, autonomic neuropathy promotes anhidrosis, leading to dryness of skin and fissures, which increase the risk for infection.

123. d) The Semmes-Weinstein 5.07 monofilament nylon wire exerts a standardized 10 gm of force against the skin of the foot to test for loss of sufficient protective sensation. Loss of this protection is common in diabetics with foot ulcers, and it should always be on the mind of the clinician taking a history and conducting a physical on a diabetic patient. Note that among diabetic and nondiabetic patients there may be other causes of sensory neuropathy, such as vitamin B12 deficiency and hypothyroidism.

124. d) Although none of the studies listed are as invasive as a traditional angiogram, the most cost-effective next level of information can often be achieved by determining the ABIs. All that is required is a blood pressure cuff for the arms, a blood pressure cuff of suitable size for ankle diameters, and a Doppler. Ultrasound is noninvasive and may become relevant to this patient; however, it costs more and likely requires a separate appointment time. Ultrasound of the veins can play a central role in determining whether a patient with venous ulcer disease has superficial venous reflux, but it is not relevant for the patient presented here. A CT angiogram may be needed as part of a larger work up in the hands of a vascular specialist, but it is more expensive and also exposes the patient to imaging contrast, which may tax the kidney reserve of patients with diabetic nephropathy.

125. e) Both off-loading and callus debridement are key to optimizing the safe healing of neuropathic ulcers. There are a number of off-loading devices, including special shoes and total contact casts. Whatever device is used, callus debridement must also be routinely accomplished, and it is usually done sharply (with the qualified clinician taking care not to cut deeply enough to injure the underlying tissues).

126. c) Although most diabetics do have compressible pedal

arteries, busy diabetes clinics and wound care centers are not surprised to come across a diabetic patient whose vessels are non-compressible. Typically, the lack of compressibility is due to calcification of the arterial wall. In this context, either the ABI will be higher than 1.2 or 1.3 or not calculable at all, as in the case presented here. Note that, from time to time, clinicians who do a high volume of ABIs come across nondiabetics whose pedal arteries cannot be compressed.

127. e) When working up a patient for whom you cannot determine useful ABIs, vascular labs can conduct toe-brachial indices, pulse-volume recordings (PVRs), and TcPO$_2$ studies. All of these can be extremely helpful in assessing the patient's arterial status, and they are often used together.

128. b) An exaggerated popliteal pulse suggests aneurysm of the popliteal artery. Note that this condition is often bilateral and that a patient with a popliteal aneurysm has a 30-50% chance of having an abdominal aortic aneurysm as well (refer to Chapter 16 on Arterial Insufficiency Ulcers).

129. e) Popliteal aneurysms are important because they can cause embolism of thrombotic material, leading to acute ischemia of any distal part of the lower extremity. They can also thrombose suddenly, leading to a limb threatening crisis, manifest by the 5 P's: pulseless, pallor, pain, paresthesias, and paralysis.

130. e) Because the thromboembolic complications of popliteal aneurysms can occur without prior warning, patients thought to have a prominent popliteal pulse should be worked up expediently. Depending on how the medical community in your area works, it would be reasonable to begin with a diagnostic ultrasound, and then refer the patient to a vascular surgeon or directly to the vascular specialist.

NOTES

NOTES

INDEX